Hospitals in Communities of the Late Medieval Rhineland

Hospitals in Communities of the Late Medieval Rhineland

Houses of God, Places for the Sick

Lucy C. Barnhouse

Routledge
Taylor & Francis Group
LONDON AND NEW YORK

First published in 2023 by Amsterdam University Press Ltd.

Published 2025 by Routledge
4 Park Square, Milton Park, Abingdon, Oxon OX14 4RN
605 Third Avenue, New York, NY 10158

Routledge is an imprint of the Taylor & Francis Group, an informa business

ISBN: 9789463720243 (hbk)
ISBN: 9781041181019 (pbk)
ISBN: 9781003697497 (ebk)
NUR 684

Cover illustration: Tympanum over portal to the Gotthard-Kapelle; photographer Stefan Dumont. Image provided by Dom- und Diözesanmuseum, Mainz
Cover design: Coördesign, Leiden

DOI 10.5117/9789463720243

For Product Safety Concerns and Information please contact our EU representative:
GPSR@taylorandfrancis.com
Taylor & Francis Verlag GmbH, Kaufingerstraße 24, 80331 München, Germany

To Joseph P. Huffman, mentor, teacher, and friend

Table of Contents

List of Figures

Acknowledgements

Acknowledging the personal and academic debts incurred in writing a book is perhaps the pleasantest part of preparing the manuscript. Conversations with Simon Forde encouraged me to submit this work for publication with Amsterdam University Press, and Shannon Cunningham, Victoria Blud, and Jasmijn Zondervan have been supportive and responsive in the process of preparing it. I am also grateful to AUP's three external readers. Helpful bibliographic suggestions were given anonymously; Anna Peterson, a valued friend and colleague, provided both thorough commentary and helpfully provocative questions. I am particularly appreciative of the generosity of spirit with which Sethina Watson responded to a work that makes clear the points where our scholarship concerning hospitals in medieval canon law reaches profoundly differing conclusions. Thanks are owed to my Doktorvater, Wolfgang Mueller, who first suggested the medieval hospital to me as a topic where I might productively explore my interest in late medieval religious life and how it was understood in legal and social terms. His rigor has always challenged me to understand and articulate my own thought better. I am indebted to him for his personal encouragement and scholarly counsel as I prepared this book for publication. Maryanne Kowaleski not only strengthened an early version of this work with her insightful comments, but supported my development as a scholar throughout my graduate career. In criticism and encouragement, she has been a model of generosity, for which I am deeply grateful. Richard Gyug's imaginative and rigorous engagement with primary sources has stimulated and inspired me. I am also indebted to the Fulbright Commission for funding the archival research on which this work depends, and to Prof. Dr. Michael Matheus for sponsoring me as a visiting scholar of the Johannes-Gutenberg Universität during my time in Mainz.

This work was also facilitated by the staff of the many archives and libraries on whose resources I have relied. Fordham University's interlibrary loan staff provided invaluable support, not only in obtaining a remarkable range of obscure German periodicals, but in their friendliness, a support and stay. The history department of the Johannes-Gutenberg Universität provided a generous welcome, as well as an impressive and valuable collection of scholarship on the middle Rhine region. I am grateful to the staff of the department for smoothing the bureaucratic processes associated with my stay, and to the medievalists there for their collegiality. Dr. Wolfgang Dobras, of Mainz's Stadtarchiv, has provided invaluable help in sharing his extensive knowledge of Mainz's sources and of relevant secondary literature, and provided a gracious welcome to the study of Mainz. The staff and regulars of the Stadtarchiv of Mainz became to me a valuable community in the academic year of 2013–2014. I am grateful to them for their expertise, their assistance, and their good humor. I am also particularly obliged to Herr Michael Scholz, of the Hessisches Staatsarchiv Darmstadt, for his aid in helping me view original documents, and his initiative in connecting me to Dr. Helmut Heinemann, who shared his long experience with the Cistercian records of the region.

Not least, I am indebted to friends and colleagues. I am grateful both to and for Rachel Clark, who helped and consoled me when, due to injury and bereavement, I couldn't work on the book, and who laughed at me when I simply didn't. Esther Cuenca has been a dear friend since the beginning of my time at Fordham University, and an indefatigable organizer of online writing groups. Christina Bruno, my Doktorschwester, has frequently commiserated with me on the complexities of canon law, and helped me grapple with the same. Allison Edgren, fellow Fulbright Scholar, has provided companionship, cheer, and clarification of obscure medieval German. Elma Brenner has stimulated my thinking on medieval leprosy, particularly, since the early days of this project, and has been generous both with encouragement and practical suggestions. Christina Welsch, Margaret Wee-Siang Ng, and Jordan Biro Walters, of the College of Wooster, graciously read drafts of several of these chapters as they were under revision. My writing is better for their questions and suggestions. While Monica Green has not read this manuscript, she has shown scholarly generosity and modeled scholarly rigor in ways that have aided my work on it.

Finally, this book would certainly not exist without the mentorship of Joseph P. Huffman. From the time I sat in his office as a prospective undergraduate student, he has offered both moral and practical support for my development as a medievalist. He supported the development of my German and Latin in coursework and beyond; he warned me about the uncertainties and challenges of graduate study, and supported my PhD applications when I proved resistant to dissuasion. Subsequently, through email exchanges and over cups of tea, he has continuously encouraged my professional development. He has also exemplified commitment to that profession as a humane endeavor, in the face of institutional and cultural devaluation of the humanities. In his own research and scholarship, he has modeled rigor and generosity of thought. He has, through upheavals personal and professional, been a friend in the fullest sense. It is to him that this work is dedicated.

Introduction

Abstract
The introduction situates this monograph in relation to the historiography, identifies the archival documents on which it relies, and lays out its argument. I aim to show how legal status was debated and utilized by hospital communities, ecclesiastical and civic authorities, and, not least, the laity who were the donors and neighbors, and sometimes the administrators, of urban and periurban hospitals. Hospitals' entitlement to the legal privileges of religious status, and their subjection to ecclesiastical jurisdiction, were tendentious questions. This fueled the needs of hospitals to assert and defend their legal rights, but also enabled negotiation of their institutional identity. This book argues that the canon law governing hospitals served as an engine of their late medieval development.

Keywords: canon law, medieval history, urban history, religious houses

Today, the Heilig Geist in Mainz is an airy restaurant, a few blocks away from the Rhine. For centuries, however, this building, located between the cathedral and the city hall, was devoted to the care of the sick. The earliest list of those who resided in Mainz's oldest hospital dates to 1487, two decades after the hospital had been returned to the control of the cathedral chapter in the aftermath of a bitter dispute over the archiepiscopal see. The hospital master and the chaplain are listed first, followed by Peter, "a poor priest," and one man and a married couple who had purchased corrodies in the house, ensuring that they would be cared for in their old age. The six other men listed by name appear to have been vowed staff. There were also six sick persons receiving care, three laywomen who cared for them, and a man to bury the dead.[1] What bound those people together in that place?

1 StAM 33/9.

Barnhouse, Lucy C. *Hospitals in Communities of the Late Medieval Rhineland. Houses of God, Places for the Sick.* Taylor & Francis Group, 2023
DOI: 10.5117/9789463720243_INTRO

The complexity of medieval hospital history has been the subject of frustration and confusion, as well as admiration.[2] The late medieval intensification of debates over hospital administration has been observed by numerous historians, but it has rarely been interpreted as a sign of tension over hospitals' status in canon law, and the implications of that status.[3] Comparative work on late medieval hospitals can be facilitated by an examination of how hospitals' religious status was understood and debated. While the scholarship on medieval hospitals has burgeoned in recent years, examinations of their social function have rarely taken their legal identity into account. Centering hospitals' status in canon law enables comparison of *leprosaria* with multipurpose hospitals, and makes sense of the chronology of hospitals' late medieval institutional development. Rejecting the isolation of the historiography of leper hospitals from that of comparable institutions, moreover, provides a more comprehensive picture of how hospitals functioned in the later Middle Ages. Hospitals' contested legal status as religious houses is key to understanding how their functions were debated, and what participation in hospital communities could mean.

Using largely unexamined primary source material from the central Rhineland, I examine four types of hospital, representative of common institutional trajectories of the later Middle Ages. The oldest hospital of Mainz is typical of many institutions in its development under the aegis of the archbishop, and the transfer of rights of administrative appointment to the city council in the first third of the thirteenth century. Comparison to other civic hospitals in the Rhineland shows how the development of these prosperous urban institutions was connected to the evolution of canon law as well as local politics. The formation of a new community by Mainz's hospital sisters in the mid-thirteenth century, subject of the third chapter, follows a narrative common to mixed-gender hospitals, but one that has not been examined as a trend. This work compares the richly documented leper hospital of St. Georg to the multipurpose hospitals of Mainz, as well as to other *leprosaria* in the region, including the leper hospitals of Worms

2 Michel Pauly, "Für eine raumbezogene Hospitalgeschichte: Einführende Bemerkungen," in: *Einrichtungen der sozialen Sicherung im mittelalterlichen Lotharingien*, Actes des 13es Journées Lotharingiennes, 12–15 October 2004, ed. Michel Pauly (Linden: Section Historie de l'Institut Grand-Ducal, 2008), 9–14; Thomas Frank, *Heilsame Wortgefechte. Reformen europäischer Hospitäler vom 14. bis 16. Jahrhundert* (Göttingen: V&R Unipress, 2014), 14–15.

3 See Benjamin Laqua, *Bruderschaften und Hospitäler während des hohen Mittelalters: Kölner Befunde im westeuropäisch-vergleichende Perspektive* (Stuttgart: Hiersemann, 2011), 99–108. On hospitals in canon law, cf. Gunther Risse, *Mending Bodies, Saving Souls: A History of Hospitals* (Oxford: Oxford University Press, 1999), 144–147.

and Speyer. Using this framework shows that *leprosaria* were institutions defined by many factors beyond disease, a reality that their historiography has often obscured.[4] The small hospital of St. Barbara, founded by a canon in the mid-fourteenth century, illustrates how private foundations could obtain legitimacy as religious institutions, even after the canon law on hospitals had been substantially refined over the course of the thirteenth century.

This work focuses on the archdiocese of Mainz: a territory large enough for a robust evidence base, both for prosperous and well-documented hospitals (usually urban) and for small hospitals with only scant extant records. This scope allows a study of trends in how the archbishops of this territory intervened in the regulation of hospitals and other religious institutions. Such a model could be adopted for other bishoprics and archbishoprics, overcoming the particularization which has been a common response to the apparently protean nature of the medieval hospital.[5] Although medieval hospitals have been described as a "total social phenomenon," the scholarship on them remains fragmented by disciplinary and linguistic boundaries.[6] Studying the practical implications and negotiations of hospitals' status in canon law enables both an integration of hospitals in studies of religious institutions and networks and a more coherent overview of late medieval hospital development.[7] Over a century ago, Léon Le Grand identified a "powerful movement" to create hospital statutes in the thirteenth century,

4 See Saul Nathaniel Brody, *The Disease of the Soul: Leprosy in Medieval Literature* (Ithaca, NY: Grainell University Press, 1974), 60–83 et passim. Brody's problematic use of the term "asylum" to describe leper hospitals is perpetuated by Timothy S. Miller and John Nesbitt, *Walking Corpses: Leprosy in Byzantium and the Medieval West* (Ithaca, NY: Cornell University Press, 2014), 62–63 et passim. See also Elke Weingärtner, *Das Medizinal- und Fürsorgewesen der Stadt Trier im Mittelalter und der frühen Neuzeit* (Trier: Porta Alba Verlag, 1981), 77-79; Martin Uhrmacher, "Entstehung und Verbreitung von Leprosorien im Westen des Reiches," in Einrichtungen der sozialen Sicherung, ed. Pauly, 463; Elinor Lieber, "Old Testament 'Leprosy,' Contagion and Sin," in: *Contagion: Perspectives from PreModern Societies*, eds. Lawrence I. Conrad and Dominik Wujastyk (Aldershot: Ashgate Press, 2000), 99–136.

5 For valuable panEuropean surveys see Gisela Drossbach, ed., *Hospitäler in Mittelalter und früher Neuzeit: Frankreich, Deutschland und Italien: eine vergleichende Geschichte = Hôpitaux au Moyen Âge et au temps modernes: France, Allemagne et Italie: une histoire comparée* (Munich: R. Oldenbourg Verlag, 2007); Michael Matheus, ed., *Funktions- und Strukturwandel spätmittelalterlicher Hospitäler im europäischen Vergleich*, Geschichtliche Landeskunde 56 (Stuttgart: Franz Steiner Verlag, 2005).

6 Pauly, "Einleitung," *Einrichtungen der sozialen Sicherung*, 14. Siegfried Reicke, *Das deutsche Spital und sein Recht im Mittelalter*, vol. 1 (Stuttgart: Enke, 1932), vii, identifies the hospital (alongside "church, canonry, and cloister") as one of the major ecclesiastical institutions of the Middle Ages.

7 The desirability of such work is noted by John R. Guy, "Of the Writing of Hospital Histories There Is No End," *Bulletin of the History of Medicine* 59 (1985), 416; Drossbach, "Introduction," in: *Hospitäler in Mittelalter*, 9–24.

but did not identify canon law as an impetus; as noted by Sethina Watson, this model does not work for English hospitals.[8] Similarly, Benjamin Laqua has observed an early thirteenth-century vogue for the creation of charters and *vitae* implying ancient antecedents for the pious purposes and dedicated care of hospitals, but the fact that these aligned with the newly defined criteria for a hospital to receive the privileges of a religious institution has not been the subject of analysis.[9] While mentions of hospitals in church councils of the early thirteenth century have been noted, the impact of these councils has been neglected or dismissed.[10]

Regulated as religious institutions—and resented or supported as such—hospitals were hubs of activity, spaces of therapeutic care both spiritual and physical, and landmarks in physical and symbolic landscapes.[11] Hospital communities used their religious status strategically in forming their policies and relationships. The hospitals of the central Rhineland were active participants not only in the socioeconomic networks of the city and its hinterland, but in its religious networks. In addition to providing spiritual as well as physical care, hospitals were places where the laity attended and endowed Masses. Hospitals' functional similarity to monasteries has been commented on for decades, but their legal parity has not.[12]

8 Léon Le Grand, *Statuts d'hôtels-Dieu et de léproseries: recueil de textes du XIIe au XIVe siècle* (Paris: Alphonse Picard et Fils, 1901), xii-xiii; Sethina Watson, *Fundatio, Ordinatio, and Statuta: The Statutes and Constitutional Documents of English Hospitals to 1300* (Oxford: D.Phil., 2003), 280.

9 Laqua, *Bruderschaften und Hospitäler während des hohen Mittelalters*, 33–34.

10 Walter De Keyser, "Le 'dépistage' de la lèpre en Hainaut. De l'expertise pratiquée par les lépreux à l'examen médical (XIV-XVI siècles,)" in: *Einrichtungen der sozialen Sicherung*, 93–95, analyzes the implications of life in a hospital for the status of medieval lepers without any reference to religious privileges and obligations; idem, "L'évolution interne des léproseries," in: *Lépreux et sociabilité du Moyen Âge aux temps modernes*, ed. Bruno Tabuteau (Rouen: Publications de l'Université de Rouen, 2000), 13; Sethina Watson, *On Hospitals: Welfare, Law, and Christianity in Western Europe, 400–1320* (Oxford: Oxford University Press, 2020), 261–294. See also Adam J. Davis, *The Medieval Economy of Salvation: Charity, Commerce, and the Rise of the Hospital* (Ithaca, NY: Cornell University Press, 2019), 109–110.

11 Studying hospitals as part of social topographies has been highlighted as a desideratum: Christian Hoffarth, pers. comm., Medieval History Seminar, German Historical Institute, 15 October 2015; Christine Jéhanno, "The Medieval Hospital as Epistemological Laboratory," University of Ghent, 15 April 2016. Michel Pauly und Martin Uhrmacher, "Die Koblenzer Hospitäler in zentralörtlicher Perspektive," in *Zwischen Maas und Rhein: Beziehungen, Begegnungen und Konflikte in einem europäischen Kernraum von der Spätantike bis zum 19. Jahrhundert*, ed. Franz Irsigler (Trier: Universität Trier, 2006), 334–340. For an overview of the theoretical complexities of considering historical landscapes, see Karl-Georg Faber, "Was ist eine Geschichtslandschaft?" in *Festschrift Ludwig Petry, Teil I*, ed. Johannes Bärmann (Wiesbaden: F. Steiner, 1968), 20–23.

12 Sheila Sweetinburgh, *The Role of the Hospital in Medieval England: Gift-Giving and the Spiritual Economy* (Portland, OR: Four Courts Press, 2004), 21–23. See also, for example, Miri Rubin,

Medieval Hospitals and their Legal Status

The debate on how legal status ought to affect hospitals' internal organization and external relationships began in the twelfth century, and remained active throughout the later Middle Ages.[13] From the second half of the twelfth century onwards, the legal status of hospitals as religious houses was invoked by hospital communities seeking privileges. The privileges of exemption from taxation conferred on hospitals and their vowed residents by religious status frequently appear in disputes over the administration and rights of urban hospitals. Medieval hospitals have, however, rarely been analyzed as religious institutions.[14] Recent years have seen increasing acknowledgment of the fact that, even after the watershed of Lateran IV, religious identity could be labile, and religious status contested, with religious communities able to "persist indefinitely in a state of fluidity."[15] The legal evolution of religious status from the twelfth through fourteenth centuries was not a top down process, conformed to—or resisted—by individual institutions. Rather, the multiplication of texts on religious

"Imagining Medieval Hospitals: Considerations on the Cultural Meaning of Institutional Change," in *Medicine and Charity Before the Welfare State*, eds. Jonathan Barry and Colin Jones (London: Routledge, 1991), 18; Carole Rawcliffe, *Leprosy in Medieval England* (Woodbridge: Boydell & Brewer, 2006), 322–337; Margaret A. Seymour, "The Organization, Personnel, and Functions of the Hospital in the later Middle Ages," *The Bulletin of the Institute for Historical Research* 21 (1948), 249.

13 Oliver Auge, "Ne pauperes et debiles in...domo degentes divinis careant." Sakralreligiöse Askpete der mittelalterlichen Hospitalgeschichte," in *Sozialgeschichte mittelalterlicher Hospitäler*, eds. Neithard Bulst and KarlHeinz Spiess (Ostfildern: Jan Thorbecke Verlag, 2007), 77. On hospitals as spaces of moral and moralized care in later periods, see for example John Chircop, "Management and Therapeutic Regimes in Lunatic Asylums," in *Hospital Life: Theory and Practice from the Medieval to the Modern*, eds. Laurinda Abreu and Sally Sheard (Oxford: Peter Lang, 2013), 179–208; Victoria Sweet, *God's Hotel: A Doctor, A Hospital, and a Pilgrimage to the Heart of Medicine* (New York, NY: Riverhead Books, 2012), 2–10, 62–67, 106–114.

14 Benjamin Thompson, "From 'Alms' to 'Spiritual Services:' The Function and Status of Monastic Property in Medieval England," in *Monastic Studies, II. The Continuity of Tradition*, ed. Judith Loades (Bangor, Gwynedd: Headstart History, 1991), 227–261. Risse, *Mending Bodies, Saving Souls*, 180. Laqua, *Bruderschaften und Hospitäler*, 16–32, and Sweetinburgh, *The Role of the Hospital*, 133–6, acknowledge the importance of religious identity for the material support of hospitals.

15 Jennifer Kolpacoff Deane, "Geistliche Schwestern: The Pastoral Care of Lay Religious Women in Medieval Würzburg," in *Partners in Spirit: Women, Men, and Religious Life in Germany, 1100–1500*, eds. Fiona J. Griffiths and Julie Hutchin (Turnhout: Brepols, 2014), 237. See also *Labels and Libels: Naming Beguines in Northern Medieval Europe*, eds. Letha Böhringer, Jennifer Kolpacoff Deane, and Hildo van Engen (Turnhout: Brepols, 2014); Sherri Franks Johnson, *Monastic Women and Religious Orders in Late Medieval Bologna* (Cambridge, Cambridge University Press, 2014) 1–2, 10–11, et passim.

status was in large part the result of hospitals and monastic institutions defending or claiming legal privileges, usually of exemption for persons or properties.

In the early twentieth century, Siegfried Reicke devoted a magisterial work to how hospitals in medieval German lands were legally defined and regulated.[16] Thomas Frank has explored the appearance of hospitals in thirteenth- and fourteenth-century commentaries on the classic texts of canon law.[17] But analysis of connections between juristic discussions of theory and the practice of hospital reform remains a desideratum, despite the recent work of Sethina Watson.[18] The present study examines how religious status was negotiated and utilized by hospital communities, ecclesiastical and civic authorities, and, not least, the laity who were the donors and neighbors, and sometimes the administrators, of urban and periurban hospitals. Over the course of the later Middle Ages, hospital administrators, ecclesiastical and civic authorities, and those who interacted with hospitals as donors and tenants all responded to the changing criteria for religious status, which was intimately connected to hospitals' policies and relationships.

By the early thirteenth century, the teaching of canon law had expanded to all major universities; and those educated in the law, in turn, to numerous ecclesiastical hubs, including Mainz.[19] The Fourth Lateran Council, building on regional synods, was also of enormous influence on how religious institutions were defined and regulated.[20] Documents of practice often echo synodal and conciliar language, demonstrating that such prescriptive texts were hardly isolated from social realities. Hospitals, as individual houses, were at the lower end of the hierarchy of ecclesiastical corporations. Thus, formal observance was relatively unlikely to be of importance to the papal curia, and perhaps even to local authorities, unless significant resources were involved.[21] Grants of exemption could make religious houses answerable to

16 Reicke, *Das deutsche Spital und sein Recht*, vii-xi et passim.

17 Thomas Frank, "Spätmittelalterliche Hospitalreformen und Kanonistik," *Reti Medievali Rivista* 11 (2010), 2 et passim.

18 Watson, *On Hospitals* (see above, note 10).

19 Kenneth Pennington, "The Decretalists 1190 to 1234," in *The History of Medieval Canon Law in the Classical Period, 1140–1234: From Gratian to the Decretals of Pope Gregory IX*, eds. Wilfried Hartmann and Kenneth Pennington (Washington, DC: Catholic University of America Press, 2008), 242–245.

20 Paul B. Pixton, *The German Episcopacy and the Implementation of the Decrees of the Fourth Lateran Council 1216–1245: Watchmen on the Tower* (Leiden: Brill, 1995), 225–282; Anne J. Duggan, "Conciliar Law 1123–1215," in *The History of Medieval Canon Law*, 359–366.

21 James A. Brundage, *Medieval Canon Law* (New York: Longman, 1995), 98.

the pope rather than to local authorities.[22] Moreover, the majority of hospitals in late medieval Europe belonged to no order. The status of a hospital relative to the ecclesiastical hierarchy might thus be ambiguous. And ecclesiastical authorities might be more interested in formalities—and their legal and economic implications—than the exactitude of observance.[23] Bound by rules, wearing habits, and vowed to the service of the sick, hospital staff were visibly religious persons, and committed to preserving that status in law.

The Historiographies of Medieval Hospitals

The scholarship on medieval hospitals remains fragmented as well as voluminous. Sethina Watson has pithily described medieval hospitals as the "oddly elusive subject of a great deal of study." Michel Pauly's question of whether it is possible to define the medieval hospital has been echoed tacitly, if not explicitly, in many recent works.[24] Gisela Drossbach has called for a "deconstruction of the historiography"; such a bringing together of research traditions appears more than ever desirable as the study of medieval medicine and health continues to grow as a subfield.[25] The early legal focus of German studies has remained separate from the movements towards social and economic history that characterized many studies of medieval hospitals in the 1960s and 1970s.[26]

22 Brundage, *Medieval Canon Law*, 43, has asserted that exempt houses "for practical purposes enjoyed immunity from any outside supervision whatever."

23 Frank, *Heilsame Wortgefechte*, 69–73.

24 Watson, *Fundatio, Ordinatio, and Statuta*, iii. Pauly, ed., *Einrichtungen der sozialen Sicherung*, 9–14. Walter Schneider, "Die Hospitäler im Raum Alt-Tirol: Probleme einer Pass- und Übergangsregion," in *Funktions- und Strukturwandel spätmittelalterlicher Hospitäler im europäischen Vergleich*, ed. Michael Matheus (Stuttgart: Franz Steiner Verlag, 2005), 61–62; Christine Vanja, "Offene Fragen und Perspektiven der Hospitalgeschichte," in *Europäisches Spitalwesen. Institutionelle Fürsorge in Mittelalter und Früher Neuzeit*, ed. Martin Scheutz, Andrea Sommerlechner, Herwig Weigl, and Alfred Stefan Weiß (Munich: R. Oldenbourg Verlag, 2008), 19–41. On comparative studies as a desideratum, see also Bettina Toson, *Mittelalterliche Hospitäler in Hessen zwischen Schwalm, Eder, und Fulda* (Darmstadt: Hessiche Historische Kommission, 2012), 16–19; Peregrine Horden, "A Discipline of Relevance: The Historiography of the Later Medieval Hospital," *Social History of Medicine* 1 (1988), 365.

25 Drossbach, "Introduction," *Hospitäler in Mittelalter*, 22–24.

26 Jürgen Sydow, "Spital und Stadt in Kanonistik und Verfassungsgeschichte des 14. Jahrhunderts," in *Der deutsche Territorialstaat im 14. Jahrhundert*, ed. Hans Patze (Frankfurt am Main: Thorbecke, 1970), 175–195. For examples of social and economic history, see Ulrich Knefelkamp, *Das Gesundheits- und Fürsorgewesen der Stadt Freiburg im Breisgau im Mittelalter* (Freiburg im Breisgau: Herder, 1981), 30–42; Ulrich Knefelkamp, *Das Heilig-Geist-Spital in Nürnberg vom 14–17.*

I analyze the varied ways in which hospitals of all types—including leper hospitals—fit into socioeconomic and religious networks as religious institutions. In studying the legal status of medieval hospitals, this work follows Siegfried Reicke's monumental *Das deutsche Spital und sein Recht im Mittelalter*. Reicke's work was based entirely on printed material, however, and few subsequent studies have examined the effects of hospitals' legal status.[27] Recent scholars have been understandably chary of Reicke's division of medieval hospitals into ecclesiastical and civic institutions, which tends to obscure the complexities of hospitals' institutional development.[28] The religious characteristics of hospital life have too often been treated as an outgrowth of charitable impulses, rather than a consequence of hospitals' legal status.[29] When commonalities between hospitals and monastic houses

Jahrhundert: Geschichte, Struktur, Alltag (Nürnberg: Verein für Geschichte der Stadt Nürnberg, 1989), 25–41; Brigitte Pohl-Resl, *Rechnen mit der Ewigkeit: Das Wiener Bürgerspital im Mittelalter* (Munich: Oldenbourg Verlag, 1996), 22–33; Beate Sophie Gros, *Das Hohe Hospital in Soest (ca. 1178 –1600). Eine prosopographische und sozialgeschichtliche Untersuchung* (Münster: Aschendorff, 1999), 58–64 et passim; Ernst-Adolf Meinert, *Die Hospitäler Holsteins im Mittelalter: Ein Beitrag zur mittelalterlichen Stadtgeschichte* (Neumünster, Wachholtz Verlag, 1997), 9–11.

27 An exception is Jürgen Sydow, "Kanonistische Fragen zur Geschichte des Spitals in Südwestdeutschland," *Historisches Jahrbuch* 83 (1964), 54–68. Sydow sees the history of the medieval hospital as ending in communalization, a teleological process which I question. Gisela Drossbach, *Christliche caritas als Rechtsinstitut: Hospital und Orden von Santo Spirito in Sassia 1198–1378* (Paderborn: Ferdinand Schöningh, 2005), focuses on the history of the papally founded Order of the Holy Spirit, without exploring the wider context of the questions of legal and social identity that her work engages with as they affected the hospital in Rome and its daughter houses. Gisela Drossbach, "Das Hospital—eine kirchenrechtliche Institution? (ca. 1150–1350,)" *Zeitschrift der Savigny – Stiftung für Rechtsgeschichte: Kanonistische Abteilung* 118 (2001), 510–522, raises the question of whether or not the medieval hospital was governed by canon law in the twelfth through fourteenth centuries, but does not touch on the social implications of the question.

28 Reicke, *Das deutsche Spital*, v-xi. This model inspired numerous studies, especially in Germany, where a wave of scholarship in the 1960s and 1970s focused on the socioeconomic development of individual urban hospitals; see for example Knefelkamp, *Das Gesundheits- und Fürsorgewesen der Stadt Freiburg*, 30–42; Knefelkamp, *Das Heilig-GeistSpital in Nürnberg*, 265–275; PohlResl, *Rechnen mit der Ewigkeit*, 22–33; Meinert, *Die Hospitäler Holsteins im Mittelalter*, 9–11.

29 Rudolf Virchow, "Der Hospititaliter-Orden des Heiligen Geist, zumal in Deutschland," in *Monatsberichte der Königlich Preussischen Akademie der Wissenschaften zu Berlin* 43 (1878), 341–342, pointed out that the hospitals of the Islamicate world in the Middle Ages were numerous and well appointed, and similar institutions existed under Buddhism, but generalizations about hospitals and Christian charity persist. See MarieLouise Windemuth, *Das Hospital als Träger der Armenfürsorge im Mittelalter* (Stuttgart: Franz Steiner Verlag, 1995), 13; Monika Eschner-Apsner, "Karitativsoziale Leistungen bruderschaftlicher Organisationen im hohen und späten Mittelalter," in *Einrichtungen der sozialen Sicherung im mittelalterlichen Lotharingien, Actes des 13es Journées Lotharingiennes (12--15 Oct. 2004)* (Linden: Section Historie de l'Institut Grand-Ducal, 2008), 178–180; Gerhard Aumüller, Kornelia Grundmann, and Christina Vanja, eds., *Der Dienst am Kranken: Krankenversorgung zwischen Caritas, Medizin und Ökonomie vom*

have been discussed, it has often been in the context of contrasting medieval hospitals with modern clinical institutions; preconceptions about medieval attitudes towards health, medicine, and hygiene have particularly shaped studies of leper hospitals.[30] Attempts to analyze medieval hospitals using modern clinical categories of care and cure have often brought more frustration than insight.[31] Peregrine Horden and others have sought to shift scholarly debate from a teleological, practitioner-centered view of gradual medicalization towards more nuanced assessments of therapeutic care in medieval hospitals.[32]

Struggles between ecclesiastical and civic authorities have often been taken as an explanation for conflicts over hospital administration, without being adequately explained themselves. The ascendency of municipal leadership groups, in such interpretations, becomes both cause and effect for the transfer of hospitals from the supervision of bishops or cathedral chapters.[33] Treating

Mittelalter bis zur Neuzeit (Marburg: Elwert, 2007); Jean Imbert, *Histoire des hôpitaux français: contribution à l'étude des rapports de l'église et de l'état dans le domaine de l'Assistance Publique: les hôpitaux en droit canonique du décret de Gratien à la sécularisation de l'administration de l'Hôtel-Dieu de Paris en 1505* (Paris: J. Vrin, 1947), 9–10.

30 Kay Peter Jankrift, *Mit Gott und schwarzer Magie: Medizin im Mittelalter* (Stuttgart: Konrad Theiss Verlag, 2005), 14: Jankrift describes a "medical Middle Ages" as lasting through the late sixteenth century; Karl W. Heyden, "Die Hospitäler in Oppenheim," *Oppenheimer Hefte* 1 (1990), 14–15, repeats numerous stereotypes about medieval cities.

31 Katharine Park, "Healing the Poor: Hospitals and Medical Assistance in Renaissance Florence," in *Medicine and Charity Before the Welfare State*, eds. Jonathan Barry and Colin Jones (London: Routledge, 1991), 26; Monika Eschner-Apsner, "Geistliche Institutionen und Hospitäler," in *Caritas im Bistum Trier: Eine Geschichte des Helfens und Heilens*, ed. Roland Ries and Werner Marzi (Trier: Kliomedia Verlag, 2006), 78–79. Nicholas Orme and Margaret Webster, *The English Hospital 1070–1570* (New Haven: Yale University Press, 1995), 1–9, 49; Edward J. Kealey, *Medieval Medicus: Physicians and Health Care in England, 1100–1154* (Baltimore: Johns Hopkins University Press, 1981), 100–106, has drawn attention to the persistence of a care-or-cure dichotomy in evaluating medieval hospitals; Kay Peter Jankrift, "Herren Kranke, arme Siechen. Medizin im spätmittelalterlichen Hospitalwesen," in *Sozialgeschichte mittelalterlicher Hospitäler*, 149–167, seems to echo cited early modern critics who saw in medieval establishments nothing worthy of the name of a hospital; Jennifer Stemmle, "From Cure to Care: Indignation, Assistance, and Leprosy in the High Middle Ages," in *Experiences of Charity, 1250–1650*, ed. Anne M. Scott (Farnham: Ashgate, 2015), 61; Rubin, "Imagining Medieval Hospitals," 14–15.

32 Horden, "A Discipline of Relevance," 372–74. For teleological views, see for example Riegel, *Lepra, Pest, und andere Seuchen*, 27; John Henderson, *The Renaissance Hospital: Healing the Body and Healing the Soul* (New Haven: Yale University Press, 2006), 1–13; Joel Agrimi and Chiara Crisciani, "Charity and Aid in Medieval Christian Civilization," in *Western Medical Thought from Antiquity to the Middle Ages*, ed. Mirko D. Grmek (Cambridge, MA: Harvard University Press, 1998), 182–192; C.H. Talbot, *Medicine in Medieval England* (London: Oldbourne, 1955), 176–180.

33 For examples, see Franz Meffert, *Caritas und Krankenwesen bis zum Ausgang des Mittelalters* (Freiburg im Breisgau: Caritas Verlag, 1927), 312–313; Jesko von Steynitz, *Mittelalterliche Hospitäler der Orden und Städte als Einrichtungen der Sozialen Sicherung* (Berlin: Duncker und

hospitals merely as symbolic pawns in such conflicts, however, leaves important elements in their history unexplained. A desire to curb or channel hospitals' institutional privilege often, as in Mainz, provided grounds for collaboration between civic and ecclesiastic leaders. Examining hospitals as religious institutions provides grounds for comparing multipurpose institutions with leper hospitals, and hospitals of all types with monastic houses. Well into the fourteenth century, the understanding of hospitals as religious institutions was independent of established orders. The provision of canonically valid rules for their shared life, however, became increasingly important. This is demonstrated by the inclusion of hospitals in Mainz and beyond in archiepiscopal attempts to regulate religious observance within their archdiocese.

The Sources and Hospitals of the Archdiocese of Mainz

This work examines both the urban and rural hospitals of the Archdiocese of Mainz. Its source base, like the archdiocese itself, is centered on the city of Mainz itself. Mainz boasted five independent hospitals in the later Middle Ages. These were the oldest hospital (sometimes called the Heilig Geist Spital,) the "new hospital" managed by St. Agnes, St. Barbara, and the leper hospital of St. Georg, as well as the hospital of St. Katherine in Vilzbach, just outside the city. While Ludwig Falck has identified as many as nine independent hospitals, I have been unable to find evidence for the existence of more than these.[34] Other hospitals in the city were associated with monastic institutions, and thus did not have legal status as religious institutions in their own right. The relevant records are concentrated in two archives: the Stadtarchiv of Mainz and the Hessisches Staatsarchiv of Darmstadt. The records of Mainz's cathedral chapter, long believed to have administered a hospital, were consulted both in the Martinus-Bibliothek of Mainz, and the Bayerisches Staatsarchiv of Würzburg.[35] The relevant records of Eberbach, the Cistercian house theoretically

Humblot, 1970), 103–105; Meinert, *Die Hospitäler Holsteins im Mittelalter*, 17–23; Mathias Kälble, "Sozialfürsorge und kommunale Bewegung. Zur Bedeutung von Hospitälern fur die politische Gruppenbildung in der Stadt," in *Sozialgeschichte mittelalterlicher Hospitäler*, eds. Neithard Bulst and KarlHeinz Spiess (Ostfildern: Jan Thorbecke Verlag, 2007), 254–261; Ulrich Knefelkamp, "Stadt und Spital," in *Städtisches Gesundheits und Fürsorgewesen vor 1800*, ed. Peter Johanek (Köln: Böhlau Verlag, 2000), 30–40.

34 Ludwig Falck, *Mainz in seiner Blütezeit als Freie Stadt (1244–1328)*, Geschichte der Stadt Mainz III (Düsseldorf: Verlag Rau, 1973), 52.

35 No records of relevant import survive in the Dom- und Diözesanbibliothek, despite indications in Wolfgang Wann, "Die alten Mainzer Archive," *Archivalische Zeitschrift* 60 (1964), 101, 115, and

responsible for supervising the convent formed by Mainz's hospital sisters, survive in Wiesbaden and Oxford; collections of canon law and medical compilations created and used in the region surrounding Mainz are now in the Stiftsbibliothek Aschaffenburg and the Bodleian Library, Oxford.[36] In addition to these materials, and those of civic and state archives throughout the former archdiocese, I have made use of antiquarians' collections of sources copied out or summarized in the seventeenth and eighteenth centuries.[37]

In comparison to cities of similar size and influence, Mainz remains patchily covered by modern historiography. In part, this is attributable to the state of the extant sources.[38] Due to the frequent redrawing of political boundaries, and the responsibilities both secular and ecclesiastical of Mainz's powerful archbishops, relevant materials are widely scattered, as well as fragmentary.[39] The losses sustained when still active religious houses and hospitals were secularized under Napoleonic Law pose a particular challenge; many sources were moved, and more still destroyed, their administrative usefulness being at an end.[40] Moreover, Bodmann, the archivist and antiquarian, was himself responsible for the sale and loss of many documents, and for the removal of many seals; I have seen numerous charters missing their last lines as a result, and it is there, rather than in the *arengae*, that the date formulation is often contained.[41] The bulk of Mainz's losses had occurred before the First and Second World Wars; but burnings, bombings, and occupation resulted in further destruction of documents, to

Bundeskonferenz der kirchlichen Archive in Deutschland, ed., *Führer durch die Bistumsarchive der katholischen Kirche in Deutschland* (Siegburg: Franz Schmitt Verlag, 1991), 137–138.

36 Ludwig Falck, "Sammlung und Erschliessung der Quellen zur Mainzer Geschichte, vornehmlich des Mittelalters. Ein Zwischenbericht," *Mainzer Zeitschrift* 96/97 (2001/2002), 50, has a fuller list of cities with archives containing materials from Mainz: Marburg, Karlsruhe, Stuttgart, Wien, Koblenz, and many other state, communal, ecclesiastical and private archives in and outside Germany.

37 Valentin Ferdinand Gudenus, *Codex diplomaticus: exhibens anectoda ab anno DCCCLXXXI ad MCCC Moguntiaca, ius Germanicum, et S.R.I. historiam illustrantia* I, (Göttingen: Sumptu Regiae Officinae Librar. Academ., 1743); Stephan Alexander Würdtwein, *Dioecesis Moguntina*, vol. I (Mannheim: Typis Academicis, 1768); Franz Joseph Bodmann, *Rheingauische Alterthümer oder Landes und Regimentsverfassung des westlichen oder Niederrheingaues im Mittlern Zeitalter*, (Mainz: Florian Kupferberg, 1819); Ludwig Baur, *Hessische Urkunden: Die Provinz Rheinhessen von 963–1325*, vols. 1–2 (Darmstadt: Der historische Verein für das Grossherzogthum Hessen, 1862.

38 Falck, "Sammlung und Erschliessung der Quellen," 49

39 Wann, "Die alten Mainzer Archive," 115–121.

40 Falck, "Sammlung und Erschliessung der Quellen," 49–50. Legally, all the foundations' records became the property of the state, but in practice, much was lost.

41 Wann, "Die alte Mainzer Archive," 101; Dr. Wolfgang Dobras, pers. comm.; Herr Michael Scholz, pers. comm.

an extent impossible to calculate precisely.[42] The projected multi-volume series on the history of Mainz begun in the 1970s was never completed, leaving the pivotal thirteenth and fourteenth centuries neglected.[43] While regional publications contain valuable studies of the political and economic life of Mainz, the history of the hospitals of the city and archdiocese remains substantially unwritten.[44]

Mainz's hospitals were deeply embedded in the city's socioeconomic and religious networks. In this, they were typical of the hospitals that emerged as independent institutions in the twelfth and early thirteenth centuries across Europe. Of other cities in the archdiocese, Worms and Speyer boast comparatively well documented hospitals; I draw on their surviving account books and statutes, as well as on extant legal records relating to hospitals throughout the region.[45] Most of these records have hitherto been unstudied. I have drawn on a range of source genres in order to give as full a picture as possible of how hospitals functioned in their communities, and how the vocabulary and privileges of canon law affected these functions. Particularly in the case of leper hospitals, using documents of practice alongside normative texts shows the extent to which these institutions and their residents were integrated with their social environment. The focus on Mainz is largely due to the fact that the city's hospitals have richer surviving records than do those of Worms and Speyer. Even comparison of the edited charters of the three cities shows a marked difference.

42 Wann, "Die alten Mainzer Archive," 122–130.

43 Franz Dumont, Friedrich Schütz, and Ferdinand Scherf, eds., *Mainz: Eine Geschichte der Stadt, Mainz: die Geschichte der Stadt* (Mainz: P. von Zabern, 1998) is a valuable survey, but more focused studies remain a desideratum.

44 Dieter Demandt, *Stadtherrschaft und Stadtfreiheit im Spannungsfeld von Geistlichkeit und Bürgerschaft in Mainz (11–15 Jahrhundert)* (Wiesbaden: Franz Steiner Verlag 1977), 76–82 et passim; Falck, *Mainz in seiner Blütezeit*, 3–9 et passim; Michael Matheus, "Vom Bistumsstreit bis zur Mainzer Stiftfehde: Zur Geschichte der Stadt Mainz 1328–1459," in *Mainz: Eine Geschichte der Stadt*, 171–204. Franz Dumont, "Helfen und Heilen," in *Mainz: Die Geschichte der Stadt*, 771–774; Ludwig Falck, "Mainzer Hospitäler im Mittelalter," in *Moguntia Medica: Das medizinische Mainz von Mittelalter bis ins 20. Jahrhundert*, ed. Franz Dumont (Wiesbaden: B. Wylicil, 2002), 409–417; Ute Mayer and Rudolf Steffens, *Die spätmittelalterliche Urbare des Heiliggeist-Spitals in Mainz* (Stuttgart: Franz Steiner Verlag, 1992), provide an overview of the late medieval economic history of the city's oldest hospital.

45 See Alfred Hilgard, ed., *Urkunden zur Geschichte der Stadt Speyer* (Strassburg: Trübner, 1885), 72,18, 117,30, 133,29ff, 142,13, 143,29, 150,41, 151,22, 159,17, 161,37, 163,2, 166,14, 167,31, 172,26, 180,23, 188,24, 196,3, 199,32–41, 216,42, 254,2, 265,19, 282,8, 289,16, 380,40, 390,2, on the civic hospital, many of the references being topographical.

Mainz in the Later Middle Ages

Late medieval Mainz was an economic, political, and religious hub. *Aurea Moguntia*—golden Mainz—was a center for trade, with its prosperous burghers making use of the Rhine, as well as the surrounding vineyards and arable land. With archbishops drawn from powerful elites, and serving as prince electors in the Holy Roman Empire, it was, often with explosive results, a city of considerable political significance. It was also a center of ecclesiastical authority, with the archbishops exercising jurisdiction over the nearby bishoprics of Worms, Speyer, and Würzburg, and over an ecclesiastical province stretching from Strasbourg to Prague. The city itself served both as a space for the performance of archiepiscopal power, and as a locus of resistance to it.

Accounts of religious activity in Mainz often begin with the influential Archbishop Willigis (r. 975–1011). Not only was the city's great cathedral constructed under his leadership, but his tenure as archbishop also saw the creation of numerous religious foundations.[46] It is from the time of Willigis, too, that the first record of care for the sick-poor in Mainz dates. The prosperous canonry of Liebfrauen, that initially supervised the St. Barbara hospital, dates from the latter eleventh century; this period, too, contains the first mentions of a community at Heilig Kreuz, where the leprous would later gather.[47] By the twelfth century, Mainz was already a great and powerful city, according to the chronicler Otto von Freising.[48] Several twelfth-century archbishops—notably Adalbert I and Marcolf—took an active interest in the religious institutions of the city and its environs, providing patronage or intervening in administration.[49] This period saw increasing political tensions between the burghers of Mainz and the archbishops. Consequently, the bishop's council, composed of burghers and clergy, dissolved. In the aftermath, the cathedral chapter, the burghers of Mainz, and the archbishop

46 Ludwig Falck, "Die Erzbischöfliche Metropole, 1011–1244," in *Mainz: Die Geschichte der Stadt*, edited by Franz Dumont, Friedrich Schütz, and Ferdinand Scherf, (Mainz: Philipp von Zabern, 1998), 113–114. The foundations first recorded under Willigis include St. Stephan, St. Victor, St. Alban, and Altmünster.

47 Falck, "Die Erzbischöfliche Metropole," 114. Michael Kläger, "Das Stadtbild im Wandel," in *Beiträge zur Mainzer Geschichte* 28 (1988), 17–18, notes that Liebfrauen was located in the center of Mainz's early medieval settlement area.

48 Adolf Hofmeister, ed., *Ottonis Episcopi Frisingensis Chronica: Sive, Historia De Duabus Civitatibus*, *MGH SS rer. Germ. 45* (Hanover: Hahn, 1912), 329.

49 Josef Semmler, "Vita Religiosa und Bischof bis gegen 1200," in: Handbuch der Mainzer Kirchengeschichte: Christliche Antike und Mittelalter, ed. Friedhelm Jürgensmeier (Würzburg, Echter Verlag, 2000), 631–640.

were rivals for influence in matters both ecclesiastical and civic.[50] In the latter half of the twelfth century, the archbishops were conspicuously caught up in the power struggles between pope and emperor; their engagement in the administration of Mainz and its archdiocese is less visible.[51] While archiepiscopal and civic factions were rivals for power, religious leaders and institutions often pursued independent policies.

From the thirteenth century onwards, the city grew in political independence, economic power, and religious complexity. Political activity under the archbishops Siegfried II and Siegfried III made Mainz an influential hub, but also gave rise to conflict within the city, and demands on the part of civic leadership for independence from the potentially polarizing policies of the archbishop.[52] Ludwig Falck has described the civic liberties obtained from the archbishop in 1244 as "purchased" through the city's support of the papal rather than the imperial interest, in contrast to most of the urban centers along the Rhine.[53] The thirteenth century also saw Mainz expanding its territories and its trade. The religious networks of the city and its environs diversified and grew, as new orders and movements found a home in Mainz. In addition to a center of ecclesiastical and religious activity, the city was also a favored location for synods.[54] Under Archbishop Siegfried III, houses such as Altmünster in Mainz, and Nonnenmünster in Worms, were brought under Cistercian observance.[55]

50 Demandt, *Stadtherrschaft und Stadtfreiheit*, 50–68; see also Semmler, "Vita Religiosa und Bischof," 644–645. On the political developments of the twelfth century see also Falck 138–160. Thomas Just and Herwig Weigl, "Spitäler im südöstlichen Deutschland und in den österreichischen Ländern im Mittelalter," in *Europäisches Spitalwesen. Institutionelle Fürsorge in Mittelalter und Früher Neuzeit*, eds. Martin Scheutz, Andrea Sommerlechner, Herwig Weigl, and Alfred Stefan Weiß (Munich: R. Oldenbourg Verlag, 2008), 158, argue that Demandt's analysis of power relationships is an oversimplification.

51 Semmler, "Vita Religiosa und Bischof," 644–669, esp. 667–669; Falck, "Die Erzbischöfliche Metropole," 123–128.

52 Falck, "Die Erzbischöfliche Metropole," 129–136. See also Jennifer Kolpacoff Deane, *Papal Schism, Archiepiscopal Politics and Waldensian Persecution (1378–1396): The Ecclesiopolitical Landscape of Late Fourteenth-century Mainz* (Ph.D. diss., Northwestern University, 2000), 50–58.

53 Ludwig Falck, "Die Freie Stadt in ihre Blütezeit," in *Mainz: Die Geschichte der Stadt*, eds. Franz Dumont, Friedrich Schütz, and Ferdinand Scherf (Mainz: Philipp von Zabern, 1998), 143.

54 Falck, "Die Freie Stadt in ihre Blütezeit," 143–148. Michael D. Bailey, *Battling Demons: Witchcraft, Heresy, and Reform in the Late Middle Ages* (University Park, PA: Pennsylvania State University Press, 2003), 71, discusses the influence of the 1318 synod.

55 Brigitte Flug, "Mainz, Altmünster," in *Die Männer – und Frauenklöster der Benediktiner in Rheinland – Pfalz und Saarland,* edited by Friedhelm Jürgensmeier, *Germania Benedictina*, vol. 9 (St. Ottilien: EOS Verlag, 1999), 398–425, esp. 404–405; Christine Kleinjung, "Nonnen und

The Premonstratensians and Augustinians also formed communities in Mainz. Both mendicant orders were present in the city by the mid-thirteenth century, but never became as influential as in many other urban centers. The fact that a Franciscan mission from Mainz to Thuringia made stops in multiple hospitals along the way suggests that Mainz's thriving hospital may have been seen—by the mendicants themselves, by donors, or both—as fulfilling the functions of providing charitable and liturgical services which were often undertaken by these orders.[56] Both mendicant orders were the recipients of patronage from Mainz's prosperous civic elites, but were not as active in the city's socioeconomic networks as its hospitals.[57] In this, Mainz forms a notable contrast with other cities in the region and beyond.[58]

Mainz's oldest hospital, known as the Heilig Geist Spital, was granted its first statutes, and thus its institutional independence, in 1236. Just over two decades later, the sisters of the hospital departed. Instead of joining the Cistercian Order as foreseen by the religious and civic officials overseeing the division of the hospital staff, the women formed an independent community, eventually managing a hospital of their own in a semiagricultural belt along the river Ambach.

The origins of the city's leper hospital, St. Georg, are unclear, but it was an established institution by the midfourteenth century. With numerous properties inside as well as outside the city walls, St. Georg was a landmark in the city, and a community with active social ties to its neighbors and donors. When a canon of Liebfrauen created the hospital of St. Barbara as a private foundation in the mid-fourteenth century, he was careful to obtain for it the privileges of a religious institution. Each of these hospitals was

Personal, Familie und Stifter," in *Norm und Realität: Kontinuität und Wandel der Zisterzienser im Mittelalter*, eds. Franz Josef Gelten and Werner Rösener (Münster: LIT Verlag, 2009), 229–240; Wolfgang Seibrich, "Monastisches Leben von ca. 1200 bis zur Reformation," in *Handbuch der Mainzer Kirchengeschichte: Christliche Antike und Mittelalter*, edited by Friedhelm Jürgensmeier, vol. 2 (Würzburg: Echter Verlag, 2000), 688–698, esp. 695–696; Brigitte Flug, "Mainz, Dalen," in *Die Männer – und Frauenklöster der Benediktiner in Rheinland – Pfalz und Saarland*, edited by Friedhelm Jürgensmeier, *Germania Benedictina*, vol. 9 (St. Ottilien: EOS Verlag, 1999), 426–444, esp. 428–433 on Dalen's flexible affiliation and on its history as a mixed gender house until 1251.

56 Thomas Berger, "Die Bettelorden," in *Handbuch der Mainzer Kirchengeschichte: Christliche Antike und Mittelalter*, edited by Friedhelm Jürgensmeier, vol. 2 (Würzburg: Echter Verlag, 2000), 805.

57 Berger, "Die Bettelorden," 805–817.

58 See Heyden, "Die Hospitäler in Oppenheim," 19–20; Charlotte A. Stanford, *Commemorating the Dead in Late Medieval Strasbourg: The Cathedral's Book of Donors and its Use (1320–1521)* (Farnham: Ashgate, 2011), 285–291; Angela Montford, *Health, Sickness, Medicine and the Friars in the Thirteenth and Fourteenth Centuries* (Aldershot: Ashgate, 2004), 134–160.

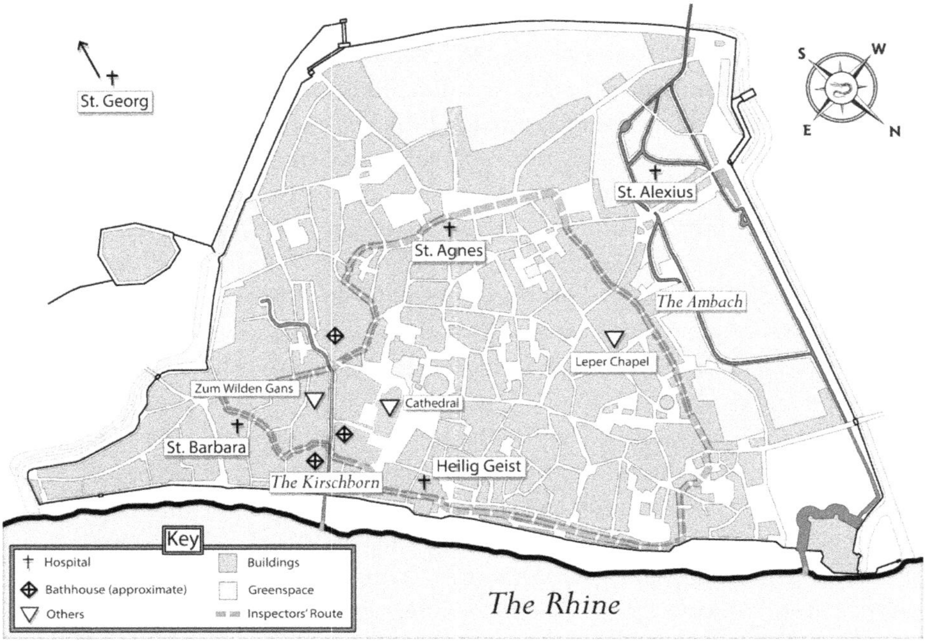

Figure 1: Hospitals of Mainz in the 14th century (J.W. Greenlee)

integrated in Mainz in ways shaped by their legal status, as well as by their socio-spatial locations in the city. After the conflict over the archiepiscopal see between Dieter von Isenburg and Adolf von Nassau, from 1461–1463, Mainz's Heilig Geist Spital, having supported Dieter's losing party, passed back into the control of the cathedral chapter after centuries of independence. In the aftermath of that episode, we see responses from Mainz's other hospitals. The women's community which managed the city's "new hospital" appears to have sought a relationship with the nearby Cistercian cloister of Eberbach. The hospital of St. Katherine had its statutes written down in 1471. The leper hospital of St. Georg started making copies of its charters, and received several sets of statutes in quick succession in the 1480s–1490s. This study takes this wave of political and legal change, in the second half of the fifteenth century, as its chronological endpoint.

The Vocabulary of this Work

Charters make clear that the sick who resided in hospitals, and the staff who were vowed to service there, were viewed as members of the hospital community. The medieval vocabulary applied to hospitals and to men and women who had taken religious vows is both labile and diverse. The vocabulary scholars have used in assessing the routines and statutes of hospitals has often been qualified—quasimonastic, quasireligious—in ways that obfuscate the issue of hospitals' legal identity.[59] The religious privileges of Mainz's hospitals, while sometimes contested, were retained throughout the period under study. I am, therefore, referring to the hospitals that are the subject of this work as religious institutions, without qualification. The medieval vocabulary for hospitals, too, includes them as a category of religious house. One of the most specific terms for hospital is *domus dei*, a house of God. But as the first chapter will discuss in more detail, they are also referred to as a type of monastery, and included as such in canonical legislation.

Echoing the language of documents created by and for medieval hospitals, I refer to the vowed men and women who served in them as brothers and sisters. The presence of permanently resident lay staff is not clearly indicated for the hospitals of Mainz and the central Rhineland, though some non-resident servants were responsible for the supervision of gardens and bathhouses, essential to the provision of therapeutic care.[60] Also significant is the question of vocabulary for those whose care provided hospitals with their distinctive social function and legal purpose. For those whose infirmities are not specified in the surviving records, I have chosen to use Sheila Sweetinburgh's term "the sick-poor" to approximate the connotations of *pauperes*. The medieval *pauperes* were a vast and broadly construed group including those affected by all sorts of sickness, weakness, and social vulnerability.[61] I refer to the sick-poor of hospital communities simply as

59 Jean Avril, "Le troisième concile de Latran et les communautés de lépreux," *Revue Mabillon* 60 (1981), 65; Reicke, *Das deutsche Spital und sein Recht*, 57–63, 87; Françoise Bériac, "Les fraternités de lépreux et lépreuses," in *Doppelklöster und andere Formen der Symbiose männlicher und weiblicher Religiosen im Mittelalter*, ed. Kaspar Elm and Michel Parisse (Berlin: Duncker und Humblot, 1980), 203–211. De Keyser, "L'évolution interne des léproseries," in *Lépreux et sociabilité*, 15–16. Risse, *Mending Bodies, Saving Souls*, 153, describes the medieval hospital as a "substitute monastery." Meinert, *Die Hospitäler Holsteins im Mittelalter*, 28–30, 47–50.

60 On lay servants, see Robert F. Berkhofer, *Day of Reckoning: Power and Accountability in Medieval France* (Philadelphia: University of Pennsylvania Press, 2004), 123–156; Odo Rigaldus, *Registers of Eudes of Rouen*, trans. Sydney M. Brown, ed. J. F. Sullivan (New York: Columbia University Press, 1964), 462, 514, 564, 569, 682–629, 671, 676; Falck, "Mainzer Hospitäler im Mittelalter," 410; Meffert, *Caritas und Krankenwesen*, 204–206, 260–269; Orme and Webster, *The English Hospital*, 80–83; Pohl – Resl, *Rechnen mit der Ewigkeit*, 134; Reicke, *Das deutsche Spital und sein Recht*, vol. 2, 111–116; Le Grand, *Statuts d'hôtels-dieu*, 7–15, 18–21, 49, 64–66, 120.

61 Sweetinburgh, *The Role of the Hospital*, 1–18 et passim. On the many meanings of the term "pauper," and its employment for hospital residents, see for example Wolfgang W. Schürle,

"residents," since the vocabulary of the "patient" presumes an anachronistic clinical relationship.[62]

Lastly, special attention is warranted by the terms "leprosy" and "lepers." As has been widely observed, it would be misleading to treat Hansen's Disease and medieval leprosy as identical; it is also inappropriate to assume continuity between ancient and medieval attitudes towards conditions identified as "leprosy."[63] The nature and effects of a diagnosis of leprosy in the Middle Ages have been much debated.[64] The visible, sometimes disfiguring, symptoms of lepromatous leprosy may have affected its popularity as a literary trope as well as social responses.[65] But this disease, so easily

Das Hospital zum Heiligen Geist in Konstanz; ein Beitrag zur Rechtsgeschichte des Hospitals im Mittelalter (Sigmaringen: Jan Thorbecke Verlag, 1970), 25–28; P.G. Caron, "L'evoluzione dalla quarta pauperum alla pia fundatio a scopo ospedaliero in alcuni testi della letteratura decretistica," *Il diritto ecclesiastico* 73 (1962), 137–159; Joseph P. Huffman, "Potens et pauper: charity and authority in jurisdictional disputes over the poor in medieval Cologne," in *Plenitude of Power: The Doctrines and Exercise of Authority in the Middle Ages. Essays in Honor of Robert Louis Benson* (Aldershot: Ashgate, 2006), 108. Michael Rogers McVaugh, *Medicine Before the Plague: Practitioners and their Patients in the Crown of Aragon, 1285–1345* (Cambridge: Cambridge University Press, 2002), 230–240; Michel Pauly, *Peregrinorum, pauperum ac aliorum transeuntium receptaculum: Hospitäler zwischen Maas und Rhein im Mittelalter* (Stuttgart: Franz Steiner Verlag, 2007), 16.

62 On the assumption of an anachronistic clinical relationship, and the perils of implying the participation of medieval hospitals in a teleological narrative culminating in the contemporary, Western clinical environment, see Rubin, "Imagining Medieval Hospitals," 14–15; Fay Skevington, "The Unhal and the Semantics of Anglo-Saxon Disability," in *Social Dimensions of Medieval Disease and Disability*, eds. Sally Crawford and Christina Lee (Oxford: Archaeopress, 2014), 7–14; Peter Murray Jones, "Image, Word, and Medicine in the Middle Ages," in *Visualizing Medieval Medicine and Natural History, 1200–1550* (Farnham: Ashgate, 2006), 1–2; Rawcliffe, *Leprosy in Medieval England*, 13–43.

63 For claims of such continuity, see Stephen Ell, "Blood and Sexuality in Medieval Leprosy," *Janus* 71 (1984), 155; Courtney Krolikoski, "Saints and Sinners: The Role of the Saint in the Life of the Leper Before the Thirteenth Century," *Annual of Medieval Studies at CEU* 18 (2012), 66–67, asserts that the Vulgate use of *lepra* for *za'arath* meant that the medieval leper "was stripped of his or her previous life and set outside the boundaries of his or her previous society." For more on Jerome's use of *lepra*, see Luke Demaitre, *Leprosy in Premodern Medicine: A Malady of the Whole Body* (Baltimore: Johns Hopkins University Press, 2007), 83–86.

64 Risse, *Mending Bodies, Saving Souls*, 167–172. Charlotte A. Roberts, "The Antiquity of Leprosy in Britain: The Skeletal Evidence," in *The Past and Present of Leprosy: Archaeological, Historical, Palaeopathological and Clinical Approaches*, ed. Charlotte A. Roberts, Mary E. Lewis, and Keith Manchester (Oxford: Archaeopress, 2000), 214–215, Simon Roffey sounds a more moderate note in "Medieval Leper Hospitals in England: An Archaeological Perspective," *Medieval Archaeology* 56 (2012), 203–233. Catherine Peyroux, "The Leper's Kiss," in *Monks and Nuns, Saints and Outcasts: Religion in Medieval Society*, eds. Sharon Farmer and Barbara Rosenwein (Ithaca: Cornell University Press, 2000), 174.

65 Demaitre, *Leprosy in Premodern Medicine*, 67–74, 175–195; Fritz Dross and Annemarie Kinzelbach, "'Nit mehr alls sein burger, sonder alls ein frembder.' Fremdheit und Aussatz in

recognizable in the stylized form given to it by the authors of romances, sermons, and saints' lives, often defied precise classification by those charged with medical diagnosis.[66] Many scholars have claimed that fear of such ambiguity drove medieval communities to ensure that the leprous would be identified—and set apart—by distinctive clothing, and by membership, constrained if necessary, in leper hospitals.[67] The evidence from the archdiocese of Mainz does not bear out such claims.

Medieval vocabulary for the disease and those deemed to be afflicted with it was frustratingly labile. *Lepra* and *elephantiasis* were both used; sometimes, it is only context that tells us *infirmi* were thought to be suffering from this disease. *Misellus/a* entered European vernaculars as *mesel/meselle*; those affected by the disease might be known as *leprosi* or simply *infecti*. In Middle High German, the sick could be *Aussätzige*, but were often simply *die armen Siechen,* or, still more ambiguously, *die armen Kinder Gottes*.[68] The latter term was frequently used for informal communities established at crossroads.[69] In this work, I focus on the development of formally established leper hospitals, which were affected more signally by debates around religious status for institutions and individuals than by the diagnosed disease of their residents. When possible, I follow Elma Brenner's

frühneuzeitlichen Reichsstädten," *Medizinhistorisches Journal* 46 (2011), 1–23; Miller and Nesbitt, *Walking Corpses*, 1–3.

66 Lucy C. Barnhouse, "Examining for Leprosy in the Fifteenth Century," in *Medieval Disability Sourcebook: Western Europe,* ed. Cameron Hunt McNabb (Earth, Milky Way: punctum books, 2020), 76–93.

67 Peter Richards, *The Medieval Leper and His Northern Heirs* (Woodbridge: Boydell, 2000), 31–32 et passim; Robert Jütte, "Stigma – Symbole: Kleidung als identitaetstiftendes Merkmal bei spätmittelalterlichen und frühneuzeitlichen Randgruppen (Juden, Dirnen, Aussätzige, Bettler,)" *Saeculum* 44 (1993), 65–89. Sheila Zimmerman, "Leprosy in the Medieval Imaginary," *Journal of Medieval and Early Modern Studies* 38 (2008), 561, argues that leprosaria afforded "a curious mixture of protection and humiliation."

68 Demaitre, *Leprosy in Premodern Medicine*, 81–83; Knefelkamp, *Gesundheits- und Fürsorgewesen der Stadt Freiburg*, 54; Miller and Nesbitt, *Walking Corpses*, 32–43; Rawcliffe, *Leprosy in Medieval England*, 72–78, offers a survey of leprosy in ancient and medieval medical texts; Antje Schelberg, "Unification des recherches sur la lèpre et les lépreux sous le nom de 'léprographie'? Une réponse," in *Lépreux et sociabilité du Moyen Âge aux temps modernes* ed. Bruno Tabuteau (Rouen: GRHIS, 2000), 93–98; Anna M. Peterson, "Connotation and Denotation: The Construction of the Leper in Narbonne and Siena Before the Plague," in *Leprosy and Identity in the Middle Ages: From England to the Mediterranean,* eds. Elma Brenner and François-Olivier Touati (Manchester: Manchester University Press, 2021), 327–329.

69 See Lucy C. Barnhouse, "Good People, Poor Sick: The Social Identities of Lepers in the Late Medieval Rhineland," in *Leprosy and Identity in the Middle Ages: From England to the Mediterranean,* eds. Elma Brenner and François-Olivier Touati (Manchester: Manchester University Press, 2021), 183–207.

use of "the leprous" to refer to those diagnosed with leprosy. I also use the term "leper," despite its contemporary social stigma, because of the ways in which this identity was significant in medieval Europe.[70]

The Form of this Work

Following chapters on canon law, civic hospitals, hospitals run by women, and *leprosaria*, there are two comparative chapters, one concerning small hospitals in the central Rhineland, for which few records survive, and one examining the participation of hospitals of all types in the religious and socioeconomic networks of the city. In the first chapter, I discuss the evolution of canon law related to hospitals as religious institutions from the twelfth to the fourteenth centuries. Hospital communities were active in claiming and maintaining their legal privileges, and the social and economic implications of these privileges often drove local and regional interactions with hospitals. The ecclesiastical province of Mainz has often been recognized as a hub of synodal legislation; this chapter examines the implications of that legislation for hospital communities in the region and around Europe. From the Third Lateran Council (1179) to the Council of Vienne (1311–1312), the meaning of religious status for hospitals was actively negotiated and debated. While law concerning hospitals did not stagnate in the fourteenth century, Vienne marked a culmination of thirteenth-century negotiations and conflicts over appropriate hospital administration.

The second chapter examines the formation of Mainz's oldest hospital as an independent institution, from its presumptive episcopal foundation, to twelfth-century tensions over its administration, through the mid-thirteenth century, with its move to a new location and its transfer to the administration of the council as part of the city's assertion of legal independence from the archbishop. This contributes to historiographical debates on the emergence of hospitals as independent institutions in the twelfth and thirteenth centuries, and what this meant for their position in relation to ecclesiastical and civic authorities. This chapter also reassesses the question of how and why civic involvement in hospital administration grew in the mid-thirteenth century. From the 1220s to 1250s, hospitals across Europe

70 On debates concerning terminology, see Elma Brenner and François-Olivier Touati, "Introduction," in *Leprosy and Identity in the Middle Ages: From England to the Mediterranean,* eds. Elma Brenner and François-Olivier Touati (Manchester: Manchester University Press, 2021), 6–7; Peterson, "Connotation and Denotation," 323.

underwent transformations paralleling those of monastic houses: they received new statutes governing their common life, and in many cases, mixed-gender houses were forced to divide, with the women often joining established orders. Such transformations have not, however, been analyzed as a coherent phenomenon reacting to legal changes.[71]

The third chapter is dedicated to the community formed by the vowed women who were forced to leave Mainz's oldest hospital in 1259. Studying the development of the hospital sisters' independent community sheds light both on hospitals, where the voluminous historiography on religious women can be usefully applied, and on the fraught question of religious status in the later Middle Ages.[72] The ambiguities of religious status remain better examined for female than for male communities. In the rich literature on religious status, moreover, hospitals have barely been mentioned.[73] Including mixed-gender hospital communities in studies of how religious status was defined and regulated can illuminate both the history of hospitals, and of women in the religious life. As the case of St. Agnes demonstrates, the legal

71 Franz Josef Felten, "Abwehr, Zuneigung, Pflichtgefühl. Reaktionen früher Zisterzienser auf den Wunsch religiöser Frauen, zisterziensisch zu leben," in *Female vita religiosa between Late Antiquity and the High Middle Ages: Structures, Developments, and Spatial Contexts*, eds. Gert Melville and Anne Müller (Berlin: LIT, 2011), 410–412; "Die Zisterzienserorden und die Frauen," in *Vita religiosa sanctimonialium: Norm und Praxis des weiblichen religiösen Lebens vom 6. bis zum 13. Jahrhundert*, ed. Christine Kleinjung (Korb: Didymos Verlag, 2011), 222–229. On the complexities of hospitals' position in canon law, see Drossbach, "Das Hospital—eine kirchenrechtliche Institution?" 510–522.

72 See, still influentially, Herbert Grundmann, *Religious Movements in the Middle Ages: The Historical Links Between Heresy, the Mendicant Orders, and the Women's Religious Movement in the Twelfth and Thirteenth Century, with the Historical Foundations of German Mysticism*, trans. Steven Rowan (Notre Dame, IN: University of Notre Dame Press, 1995). For recent literature complicating the typology of religious movements and communities as orthodox or heretical, see e.g. Elizabeth M. Makowski, *A Pernicious Sort of Woman: Quasi-Religious Women and Canon Lawyers in the Later Middle Ages* (Washington, DC: Catholic University of America Press, 2005); Jennifer Kolpacoff Deane, "From Case Studies to Comparative Models: Würzburg Beguines and the Vienne Decrees," in *Labels and Libels: Naming Beguines in Northern Medieval Europe*, ed. Letha Böhringer (Turnhout: Brepols, 2014), 53–82. Anne E. Lester, "Cares Beyond the Walls: Cistercian Nuns and the Care of Lepers in Twelfth and Thirteenth- Century Northern France," in *Religious and Laity in Western Europe 1000––1400: Interaction, Negotiation, and Power*, ed. Emilia Jamroziak and Janet Burton (Turnhout: Brepols, 2006), 197–224, begins to redress this. See also Barbara Rosenwein, "Views from Afar: North American Perspectives on Medieval Monasticism," in *Dove va la storiografia monastica in Europa?: temi e metodi di ricerca per lo studio della vita monastica e regolare in età medievale alle soglie del terzo millennio: atti del convegno internazionale Brescia-Rodengo, 23–25 marzo 2000*, ed. Giancarlo Andenna (Milan: Vita e pensiero università, 2001), 82–84.

73 Makowski, *A Pernicious Sort of Woman*, 36–38, 106–113, et passim; Johnson, *Monastic Women and Religious Orders*, 124–125 et passim.

status and social perceptions of hospitals were intricately intertwined.[74] The sisters' role in managing Mainz's "new hospital" has gone hitherto unacknowledged in scholarship on Mainz, falsifying the picture of the city's late medieval religious networks.[75]

In the chapter on *leprosaria*, I present an analysis of these institutions that does not assume that disease was the primary cause of change or stagnation in their medieval history. The records of Mainz's leper hospital, St. Georg, bear witness to ongoing social relationships with the hospital's neighbors. When the first extant rules for St. Georg were handed down by the archbishops (in 1488, 1493, and 1512,) questions of who had the right to examine for leprosy, and collect the fee for so doing, were prioritized over those of separation or internal regulation. Prescriptive sources and documents of practice alike envision situations where those identified as lepers, far from being segregated from urban life, retained social and economic ties to those outside the hospital.[76] The leper hospitals of Mainz and the central Rhineland were, like multipurpose hospitals and monastic houses, included in archiepiscopal reforms and favored by donors as religious institutions. Their locations were various, and their urban properties gave them social and economic visibility. This chapter looks chiefly at the *leprosaria* of Mainz, Worms, and Speyer, comparing the hospitals' spatial locations, their relationships to civic authorities, and their regulations.

The fifth chapter undertakes an analysis of the small hospitals in the archdiocese of Mainz. Such hospitals, located in small towns, were an important part of the region's social and religious networks. The relative poverty of the towns in which they were situated, however, contributed to the poor survival of such hospitals records. The extant records are too few to enable a detailed reconstruction of the institutional history of any one of these hospitals. Analyzing extant charters and court cases, however, can provide at least a suggestive look at how these hospitals, too, were affected by the thirteenth– and fourteenth-century developments in canon law. Extant charters make clear that small hospitals could also be active participants in local economic networks, and that such institutions were also the objects of episcopal regulation and of donors' charity as religious institutions.

74 Vanja, "Offene Fragen und Perspektiven der Hospitalgeschichte," 19–41.

75 Falck, "Mainzer Hospitäler im Mittelalter," 414–15; Schaab, *Geschichte der Stadt Mainz*, 230–32.

76 Guy Geltner, "Social Deviancy: A Medieval Approach," in *Why the Middle Ages Matter: Medieval Light on Modern Injustice*, eds. Celia Chazelle et al. (New York: Routledge, 2012), 29–40, esp. 31–34.

The sixth and final chapter examines how the hospitals of Mainz managed their property and relationships. I argue that communal religious status influenced hospital staff and donors, as well as external authorities.[77] A comparative study of how Mainz's hospitals cultivated connections to people and property shows both how hospital staff pursued long-term strategies as religious communities, and how hospitals' diverse social and geographic ties affected their functions in the city of Mainz and beyond. This chapter looks not only at hospitals and their property, but also their donors, analyzing which types of donors, e.g. burghers, clergy, and widows, favored which hospitals. This also demonstrates that relationships to hospitals could be multigenerational and were often multifaceted. An enormous variety of procedures used the rhetoric of donations, with the sick-poor designated as the recipients of the goods and revenues concerned. Through showing us the resources at hospitals' disposal, and the services hospitals were expected to perform, such data bring us closer to the frustratingly elusive question of how care for the sickpoor was carried out. Finally, an analysis of known hospital staff and named donors shows how hospitals remained connected to neighbors and families, an approach that can also productively be applied to late medieval monastic houses.

Conclusion

The present work fills a gap in the existing literature, and suggests a framework for further comparative study. Over the course of the later Middle Ages, the development of medieval hospitals was crucially shaped by the increasingly strict canon law governing religious status. Using largely untapped evidence from the central Rhineland, I examine multiple hospital types: independent institutions under civic oversight; foundations formed by the division of mixed-gender hospital communities; small and extra-urban communities; and leper hospitals, which have too often been historiographically isolated. In Mainz, these are exemplified by an episcopal foundation, given statutes in the 1230s, and transferred to civic control in the subsequent decade; the hospital managed by the women who were forced to leave the first hospital, and whose negotiation of religious identity lasted decades; a private foundation of the fourteenth century; and the city's leper hospital.

77 For an opposing view, see Watson, *Fundatio, Ordinatio, and Statuta*, i. Watson argues "that the early hospitalis was a recognized category of house, distinguished from a monastic house in terminology, legal statute, role, and constitutional form."

This study also draws on hitherto underexamined archival materials from hospitals of the episcopal cities of Worms and Speyer, and others from the archdiocese of Mainz. Analyzing hospitals as religious houses provides a basis for comparative study of their institutional development. Such an approach takes seriously the agency of hospitals, while also bringing a new perspective to how ecclesiastical and civic authorities sought to control them.

1 Houses of God

Abstract
This chapter, focusing on the archdiocese of Mainz, examines how hospitals were affected by the development of canon law. Legal religious status became increasingly important for hospital communities over the course of the thirteenth and fourteenth centuries, but the methods for obtaining this status were only gradually defined. Though hospitals' entitlement to the privileges of religious status could be tendentious, hospitals were not separated, legally or in the eyes of ecclesiastical authorities, from other kinds of religious institutions. Surviving documents indicate that the sick-poor and the staff who served them could be agents of legal processes. At ecumenical and provincial councils, the privileges of hospitals were repeatedly defined in terms of the service of the sick-poor.

Keywords: canon law, medieval hospitals, papal decretals, ecclesiastical councils

In 1343, Archbishop Heinrich of Mainz sent a letter in response to a request from the sizable Cistercian house of Eberbach. The suggestion that the monks would be freer to devote themselves to spiritual service at the feet of the Virgin if they were liberated from anxieties concerning temporal matters may have been taken from their petition, which no longer survives. The archbishop granted Eberbach rights over the revenues of two parish churches, specifically so that the brothers might expand the services of their hospital and encourage works of charity in the diocese.[1] In doing so, he echoed the language of the late twelfth-century papal decretal "Inter opera caritatis," and used formulae common to hospital documents.[2] "Inter

1 HStAD A2 234/49.

2 Clemens III, RPR vol. 2, pg. 572, Nr. 16627. "Inter opera caritatis non minimum reputamus debilibus, pauperibus, egenis, et laborare non valentes per Christi fidelium elemosinas misericorditer subvenire, et montes fidelium ad huiusmodi pietatis exercicium per allectanda indulgenciarum munera propensius excitare." See also Thomas Aquinas, *Summa Theologiae*,

Barnhouse, Lucy C. *Hospitals in Communities of the Late Medieval Rhineland. Houses of God, Places for the Sick.* Taylor & Francis Group, 2023
DOI: 10.5117/9789463720243_CH01

opera caritatis" is quoted and alluded to in documents created by and for hospitals and other religious houses throughout Europe.[3] Within the archdiocese of Mainz, the civic hospital of Speyer, the hospital managed by the monks of Eberbach, and the hospital sisters of St. Agnes in Mainz all preserve records which draw on this influential text.[4] All hospitals were, like the one under the oversight of Eberbach, sites for the performance of the biblical works of mercy, providing shelter and food, clothing and care, to the most vulnerable of society, the poor of Christ.[5] Many hospitals, moreover, were independent houses. These, while not affiliated with any order, were acknowledged as religious institutions, and integrated in the canon law and religious networks of medieval Europe. From the late twelfth century onwards, works of charity were not only a cultural and spiritual imperative, but were increasingly given legal definition.[6] Hospitals' function as institutional expressions of Christian charity has been often acknowledged.[7] How the language and practice of charity were used in defining and defending the status of hospitals as religious institutions, however, has been little examined. Hospitals' legal status was debated and utilized by

II:ii, Question 188.3, https://www.corpusthomisticum.org/sth3183.html, last accessed November 24, 2020.

3 See, for example, David M. Smith, *English Episcopal Acta 30: Carlisle 1133–1292* (Oxford: Oxford University Press, 2005), 69–70; Christopher Harper-Bill, *English Episcopal Acta 32: Norwich 1244–1266,* vol. 3 (Oxford: Oxford University Press, 2007), Nr. 41; James A. Brundage, *Law, Sex, and Christian Society in Medieval Europe* (Chicago: University of Chicago Press, 1987), 395–396; Nikolaus Paulus, "Die ältesten Ablässe für Almosen und Kirchenbesuch," *Zeitschrift für katholische Theologie* 33:1 (1909), 22.

4 Uses of "caritatis opera" in legal formulae are found in the 1261 rule for Speyer's civic hospital, Alfred Hilgard, ed., *Urkunden zur Geschichte der Stadt Speyer* (Strassburg: Trübner, 1885), 98, and letters of indulgence issued for the community of St. Agnes in the 1270s and 1280s, HStAD A2 115/4 and HStAD A2 115/17, as well as a letter concerning St. Agnes and other religious women, HStAD A2 118/4.

5 On the link between hospitals and the works of mercy, see for example Adam J. Davis, "Hospitals, Charity, and the Culture of Compassion in the Twelfth and Thirteenth Centuries," in *Approaches to Poverty in Medieval Europe: Complexities, Contradictions, Transformations, c. 1100–1500*, ed. Sharon Farmer (Turnhout: Brepols, 2016), 35–37.

6 See Emmanuel Bain, "Politiques des œuvres de miséricorde dans le discours scolastique (XIIe-XIIIe siècles)," in *Politiche di Misericordia tra Teoria e Prassi: Confraternite, ospedali e Monti di Pietà (XIII-XVI secolo)*, ed. Pietro Delcorno (Bologna: Il Mulino, 2018), 21–48.

7 Most recently Adam J. Davis, *The Medieval Economy of Salvation: Charity, Commerce, and the Rise of the Hospital* (Ithaca: Cornell University Press, 2019), 33–78; Carole Rawcliffe, *The Hospitals of Medieval Norwich* (Woodbridge: Boydell, 1995), 16–17; see also Sheila Sweetinburgh, *The Role of the Hospital in Medieval England: Gift-Giving and the Spiritual Economy* (Portland, OR: Four Courts Press, 2004), 1–14; Jean Manco, "The Heritage of Mercy," *Medieval History Magazine* 3 (2003), 22–29.

hospital communities, ecclesiastical and civic authorities, and, not least, the laity who were the donors, neighbors, and sometimes the administrators of urban and periurban hospitals. Religious status became increasingly important for hospital communities over the course of the thirteenth and fourteenth centuries, but the methods for obtaining this status were only gradually defined. The tendentious question of hospitals' legal identity fueled the needs of communities to assert and defend their rights, but it also meant that hospitals were able to manipulate their institutional identity. Hospitals have frequently been defined as imitating the functions of monasteries while remaining legally separate from them.[8] But the documents created by multiple stakeholders—bishops and founders, donors and administrators—indicate that hospitals were perceived and regulated like other houses of religion. In examining hospitals as governed by canon law, I arrive at different conclusions than Sethina Watson, who sees them as existing on its periphery. Watson has argued that hospitals "lay within the concerns of churchmen but beyond the claim of canon law."[9] I argue, however, that hospitals were included in ecclesiastical law as a category of religious house. Individual hospitals, moreover, expended considerable effort in asserting and defending their rights as religious institutions. Particularly in the classical period of canon law, local contexts affected the development of legal collections. The question of how ecclesiastical administrators and religious institutions alike employed the sources of medieval canon law remains a question to be investigated further.[10]

This chapter examines the evolution of canon law relevant to hospitals in the long thirteenth century, and how canon law was developed and promulgated within the archdiocese of Mainz. Before the mid-thirteenth century, Danica Summerlin has argued, "canon law was a body of changing legal concepts and approaches used or adapted locally."[11] Even as commentaries and decretal collections were, increasingly, promulgated in law codes, debate around the practical implications of religious status continued. Analyzing these debates, and the uses of law by individuals and institutions, enriches understanding of hospital communities as agents of law, as well

8 See, most recently, Sethina Watson, *On Hospitals: Welfare, Law, and Christianity in Western Europe, 400–1320* (Oxford: Oxford University Press, 2020), 232 et passim.

9 Watson, *On Hospitals*, 3.

10 Melodie H. Eichbauer and Danica Summerlin, "Introduction," in *The Use of Canon Law in Ecclesiastical Administration, 1000–1234*, eds. Melodie H. Eichbauer and Danica Summerlin (Leiden: Brill, 2019), 1–22.

11 Danica Summerlin, *The Canons of the Third Lateran Council of 1179, Their Origins and Reception* (Cambridge: Cambridge University Press, 2019), 29.

as its objects. Although individual users of canon law are rarely visible within hospital communities, and although it can be difficult to distinguish between initiative and response in hospital policy, surviving documents indicate that the sick-poor and the staff who served them initiated legal processes and negotiated legal agreements.[12] Hospital rules consistently define those serving within them as religious: governed by binding vows and distinguished by their habit. Hospitals and their staff were also defined by the service of the sick-poor. Conspicuous charitable commitment appears in conciliar texts and charters alike as helping to define hospitals' religious status. Furthermore, debate and disagreement about the parameters of religious status for individuals and institutions was anything but uncommon in the twelfth and thirteenth centuries.[13] That hospitals were the subject of such debate does not mark them out as a separate category of institution from houses of monks and canons, friars and nuns. What does make independent hospitals unusual is that, though they abided by religious rules, and their staff were bound by permanent vows, they did not belong to religious orders. Hospital orders are beyond the scope of this examination; my interest is particularly in those hospitals which—unlike that supervised by the monastery of Eberbach—enjoyed legal autonomy.

Institutional changes in late medieval hospitals are often debated in terms of moralization and medicalization. Late medieval hospital rules and public health regulations were increasingly geared towards the exclusion of certain groups of persons, whether beggars, or lepers, or simply those from outside the cities where hospitals were located.[14] This so-called decline or moralization of charity can be explained as a response to canon law. By the early fourteenth century, hospitals'

12 Thomas Frank, *Heilsame Wortgefechte: Reformen europäischer Hospitäler vom 14. bis 16. Jahrhundert* (Berlin: Vandenhoek & Ruprecht, 2014), 15.

13 On the difficulty of resolving questions of affiliation, see Ludwig Potthast, RPR Nr. 17896, "Virtutum meritis rutilans," a 1260 letter of Alexander IV; Maria Magdalena Rückert, "Zur Inkorporation südwestdeutscher Frauenklöster in den Zisterzienserorden. Untersuchungen zu Zisterzen der Maulbronner Filiation im 12. und 13. Jahrhundert," in *Studien und Mitteilungen zur Geschichte des Benediktiner-Ordens und seiner Zweige* 111 (2000), esp. 410; Johannes Helmrath, "Theorie und Praxis der Kirchenreform im Spätmittelalter," *Rottenburger Jahrbuch für Kirchengeschichte* 11 (1992), 62–66; Kenneth Pennington, *Pope and Bishops: The Papal Monarchy in the Twelfth and Thirteenth Centuries* (Philadelphia: University of Pennsylvania Press, 1984), 177–186.

14 Frank Rexroth, "Zweierlei Bedürftigkeit. Armenhäuser und selektive caritas im England des 14. bis 16. Jh.," in *Sozialgeschichte Mittelalterlicher Hospitäler,* eds. Neithard Bulst and Karl-Heinz Spiess (Ostfildern: Jan Thorbecke Verlag, 2007),11–37; Fritz Dross and Annemarie Kinzelbach, "'Nit mehr alls sein burger, sonder alls ein frembder.' Fremdheit und Aussatz in frühneuzeitlichen Reichsstädten," *Medizinhistorisches Journal* 46 (2011), 1–23.

legal status was defined in terms of the purposes, and the persons, they served. At ecumenical and provincial councils, the religious privileges of hospitals were repeatedly linked to the service of the sick. Thus, the late medieval drive to provide clearer definitions of the sick-poor could bolster or undermine the assertions of legitimacy by the institutions designed for their support and care.

The Third Lateran Council, held in 1179, forms a useful starting point for the consideration of canon law affecting hospitals because of its historiographical, as well as its historical significance. The Third Lateran Council has long been singled out as a crucial moment in the legal history of medieval leper hospitals, but its implications for multipurpose institutions have been the subject of less attention.[15] The fact that the years following the council saw the entrance of many hospitals into the documentary record suggests that they were seen as affected by the council's prescriptions.[16] Hospitals were not singled out in the canons of the council, but the fact that medical thought and practice were familiar to many there is indicated by the council's figurative language. In correcting the abuses of clerics and prelates, the council refers to an exchange of charity and grace like the balance of humors within the body: "since within the body of the Church all things ought to be drawn [*tractari*] out of charity, and as received grace is grace to be bestowed."[17] The choice of medical language suggests that the practicalities of care for the sick-poor were not unknown to those present, undermining the claim that its influential pronouncement about the care

15 Jean Imbert, *Histoire des hôpitaux français: contribution à l'étude des rapports de l'église et de l'état dans le domaine de l'Assistance Publique: les hôpitaux en droit canonique du décret de Gratien à la sécularisation de l'administration de l'Hôtel-Dieu de Paris en 1505* (Paris: J. Vrin, 1947), 156–158. Siegfried Reicke, *Das Deutsche Spital und sein Recht im Mittelalter*, vol. 2 (Stuttgart: Enke, 1932), 310–326; Martin Uhrmacher, "Entstehung und Verbreitung von Leprosorien im Westen des Reiches," in *Einrichtungen der sozialen Sicherung*, 463; Christine Boeckl, *Images of Leprosy: Disease, Religion, and Politics in European Art* (Kirksville, MO: Truman State University Press, 2011), 47–49; Martin Uhrmacher, *Leprosorien in Mittelalter und früher Neuzeit* (Köln: Rheinland Verlag, 2000), 5–6, Jean Avril, "Le troisième concile de Latran et les communautés de lépreux," *Revue Mabillon* 60 (1981), 39 et passim. Cf. Watson, *On Hospitals*, 24–35.

16 Bruno Tabuteau, "De l'expérience érémétique à la normalisation monastique: étude d'un processus de formation des léproseries aux XIIe – XIIIe siècles. Le cas d'Evreux," in *Fondations et œuvres charitables au Moyen Âge: Actes du 121e congrès national des sociétés historiques et scientifiques, section histoire médiévale et philologie, Nice, 1996* (Paris: CTHS, 1999), 95–96. Cf. Summerlin, *The Canons of the Third Lateran Council*, 40–43.

17 Joseph Alberigo, Joseph A. Dossetti, Pericles Joannou, Claude Leonardi, and Paul Prodi, eds., *Conciliorum Oecumenicorum Decreta*, 3rd ed., (Bologna: Istituto per le scienze religiose, 1973), 169.

of lepers was the result of widespread cultural fear or ignorance.[18] Though the canon has been interpreted as "urging the segregation of lepers," such a reading is not borne out by the text.[19] On the contrary, the authors of the canon appear to have assumed that communities of the leprous might exist with varying degrees of social integration.[20] Where Danica Summerlin reads commentaries on this canon as asserting the need for segregation, I read these as a commentary on ancient custom as attested by biblical and patristic texts.[21]

Communities of lepers are envisioned by Lateran III as self-sustaining—with gardens, grains, and beasts—and potentially close enough to other settlements that disputes over parish rights might arise. A hitherto unexamined possibility is that those referred to in the canon are a subgroup of the leprous population, and that "the lepers who are not able to live with the healthy, or to come to church together with others," do not represent all of those diagnosed with the disease.[22] Such a possibility is suggested by a variety of records. Édouard Jeanselme discussed a diagnosed leper's living at home as a possibility if "sufficient doctors" were on hand, using one literary example and one from the thirteenth century. That such a practice may have been more widespread than presumed is suggested by canonist and theologian Hinkmar of Reims' use of a priest's inspection of a leper's home as an elaborate analogy for the health of the church.[23]

18 Martin Uhrmacher, *Lepra und Leprosorien im rheinischen Raum vom 12. bis zum 18. Jahrhundert* (Trier: Porta Alba Verlag,) 26–28, describes the council as the springboard for the institutionalization and systematization of care for lepers; Kay Peter Jankrift, *Mit Gott und schwarzer Magie: Medizin im Mittelalter* (Stuttgart: Konrad Theiss Verlag, 2005), 18; Irven M. Resnick, "The Jews and Leprosy," in *Marks of Distinction: Christian Perceptions of Jews in the High Middle Ages* (Washington, DC: Catholic University of America Press, 2012), 107. Carole Rawcliffe, *Leprosy in Medieval England* (Woodbridge: Boydell), 252–262.

19 Irwin W. Sherman, "Leprosy, the Striking Hand of God," in *The Power of Plagues* (Washington, DC: ASM Press, 2006), 305.

20 For the model of semi-integration, see Guy Geltner, "Social Deviancy: A Medieval Approach," in *Why the Middle Ages Matter: Medieval Light on Modern Injustice*, eds. Celia Chazelle, Simon Doubleday, Felice Lifshitz, and Amy G. Remensnyder (New York: Routledge, 2012), 29–40. There are also parallels, in canon law, to provisions for the insane; see Claire Trenery, *Madness, Medicine and Miracle in Twelfth-Century England* (Abingdon: Routledge, 2019), 72–73.

21 Summerlin, *The Canons of the Third Lateran Council*, 110–112.

22 Alberigo et al, eds., *Conciliorum Oecomenicorum Decreta*, Canon 23, lines 25–26.

23 Édouard Jeanselme, "Comment l'Europe, au Moyen Âge, se protégea contre la Lèpre," *Bulletin de la Société Française d'Histoire de la Médecine* 25 (1931), 62–73; *MGH Fontes Iuris II*, 84. Imbert, *Histoire des hôpitaux français*, 1617, suggests that a framework of ecclesiastical support enabled the care of the sick-poor in their homes.

The exclusion of the leprous from the Body of Christ through a failure to provide churches for their use, priests for their ministry, and cemeteries for their need, is condemned by the council in the strongest terms as a failing of both Christian charity and clerical duty. Perhaps the most significant function of the canon is its explicit articulation of the church's authority to regulate the care of the sick-poor. This would come to affect all types of hospitals in later medieval Europe, and how these institutions and their residents were understood; notably, in collections, Canon 23 is sometimes included under canons on churches and their renovation, rather than with other materials concerning the leprous.[24] In the late twelfth and early thirteenth centuries, these canons were echoed in the privileges of individual communities, and adapted to local conditions, used and cited in the archdiocese of Mainz as elsewhere.[25] In records of the same period, hospitals appear alongside monasteries; they appear alongside oratories and churches; and they appear, also, as their own subcategory of religious house.[26] A twelfth-century chronicler, discussing the rise of new orders and how pleasing it is to God to bestow charity, lists hospitals of the poor and communities of lepers alongside Carthusians, Cistercians, and others.[27]

Foundation charters of hospitals from the twelfth and early thirteenth centuries rarely survive. This phenomenon would be strange if it were on the dispositions of founders that hospitals' legal rights depended, as has

24 Summerlin, *The Canons of the Third Lateran Council*, 164. Cf. Watson, *On Hospitals*, particularly 133–135, 212–215, for the argument that hospitals were only exceptionally seen as subject to the governance of canon rather than Roman law.

25 Summerlin, *The Canons of the Third Lateran Council*, 154, 180–182, 192–193, 225–226. One manuscript is found in the hospital library of Bernkastel-Kues.

26 See François-Olivier Touati, *Archives de la lèpre: Atlas des léproseries entre Loire et Marne au moyen âge* (Paris: Comité des Travaux historiques et scientifiques, 1996), 4041; Schneider, "Lexicographie du Latin Mediévale et Vocabulaire des Institutions," in *La Lexicographie du latin médiéval et ses rapports avec les recherches actuelles sur la civilisation du Moyen âge*, ed. Yves Lefèvre (Paris: Centre nationale de la recherche scientifique, 1981), 204–205; Bettina Toson, *Mittelalterliche Hospitäler in Hessen zwischen Schwalm, Eder, und Fulda* (Darmstadt: Hessiche Historische Kommission, 2012), 13; Monia Franzolin, "Gli ospizi lungo il tratto bellunese della Strada Regia di Alemagna," in *L'accoglienza religiosa tra tardo antico ed età moderna: Luoghi, architetture, percorsi*, eds. Silvia Beltramo and Paolo Cozzo (Rome: Viella, 2013), 129–134. Cf. Watson, *On Hospitals*, 232, 240–242.

27 Geoffroy de Vigeois, *Chronica Gaufredi prioris vosiensis*, in *Novae Bibliothecae Manuscriptorum Librorum Tomus Secundus: Rerum Aquitanicarum Presertim Bituricensium Uberrima Collectio. Historias, Chronica, Vitas Sanctorum, ac similia Antiquitatis Monumenta, nunc primum ex MSS Codicibus eruta, copiose repraesentans*, ed. Philippe Labbé (Paris: Sebastian & Gabriel Cramoisy, 1657), 296.

sometimes been argued.[28] The earliest extant records for many hospitals show them as the recipients of statutes devised by bishops, or of gifts conferred on them by lay persons: as religious institutions, concerned with their rights.[29] Lateran III's specification that *leprosaria* were to have their properties exempted from tithes, for example, is echoed in petitions directed to ecclesiastical authorities by such communities.[30] The increasingly exclusive application of "brothers and sisters" to healthy staff, and increasingly explicit identification of the sick, have been interpreted as reflecting a transition from fraternities founded by the initiative of the leprous themselves into hospitals led by healthy administrators, or from a movement characterized by charitable zeal to one determined by religious

28 See Watson, *On Hospitals*, 163–173, 310–314. Uhrmacher, *Leprosorien im Mittelalter*, 38–39; Cullum, "Leperhouses and Borough Status in the Thirteenth Century," 39–40; Thomas Just and Herwig Weigl, "Spitäler im südöstlichen Deutschland und in den österreichischen Ländern im Mittelalter," in *Europäisches Spitalwesen. Institutionelle Fürsorge in Mittelalter und Früher Neuzeit*, eds. Martin Scheutz, Andrea Sommerlechner, Herwig Weigl, and Alfred Stefan Weiß (Munich: R. Oldenbourg Verlag, 2008), 168; Kay Peter Jankrift, "Hospitäler und Leprosorien im Nordwesten des mittelalterlichen Regnum Teutonicum unter besonderer Berücksichtigung rheinisch-westfälischer Städte," in *Europäisches Spitalwesen. Institutionelle Fürsorge in Mittelalter und Früher Neuzeit*, eds. Martin Scheutz, Andrea Sommerlechner, Herwig Weigl, and Alfred Stefan Weiß (Munich: R. Oldenbourg Verlag, 2008), 301–302; Michel Pauly, *Peregrinorum, pauperum ac aliorum transeuntium receptaculum: Hospitäler zwischen Maas und Rhein im Mittelalter* (Stuttgart: Franz Steiner Verlag, 2007), 160–161; Simon Roffey, "Medieval Leper Hospitals in England: An Archaeological Perspective," in *Medieval Archaeology* 56 (2012), 212–213, points to the potential of archaeology to clarify the dating of hospitals' institutional development.

29 On early documents, see Maria Pia Alberzoni, "Norditalienische Pilgerhospize im 12. und 13. Jahrhundert," in *Wege zum Heil: Pilger und Heilige Orte an Mosel und Rhein*, eds. Thomas Frank, Michael Matheus, Sabine Reichert (Stuttgart: Franz Steiner Verlag, 2009), 279; Thomas Coomans, "Belfries, Cloth Halls, Hospitals, and Mendicant Churches: A New Urban Architecture in the Low Countries around 1300," in *The Year 1300 and the Creation of a New European Architecture*, ed. Alexandra Gajewski (Turnhout: Brepols, 2007), 185–202.

30 Jaffé, *RPR*, vol. 2, Nr. 8938 and Nr. 10858, records that the house of lepers at Grand-Beaulieu sought a dual confirmation of their possessions and privileges on 2 July 1146, and again on 29 April 1163. Ibid, Nr. 12944: "Domum infirmorum fratrum (leprosorum) de Dullendio tuendam suscepit, eorumque possessiones et privilegia confirmat" (1177 September 29); 405, nr. 14240: Fratribus Corbeiensibus (d. Ambian) concedit, ut a religiosis diversorum ordinum viris et leprosis in circuitu monasterii constitutis decimas de terris, praeterquam de novalibus eorum, exigere debeant" (7 January 1171–1181); 443, nr. 14699: "Leprosorum S. Mariae Magdalenae de Quercu possessiones confirmat" (1182 November 16); 476: "Leprosis de Fixa indulget, ne de hortis et nutrimentis animalium decimas solvant"(22 March 1182–1185); 479: "Leprosis S. Lazari Parisensibus indulget, ut de hortis, arborum pomis sive animalium nutrimentis nemini decimas solvant" (30 September 1184–1185); 591, nr. 16883: "Leprosorum S. Mariae Magdalene Exoniensium bona confirmat, iisque asserit eleemosynam, a.b.m. Bartholomaeo episcopo Exoniensi collatam" (26 May 1192).

discipline.[31] Some scholars have interpreted this shift as corresponding to a new moralization of leprosy.[32] This shift was, however, not limited to leper hospitals, but is mirrored in the language of hospital documents across Europe with increasing frequency from the first third of the thirteenth century onwards.[33] As Bruno Tabuteau has observed in the case of *leprosaria*, hospitals were institutions recognized as part of a religious landscape both increasingly diverse and increasingly regulated.[34] The distinctions made in the *Liber Extra* (1234) between the rights of episcopal and non-episcopal hospitals contributed to the fact that, over the course of the thirteenth century and beyond, bishops often intervened—on their own initiative or by request—in the affairs of hospitals.[35] Such requests were formulated by legally knowledgeable communities; research has shown that hospital libraries might often include volumes of canon law.[36]

The Legal Status of Hospitals in the Later Middle Ages

The Decretals of Gregory IX, often known as the *Liber Extra*, reflect the priorities of early thirteenth-century canon law both in form and content.[37]

31 Françoise Bériac, "Les fraternités de lépreux et lépreuses," in *Doppelklöster und andere Formen der Symbiose männlicher und weiblicher Religiosen im Mittelalter*, ed. Kaspar Elm and Michel Parisse (Berlin: Duncker and Humboldt, 1980), 205–208. Potthast, RPR, Nr. 8951, Nr. 17278, Nr. 17565, Nr. 24014, provide a survey of letters from the thirteenth century. Drossbach, "Hospitalstatuten im Spiegel von Norm und Wirklichkeit," in *Hospitäler in Mittelalter und Früher Neuzeit: Frankreich, Deutschland und Italien. Eine Vergleichende Geschichte*, ed. Gisela Drossbach (Munich: Oldenbourg, 2007), 55–63; Alberzoni, "Norditalienische Pilgerhospize im 12. und 13. Jahrhundert," 282–284.

32 François-Olivier Touati, "Les Léproseries aux XIIème et XIIIème siècles: Lieux de Conversion?" in *Voluntate Dei Leprosus: les lépreux entre conversion et exclusion aux XIIème et XIIIème siècles*, Nicole Bériou and François-Olivier Touati (Spoleto: Centro Italiano di studi Sull'altro Medioevo, 1991), 19–28; Timothy S. Miller and John Nesbitt, *Walking Corpses: Leprosy in Byzantium and the Medieval West* (Ithaca: Cornell University Press, 2014), 132–135.

33 Knefelkamp, *Gesundheits- und Fürsorgewesen der Stadt Freiburg*, 54–60.

34 Tabuteau, "De l'expérience érémétique à la normalisation monastique," 89–96.

35 Pauly, *Peregrinorum, pauperum ac aliorum* 167–171, 208–212, for leper hospitals as instruments of power in civic government; cf. Brigitte Pohl-Resl, *Rechnen mit der Ewigkeit: Das Wiener Bürgerspital im Mittelalter* (Munich: Oldenbourg Verlag, 1996), 22–33, for parallels to multipurpose institutions.

36 Nigel Ramsay and James M. W. Willoughby, eds., *Hospitals, Towns, and the Professions* (London: British Library, 2009), 96–110, 225–230, 230–233, 274–278.

37 Their publication in 1234 has often been used as a line of demarcation between periods of canonistic thought. See, for example, Robert Génestal, *Le Privilegium fori en France: du Décret de Gratian à la fin du XIVe siècle* (Paris: Éditions Ernest Leroux, 1921), 14–20; James A. Brundage,

The title *De Religiosis Domibus* addresses the questions of which houses are entitled to be known as religious houses; of their subjection to episcopal authority; and of the necessity of papal approval for the introduction of a new rule. The first heading affirms that hospitals, "xenodochia, nosocomia, and similar places," may be called religious. The declaration that visitation and reform should be undertaken exclusively by religious persons points up the potential ambiguities arising from the fact that canon law recognized the will of the founder as having legal force.[38] The repeated emphasis on the intent of the hospital founders anticipates the assertion of Hostiensis that anyone could make a valid hospital.[39] The treatment of such intent as legally binding did not obviate dispute, as numerous examples show. Founders might attempt to exclude episcopal influence; or, conversely, sign over control to the bishop if a hospital's religious status was in doubt. Supposed founders might be invoked as part of a hospital's claim to legitimacy as a religious institution, and expressed desires of founders and patrons might come into tension with the needs of surrounding communities and the attitudes of religious leaders.[40] A fifteenth-century debate from the village of Biberg exemplifies this.

Medieval Canon Law (New York: Longman, 1995), 55–69; Hartmann and Pennington, eds. *The History of Medieval Law in the Classical Period*, esp. Kenneth Pennington, "The Decretalists 1190 to 1234,"–, 211–245.

38 Toson, *Mittelalterliche Hospitäler in Hessen*, 39–45, discusses the Gudensberg Heilig Geist Spital, which enters the record in 1365, and the dispute arising after the deaths of the founding spouses; Ulrich Knefelkamp, *Das Heilig-Geist-Spital in Nürnberg vom 14–17. Jahrhundert: Geschichte, Struktur, Alltag* (Nürnberg: Verein für Geschichte der Stadt Nürnberg, 1989), 27–45, 112–115, 152–153, 223–224, discusses the disputes of a wealthy founder's descendants with hospital officials; cf. Paul Bonenfant, "Les premiers 'hospitia' de Bruxelles au XIIe siècle," *Annales de la Société belge d'histoire des hôpitaux* 11 (1973), 9–13. Sethina Watson, *Fundatio, Ordinatio, and Statuta: The Statutes and Constitutional Documents of English Hospitals to 1300* (Oxford: D.Phil., 2003), 77–128, describes founders as becoming increasingly ambitious in their visions for hospitals, but does not mention the stipulations of canon law.

39 See Nicholas Orme and Margaret Webster, *The English Hospital 1070–1570* (New Haven: Yale University Press, 1995), 35–41. On the importance of hospital founders in canon law, see for example Imbert, *Histoire des hôpitaux français*, 58–66; Reicke, *Das deutsche Spital und sein Recht*, vol. 1, 124–50; Watson, *On Hospitals*, 80–113. See Timothy S. Miller, *The Birth of the Hospital in the Byzantine Empire* (Baltimore: Johns Hopkins University Press, 1985), 104–10, on the importance of hospital founders in Byzantium.

40 Franz Josef Felten, "Zum Problem der sozialen Zusammensetzung," in *Vita religiosa sanctimonialium: Norm und Praxis des weiblichen religiösen Lebens vom 6. bis zum 13. Jahrhundert*, ed. Christine Kleinjung (Korb: Didymos-Verlag, 2011), 163–198. See also Oliver Auge, "'Ne pauperes et debiles in… domo degentes divinis careant.' Sakral-religiöse Askpete der mittelalterlichen Hospitalgeschichte," in *Sozialgeschichte mittelalterlicher Hospitäler*, eds. Neithard Bulst and Karl-Heinz Spiess (Ostfildern: Jan Thorbecke Verlag, 2007), 98; Pauly, *Peregrinorum, pauperum*

In 1497, officials from the Benedictine monastery of St. Veit conducted a third-party investigation into a dispute between the chamberlain and council of Biberg, on the one hand, and the founder of the local hospital on the other. Of primary concern were the right to appoint priests (secular or religious) and the circumstances under which Mass could be heard in the hospital. In the end, the resolution allowed the founder of the hospital in Biberg to appoint the priests, concluded that anniversary Masses could be heard there, and that non-members of the hospital community were by all means to be allowed to go there to hear Mass. If burghers sought burial in the hospital, the hospital priest was to receive a measure of wine.[41] A charter possessed by the hospital, no longer extant, is invoked in the conclusion of this record as instrumental in confirming the rights they have long held. Both prescriptive sources and documents of practice show hospitals as institutions governed by canon law. The translation of canon law into practice, as seen in the foregoing document, remained largely dependent on local and regional initiative.

In the thirteenth and fourteenth centuries, Mainz was a center of provincial ecclesiastical and religious activity.[42] This legal activity, moreover, coincided with the most active period of documentation concerning hospitals: their endowment, their rights, and their regulation. The authority of bishops and episcopal judges is highlighted by the Synod of Mainz, in 1239, with criticism of laypersons being elected to ecclesiastical office; similar concerns are addressed at the provincial council held in 1244, also in Mainz.[43] The provincial council of 1259 denounced multiple legal infractions by those with religious status. The lengthiest of the council's canons is *De statu et habitu monachorum et monialium*. This canon condemns the wearing of habits in a false color, and women "who live in the world for a time" are reproved in strong terms.[44] The enforcement of the council's prescriptions

ac aliorum transeuntium receptaculum, 113; Alberzoni, "Norditalienische Pilgerhospize," 284–292; Fritz Viktor Arens, *Die Kunstdenkmäler der Stadt Mainz* (Berlin: Deutsche Kunstverlag, 1962), 9.

41 BayHStA, Kloster St. Veit Urk 87.

42 Ludwig Falck, "Die Freie Stadt in ihre Blütezeit," in *Mainz: Die Geschichte der Stadt*, eds. Franz Dumont, Friedrich Schütz, and Ferdinand Scherf (Mainz: Philipp von Zabern, 1998), 148.

43 Giovan Domenico Mansi, *Sacrorum conciliorum nova et amplissima collectio*, vol. 23 (Florence: Antonio Zatta, 1759), 501–502, and 687–688.

44 This is echoed in the 1292 provincial council held in Aschaffenburg, Mansi, *Sacrorum conciliorum*, vol. 24, 1082–1094. The language of these canons is subtly different, indicating that they were not simply copied in on principle, but responding to still active concerns. The 1270s–1290s saw a wave of archiepiscopal reforms directed at institutions including hospitals, as later chapters shall show.

is enjoined upon "all abbots, abbesses, and other superiors of any order or condition whatsoever, and by whatever name they are called."[45] *Magister/magistra* was the title commonly used for men and women in charge of hospitals; the term's use suggests that hospitals and their staff were seen as religious, and in need of governance accordingly. The provincial synod of Mainz, in 1261, reiterates the mandate that all monastic houses should have infirmaries (*domus hospitalis*).[46] These did not have religious status in their own right. But the fact that independent hospitals did enjoy such status is further indicated by two letters of Clement V, just predating the Council of Vienne. In one, the pope grants exemptions to the brothers and superior of a house in support of their charitable works "for the poor and infirm coming to the hospital of your monastery." In the other to the same community, the terms "monastery" and "hospital" are used redundantly, as Clement refers to the community as "the magister and brothers of the hospital."[47] Records from regional councils were copied down for local use under Archbishop Peter von Aspelt in the early fourteenth century, indicating that they were anything but dead letters.[48]

The Council of Vienne, held in 1311, was intended to provide answers to many of the questions that had preoccupied canonists and ecclesiastical authorities during the previous century. *Quia contingit*, its canon on the governance and definition of hospitals, was to become a popular reference for prelates and legislators in subsequent decades. Sethina Watson has referred to this legislation as "the only sustained legal treatment of hospitals and their government" in the later Middle Ages, representing both a new attention to hospitals within canon law, and a springboard for substantial change in subsequent centuries.[49] The significance of the canon is indisputable; I view it as more closely connected to the debates and developments of the preceding century than does Watson.[50] *Quia contingit* comes directly after the canon *Cum de quibusdam* (even more frequently cited by contemporaries and historians alike) concerning the women "vulgarly called beguines."

45 Mansi, *Sacrorum conciliorum*, vol. 23, col. 997–1000, quoted at col. 1000.

46 Mansi, *Sacrorum conciliorum*, vol. 23, col. 1105.

47 Clement V, *Regestum Clementis papae V: ex vaticanis archetypis sanctissimi domini nostri Leonis XIII pontificis maximi iussu et munificentia*, vol. 5 (Rome: Vatican Press, 1887), Nr. 5105, Nr. 5112. For the text of the latter, see René Choppin, *Monasticon seu de jure coenobitarum libri duo* (Paris: Michael Sonnius, 1601), 139–140.

48 StAM 013/0001.

49 Watson, *On Hospitals*, 295–296, quoted at 295.

50 Watson, *On Hospitals*, 294, says that *Quia contingit* confirmed "the marginal, muddled, and neglected state of welfare houses" in canon law.

The primary concern with these women was that they were not under any "approved rule" of religion. Similar anxieties prevail in the canon concerning the supervision and management of hospitals.[51] What the canon identifies as prevalent misuses could easily stem from divergent understandings of what privileges should appertain to ecclesiastical property.[52] This is particularly suggested by the prohibition of granting hospitals as benefices to secular priests. In formulating *Quia contingit*, Pope Clement V may well have been influenced by the administrative complexities of hospitals in Avignon.[53]

It is not hospitals themselves that appear as the main subject of the canon (a fact neglected by modern commentators.) Rather, it is their administrators, or *rectores*, allegedly suspected of laxity. The canon becomes positively verbose in its assertions of the religious status enjoyed by hospitals, and the obligations thus conferred on their overseers. In concrete terms, the types and uses of donations to hospitals are debated and defined, and the hospital *rectores* are accused of allowing the architectural fabric of the hospitals to decay, and the gifts of the faithful to be perverted for secular uses.[54] This language is too hyperbolic to be taken at face value. It is not, however, mere euphuism; the terms in which these criticisms are couched have legal specificity. Hospital administrators are accused not only of mismanagement, but of allowing the *cura* of these places to be taken over by occupiers and usurpers.[55] These usurpers, in turn, are accused of allowing the redirection of the designated gifts of the faithful. This was prohibited under existing canon law; the fact that some hospital supervisors apparently saw re-designation as within their purview is suggestive of conflicting understandings of hospitals' religious status, or at least of what that status meant.[56]

51 For edition, translation, and interpretation of *Cum de quibusdam,* see Elizabeth Makowski, "When is a beguine not a beguine? Names, Norms, and Nuance in Canonical Literature," in *Labels and Libels: Naming Beguines in Northern Medieval Europe*, ed. Letha Böhringer (Turnhout: Brepols, 2014), 83–98. Tanya Stabler Miller, "Lay Religious Women, University Clerics, and Marguerite de Porete," (talk given at AHA, January 3, 2015,) argues that there were close ties between beguines and university clerics, and that the support given to these women by theologians and priests was one source of the ecclesiastical hierarchy's anxiety; such a theory would certainly seem to be supported by the text of the canon.

52 See Frank, *Heilsame Wortgefechte*, 40–43.

53 Frank, *Heilsame Wortgefechte*, 43–46.

54 Alberigo et al, eds., *Conciliorum Oecumenicorum Decreta*, 350.

55 Alberigo et al, eds., *Conciliorum Oecumenicorum Decreta,* 350. "Quia contingit interdum, quod xenodochiorum, leprosariarum, eleemosynarium, et hospitalium rectores, locorum ipsorum cura postposita, bona, et iura ipsorum interdum ab occupatorum et usurpatorum manibus excutere negligunt."

56 On the designation of funds, see Imbert, *Histoire des hôpitaux français,*101–104. Léon Le Grand, *Statuts d'hôtels-Dieu et de léproseries: recueil de textes du XIIe au XIVe siècle* (Paris: Alphonse

Central to the rhetoric of *Quia contingit* is the care of the sick-poor, which often appears centrally in hospital rules, particularly in the later thirteenth century. The directive of the *Liber Extra* was that only papally-approved rules should be used for religious communities, "lest confusion arise from the multiplicity of rules."[57] The translation of this prescription into fact, however, remained patchy at best throughout the thirteenth century. The statutes given by the cathedral chapter of Puy to its mixed-gender hospital in 1249, and confirmed by Innocent IV the following year, are typical in their language. The chapter declares that they issue the document in order to ensure that "no scandal is spoken of a place where the seeds of virtue should spring forth, and that the sick-poor, the members of Christ's body, may lack nothing."[58] With this as its justification, the rule is primarily concerned with the conduct of the hospital brothers and sisters, ensuring that, in accordance with canon law, they wear a hacbit, share meals, and have no personal property; the hospital priests, too, are enjoined to share the communal life of the house.[59] Similar prescriptions are found for the hospital of Troyes, the Latin rule of which is addressed to "whoever wishes to renounce the world and to serve the poor."[60] The rule limits the number of brothers and sisters to that "useful to the sick," both preserving flexibility and directly echoing canonical prescriptions. That practical and spiritual concerns were directly linked is demonstrated by the specification that the hospital is to have only one kitchen for preparing "vegetables and chicken and the other victuals of the sick-poor and the sisters."[61] Such connections between canon law and pragmatic management are not limited to rules issued by religious authorities. The Count of Saint-Pol, in 1265, issued a hospital rule which, even before the specifications that the staff should

Picard et Fils, 1901), 47, records that the hospital rule of Paris, from the 1220s, specified that designated gifts could be distributed by the donor if that was the donor's wish. See also Hans-Peter Widmann, "Das Spitalwesen," in *Spätmittelalter am Oberrhein. Große Landessausstellung Baden-Württemberg, Staatliche Kunsthalle Karlsruhe, 29. September 2001–2003. February 2002*, eds. Sönke Lorenz and Markus Dekiert (Stuttgart: Jan Thorbecke Verlag, 2002), 493.

57 UCLA Digital Library Program. *Corpus Juris Canonici (1582)*, https://digital.library.ucla.edu/canonlaw/. Last accessed November 22, 2021.

58 Le Grand, *Statuts d'hôtels-dieu*, 98. The statutes survive in a 1383 vidimus of the papal confirmation.

59 Le Grand, *Statuts d'hôtels-dieu*, 97–100.

60 Le Grand, *Statuts d'hôtels-dieu*, 104–105. "Quicumque seculo abrenunciare voluerit et servire pauperibus, primo petat assensum priori et conventus; et, exposita regula vera, si eam server voluerit et promiserit, tunc primum a priore in capitulo conventui presentetur, et tunc a priore et conventu recipiatur, ad serviendum pauperibus, remota omni specie simonye et turpi pacto."

61 Le Grand, *Statuts d'hôtels-dieu*, 112.

take vows, wear a habit, and not leave the hospital without license, defined the necessity of their practical knowledge. The hospital priests should have experience not only in administering sacraments, but in counseling the sick and administering appropriate penances; the lay brothers are to be knowledgeable in affairs so that they may manage the business of the house and provide for the poor. The sisters of the house are to be strong and capable, knowledgeable about moving the bed-ridden (*pauperes cubare et levare*) and administering to the sick according to their needs.[62] Concern with the conduct of hospital administrators should not be assumed to be evidence of laxity. Rather, such specificity testifies to the active involvement of multiple stakeholders concerned with hospitals' social functions and religious status.[63]

The Council of Vienne, then, is responding not to a lack of definition of hospitals' institutional purpose, but rather to the perceived or alleged failure of hospitals in fulfilling already normative legal obligations as religious institutions. The mismanagement of hospitals is criminal "because these places were founded and endowed with donations by the faithful in order that the poor and those infected with leprosy might be received there, and sustained with their produce."[64] The division of hospital residents into "the poor and those infected with leprosy" is intriguing for two reasons. Firstly, there is the clinical use of the language of infection, rare in hospital rules and charters. Secondly, there is the implication that the four types of hospital enumerated—*xenodochia, eleemosynaria, leprosaria*, and *hospitalia*—were imagined as collectively catering to groups comprised of lepers and *pauperes*. It would seem that the mention of the sick-poor was perceived as carrying legal weight; their invocation in this context may parallel their role in hospital rules, where the sick often appear occupying a place similar to that of saints in the rules of monastic houses.[65] In this context, the sick-poor are identified as the proper recipients of the donations of the faithful, made in keeping with the *iura* of the hospital.

62 Le Grand, *Statuts d'hôtels-dieu*, 120.

63 I owe the language of stakeholders to Anna Peterson, e.g. in "Changing Stakeholders and the Church's Approach to Accountability in Assistive Institutions in Thirteenth-Century Western Europe," unpublished paper.

64 Alberigo et al, eds., *Conciliorum Oecumenicorum Decreta*, 350–351. The relevant Latin reads: "quod loca hoc fundata et fidelium erogationibus dotata fuerunt, ut pauperes infectique lepra reciperentur inibi et ex proventibus sustentarentur illorum."

65 Gisela Drossbach, "Bild und Text im *Liber Regulae* des römischen Hospitals von Santo Spirito in Sassia," in *Sozialgeschichte Mittelalterlicher Hospitäler*, ed. Neithard Bulst and Karl-Heinz Spiess (Ostfildern: Jan Thorbecke Verlag, 2007), 125–127.

It is the *iura* itself of hospitals which is at stake, and which enables the Council of Vienne to see the foundation charters and the statutes of hospitals as belonging within their purview, the activities of their administrators as open to conciliar sanction. The administrators have (allegedly) acted inhumanely because their conduct affects the sick; damnably, because their error lies in the "conversion of the hospital's goods [*proventus*] to their own uses, though these were, through the generosity of the faithful, designated for a certain use, and are owed to that use and should be converted to none other."[66] There is a signal exception made to this rule: hospital donations may be put to other purposes at the discretion of the hospital administrators, if they receive papal approval. Appeals to the papacy by the communities of the sick-poor themselves throughout the thirteenth and fourteenth centuries demonstrate that this was not an empty illustration. Such appeals most often make appeal to ancient rights, but these rights are always being defended against a rival claim, from lay or clerical authorities. They bear witness to widespread acceptance of the Council of Vienne's assertion that the rights of hospitals are dependent upon, even as they are defended by, apostolic privilege.

In order to "healthfully reform" hospital communities, the council instates new parameters for the activities of their administrators, and new punishments for administrative violations of hospitals' rights as religious institutions. It is specified that no hospital property is to be converted into benefices for individual priests (such priests may have been counted among the "usurpers" darkly referred to in earlier canons.) Moreover, hospital *rectores* are to be deprived of their privileges if improperly using hospital goods. All of these initiatives, identified as conforming to legitimate custom and apostolic privilege, are ostensibly intended to provide for the "reception and sustenance of the poor."[67] Defining what that sustenance consisted of, and who might be included in the category of the *pauperes*, would fuel legal and social tensions over hospital care throughout the later Middle Ages.

Even in the Council of Vienne, ambiguities about the meaning and maintenance of hospitals' religious status appear. The emphasis of the canon on explaining the ways in which their property was and was not covered by exemption reveals ambiguity in the way their property was understood as ecclesiastical. The council's prohibition on converting the uses of hospital property also indicates tensions caused by the autonomy of

66 Alberigo et al., eds., *Conciliorum Oecumenicorum Decreta*, 351.
67 Alberigo et al., eds., *Conciliorum Oecumenicorum Decreta*, 351.

individual hospitals. The council enumerates several ways in which hospitals can gain religious status. Hostiensis' distinction between *loca religiosa* (communities with institutional privileges as religious houses) and *loca sacra* (communities with distinctive status, but not legal privileges) is not found in the language of the council, where hospitals appear as *pia loca*.[68] That religious status—however fraught—was significant to hospitals as communities, and in their relationships with their neighbors, is revealed in documents created by the institutions themselves. In the absence of unified papal policy concerning the legal privileges of hospitals, vocabulary concerning hospitals was shaped by communities intent on preserving or obtaining rights as religious institutions.

Papal Letters: Canon Law on Hospitals in Practice

The vast majority of documents concerning the government and rights of thirteenth-century leper hospitals were produced by the hospitals themselves, rather than by concerned officials. Hospital communities anxious to affirm or define their status as religious houses petitioned episcopal and even papal officials for records confirming their rights. The records of the papal curia shed light on the ways in which hospitals functioned and understood themselves as religious communities in the thirteenth and fourteenth centuries. The practical regulation of hospitals and their privileges was conducted largely on a case-by-case basis. The papal curia issued very few letters concerning hospitals as a distinct category of institution; when multiple hospitals are addressed, it is almost always those of a particular ecclesiastical jurisdiction. It has been argued that this is evidence that hospitals were not seen as religious houses. However, hospitals are not unique in this respect. Papal letters concerning religious houses of all orders, and hospitals both belonging to orders and established as independent institutions, are generally directed to specific institutions. From the mid-thirteenth century onwards, these letters are characterized by increasingly definite and regular vocabulary for hospitals. Many of them are addressed in response to petitions, indicating the initiative of vowed staff in acquiring and defending the collective rights associated with their religious status.

Over the course of the thirteenth century, letters seeking the confirmation of religious privileges became less frequent, while the number of requests

68 Auge, "'Ne pauperes et debiles,'" 98–102. Alberigo et al., eds., *Conciliorum Oecumenicorum Decreta*, 351.

made on the basis of such status rose. Where specific hospitals are addressed, their vowed staff are often explicitly included, with confirmation of their rights as religious persons. Significantly, the first such letters are issued shortly after the Fourth Lateran Council, that created new criteria for institutions with religious status. In confirming hospitals' rights to collect alms, moreover, the council grouped hospital communities together with other religious houses and persons.[69] The initiative of individual communities, rather than of popes or lawmakers, appears behind the majority of such records throughout the later Middle Ages. The hospitals seeking papal confirmation of their legal privileges dealt with a small cluster of issues, centered around the fluidly defined criteria of religious status. Notably, no distinction in legal status is made between leper houses and multipurpose hospitals, nor are the privileges of leper houses treated as needing particular justification or protection. Hospital staff members must either have had or sought out knowledge about issues of law.

Honorius III granted privileges to multiple *leprosaria*, confirming hospitals and their residents in their rights, and in several cases taking them under the protection of the papacy. All three letters he issued for multipurpose hospitals also responded to petitions by hospital communities. Two out of three of them granted papal protection, and thus legitimacy, to the communities in question. It is not only—or even primarily—the rights of hospitals as permanent institutions that are at stake. Rather, hospital staff request confirmation of their own rights as religious persons. The master and brothers of the *domus dei* in Brignais are confirmed in all their possessions, present and future, with specific mention of the properties with which they were endowed by their lay founder. The pope granted a similar petition for the *magister* and brothers of the hospital of St. Catherine in Paris.[70] Hospitals' right to such exemption could be contested, as indicated by the papal response to the hospital community of Bancigny, which was being harassed by a count. Numerous ecclesiastical personages—a nearby abbot, the archdeacon of Noyon, and the bishop of Artois—are mentioned

69 Alberigo et al., eds., *Conciliorum Oecumenicorum Decreta,* 223, 240–243.

70 Honorius III, Nr. 3740. The hospital of St. Catherine also had its privileges of exemption from civic jurisdiction confirmed by Innocent IV in 1253, Nr. 7172. Ut Per Litteras Apostolicas: https://clio.columbia.edu/catalog/4346120, last accessed November 22, 2021. Printed in Pietro Pressutti, *Regesta Honorii Papae III,* vol. 2 (Rome: Vatican, 1895), 34; Élie Berger, *Les Régistres d'Innocent IV,* vol. 3 (Paris: Ernest Thorin, 1911), 350. On the activities of Honorius III providing concessions and confirmations for religious houses, see Ernst Pitz, *Papstreskript und Kaiserreskript im Mittelalter* (Tübingen: Niemeyer Verlag, 1971), 154–167.

in the letter, implying that Bancigny's staff saw themselves as integrated in regional networks of religious persons and institutions.

Two letters issued by Gregory IX in the 1230s include hospitals in lists of religious institutions to be protected from the impositions of the laity. That such letters were issued points to both ongoing debates about the parameters of religious status, and to hospitals' inclusion as a category of religious house.[71] Moreover, the privileges Gregory bestowed on Speyer's leprosarium of St. Nicolaus in 1239, in response to a petition, indicate that hospitals continued to seek formal affirmation of their entitlement to religious privileges. The emphasis on legal and moral entitlement in that document suggests that such entitlement might be contested. The residents of the *leprosarium*, "the hospital in which [they] share a common life," and their communal property are all granted the protection of St. Peter.[72] Although no particular local authorities are mentioned as threatening the hospital's rights, Gregory goes on to identify vineyards and houses as being covered by this papal privilege, suggesting that the community of St. Nicolaus had written with a list of very definite concerns. These privileges were confirmed in 1240.[73] The first surviving papal letter concerning multiple hospitals is from 1255, and addresses the religious status of hospitals and their staff in the context of other infractions of canon law in the archdiocese of Rheims. The letter identifies the appointment, installation, and deposition of hospital officials as the prerogative of the archbishop and archdeacon, but specifies that the communal consent of the members of the hospital is also requisite.[74]

Throughout the thirteenth and fourteenth centuries, explicit references to hospitals' observation of a rule, or association with an order, are rare.[75] An

71 Dec 21, 1232; Feb 28, 1233. Ut Per Litteras Apostolicas: https://clio.columbia.edu/catalog/4346120, last accessed November 22, 2021.

72 StASp Zinsbuch 280–281

73 StASp U 121.

74 Registra Vaticana 24, fol. 67^{v}, c. 464. "De rectoribus vero et custodibus ponendis vel instituendis et amovendis in domibus leprosorum et aliis que Domus Dei vocantur in civitate et archidiaconatu Remensibus, ordinatum est quod archiepiscopus et archidiaconus tam per se quam per officiales suos vel alios simul communi consensu instituant et destituant rectores et custodes eosdem." Ut Per Litteras Apostolicas: https://clio.columbia.edu/catalog/4346120, last accessed November 22, 2021.

75 The only such references are: Registra Vaticana 25, fol. 95, c. 715; Reg. Vat.Registra Vaticana 12 v°; Reg. Vat. 44, c. 4Registra Vaticana2 r° (notably, in this letter of 1289, the archbishop of Vienne is attempting to reform a traditionally Augustinian hospital and bring it under a stricter observance, and his authority); Reg. Vat. 49, fol. 155, ep.Registra Vaticanaas a privately founded hospital being placed under the authority of a Dominican priory, with consent of the hospital community being necessary to the appointment of nominated officials (1299); Reg. Vat. 51, n° 383,

unusual case is provided by the 1274 confirmation of the rights and properties of the hospital in Vienne, which is described as following the same statutes (*simili jure spectante*) as the hospital of St. John in Jerusalem.[76] Another is found in an indulgence granted to sisters of an independent hospital following the customs (*instituta*) of the Dominicans. The language makes clear that the sisters receive pastoral care from a community of Dominicans but are not understood as Dominicans themselves.[77] I do not subscribe to the historiographical tradition that would have the hospital of St. John in Jerusalem serving as the dominant institutional model for European hospitals during this period. The mother house in Jerusalem, in addition to commanding more staff and resources than most European hospitals, provided a site-specific response to growing poverty in a war-torn city.[78] The material benefit of having (or claiming) identical observation was the canonical legitimacy it provided. As late as 1311, the affiliation of a hospital appears as secondary to the question of its religious status.[79] Hospitals seeking confirmation of their privileges used care for the sick-poor as an indicator of religious status more often than claims of affiliation with a rule or order. An unusually detailed example of such a letter, issued by Gregory IX in 1278, explicitly invokes the Council of Paris (1212) both in exempting the property and revenues (*reditibus et proventibus*) of a hospital from taxes, and specifying that the said income must be used exclusively to provide for the needs of the sick-poor. The exemptions of the same hospital are again

fol. 90, sees Registra Vaticanaprivately founded hospital being confirmed in its privileges (1303); Reg. Vat. 57, cap. 613, f. 157*a* (1310.) Ut PeRegistra Vaticanas Apostolicas: https://clio.columbia.edu/catalog/4346120, last accessed November 22, 2021.

76 Registra Vaticana 38, fol. 12 v°. Ut Per Litteras Apostolicas: https://clio.columbia.edu/catalog/4346120, last accessed November 22, 2021. Cf. Potthast, RPR vol. 1, Nr. 1409, providing evidence of a 1258 grant made by Alexander IV to the magister and brothers of the hospital of St. Mary (Teutonic Order) in Jerusalem, and all those of the order, that they receive general absolution for crimes committed before taking the habit.

77 Clement V, *Regestum Clementis papae V* (Rome: Vatican, 1885), Nr. 5757, refers to the prioress and sisters of a *domus Dei* who are living "secundum instituta et sub cura fratrum Praedicatorum."

78 Jessalynn Lea Bird, "Medicine for Body and Soul: Jacques de Vitry's Sermons to Hospitallers and their Charges," in *Religion and Medicine in the Middle Ages*, eds. Peter Biller and Joseph Ziegler (Rochester, NY: York Medieval Press, 2001), 101–103, provides both a historiographical overview and a counter-argument. Marie-Louise Windemuth, *Das Hospital als Träger der Armenfürsorge im Mittelalter* (Stuttgart: Franz Steiner Verlag, 1995), 66–74.

79 Registra Vaticana 58, cap. 240, f. 59*a*. Ut Per Litteras Apostolicas: https://clio.columbia.edu/catalog/4346120, last accessed November 22, 2021. An Augustinian canon, hitherto prior of a hospital but now himself in failing health, is authorized to give his resignation to the bishop of Sens, who may then confer the hospital to a monastery or other place dedicated to St. Augustine, or to another order.

under question in 1308; at issue is the question of whether its income is used to sustain the poor or the preceptor and brothers of the house.[80] Several examples of similar exemptions survive from the letters of Clement V. Perhaps the most notable of these is a letter issued in 1310, specifying that the hospital of Bordeaux is included in the general exemptions to which hospitals (including *leprosaria*) are entitled, and that its exempt incomes are to be converted for the exclusive use of the poor.[81]

Throughout the later Middle Ages, the vocabulary concerning hospitals in papal letters is both pluralistic and labile. Especially in the mid-thirteenth century, the terms "domus dei" and "leprosarium" are used to designate the same institution. References to hospitals as "domus dei" experience an uptick around the midpoint of the thirteenth century, but increase sharply in the 1320s and 1330s, following the Council of Vienne. Another remarkable spike in the 1360s–1370s may represent a response to the uncertainty cause by the Great Schism. An increase in references to individual *leprosaria* in the same period is caused primarily by a handful of ongoing legal cases, rather than petitions from a great number of institutions. The specificity of these late fourteenth-century letters makes clear that the needs of hospitals were taken into account by a curia responsive to carefully formulated petitions.

Papal letters regulating hospitals as a category of religious institutions survive in much smaller numbers than those documents generated by petitions from individual institutions. Analyzing them, however, helps complete the picture of how hospitals were regarded in legal terms. Such letters begin to appear in the 1220s, shortly after the first recorded petitions, and in the wake of the Fourth Lateran Council. The last letter concerning *hospitalium* appears in 1299, shortly before the Council of Vienne, which aimed to codify the legal status of hospitals as religious institutions. In the interim, a trend towards defining hospitals in terms of how they used their property can be perceived, as well as a trend towards emphasizing the status of the institutions themselves, rather than that of their vowed staff.

The letters issued by Gregory IX affirm the status and property of communities that have written to them, extending those rights to the hospitals under their supervision. Neither of these communities, located in Bologna

80 Registra Vaticana 55, cap. 265, f. 50*a*. Ut Per Litteras Apostolicas: https://clio.columbia.edu/catalog/4346120, last accessed November 22, 2021.

81 Registra Vaticana 58, cap. 592, f. 146*b*, printed in Clement V, *Regestum Clementis papae V*, vol. 6, Nr. 7009. See also Reg. Vat.Registra Vaticana 708, f. 173*a*, a letter for the hospital of Orléans, 1311; Reg. Vat. 59, cap.Registra Vaticana 135*a*, a letter for the hospitals of the diocese of Bazas, in southern France, 1312. Ut Per Litteras Apostolicas: https://clio.columbia.edu/catalog/4346120, last accessed November 22, 2021.

and Parma, were the mother houses of recognized orders, but rather leaders of regional networks of hospitals.[82] A similar privilege is granted by Alexander IV in 1257, exempting a hospital of Pisa from a recent union of hospitals formed by the Pisans, on the condition that it be subject to the jurisdiction of the Camaldolese hermits.[83] The existence of such networks and such petitions reflects the transitions following on Lateran IV's new criteria for religious orders and institutions. Moreover, hospitals are included alongside other religious houses, as in a letter of 1218 ordering the religious houses of the diocese of Prague to observe a papal interdict despite Siegfried II of Mainz's relaxation of the same.[84] More analysis of hospitals' participation in such networks remains a desideratum. Notably, these letters follow a very similar pattern to those provided for the Antonine friars, and for the Templar, Hospitaller, and Teutonic orders during the same decades; no clear distinction between the regular orders and less formal congregations is found in the vocabulary of the papal letters concerning them.[85]

From the 1260s onwards, a dual emphasis on the rhetoric of reform and on hospitals' exemption from tithes emerges in papal letters concerning hospitals. Urban IV appears to have been particularly concerned with hospital observance, issuing both a command for the reform of hospitals following the Augustinian Rule, and an inquiry about falsified papal letters being used by the hospitals of Altopascio.[86] The former letter, concerning the hospitals of the diocese of Langres, is particularly notable for its elaborate and exalted language of reform, claiming the dual threat of offending divine majesty and giving rise to scandal among the laity. The process of reforming hospitals and their staff is framed in terms of administering spiritual medicine. The concrete implications of this are clearly spelled out: the hospitals' liturgical performance and temporal administration is to be examined, with the

82 Letters of Gregory IX, 10 July 1228 and 18 May 1235. Ut Per Litteras Apostolicas: https://clio.columbia.edu/catalog/4346120, last accessed November 22, 2021.

83 Letter of Alexander IV, 3 November 1257. Ut Per Litteras Apostolicas: https://clio.columbia.edu/catalog/4346120, last accessed November 22, 2021. A summary is found in Potthast, RPR, Nr. 17055.

84 Letter of Honorius III, 4 March 1218, copied or repeated 27 March. Ut Per Litteras Apostolicas: https://clio.columbia.edu/catalog/4346120, last accessed November 22, 2021. Printed in Pressutti, *Regesta Honorii Papae III*, Nr. 1130, Nr. 1187.

85 Letters of Innocent IV, 13 September 1247 and 21 July 1248. Ut Per Litteras Apostolicas: https://clio.columbia.edu/catalog/4346120, last accessed November 22, 2021. Printed in Berger, *Régistres d'Innocent IV*, vol. 2, 12, 108–112.

86 Letters of Urban IV, 20 March 1263 and 23 March 1264. Ut Per Litteras Apostolicas: https://clio.columbia.edu/catalog/4346120, last accessed November 22, 2021. Printed in Jean Guiraud, ed., *Les registres d'Urbain IV (1261-1264)* (Paris: Thorin et Fils, 1899–1906.)

bishop being given full authority to intervene. The letter insists that hospital staff are to "perpetually serve their hospitals and the persons within them," only permitted to depart if joining a stricter religious observance.[87] This demonstrates that hospital vows were understood conferring religious status, and that some ambiguity about the legal implications of that status endured.[88] Other letters concerning the observance and obligations of hospitals are usually more clearly responsive to specific local concerns, or more general in what they enjoin.

Throughout the latter half of the thirteenth century, papal letters confirm the privileges of hospitals, and their obligations to the sick-poor. A letter to multiple bishops and archbishops concerning the rights of St. Antony in Vienne, for example, invokes the many sick and poor who come to the hospital and have long done so; the privileges are to apply to other churches, monasteries, and hospitals constructed in the name of the saint.[89] Martin IV, 5 June 1282 and 17 June 1283, grants indulgences to those donating to the construction of churches and hospitals; Boniface VIII, 1 August 1299, gives, almost certainly in response to a petition, specific guidelines to hospitals in the dioceses of Florence and Lucca for filling vacancies, which are not to be filled by external candidates put forward by religious authorities; Benedict XI, 31 January 1304, issues multiple letters entitling bishops to hospitality from religious houses and persons, including "hospitalium sive domorum."[90] This formulation is also found in geographically diverse locations, suggesting the influence of canon law both before as well as after the Council of Vienne.[91] While hospitals are still somewhat amorphously defined themselves, they are consistently grouped with other religious institutions.

87 Letter of Urban IV, 20 March 1263. Ut Per Litteras Apostolicas: https://clio.columbia.edu/catalog/4346120, last accessed November 22, 2021.

88 For parallels in other religious houses, see Sherri Franks Johnson, *Monastic Women and Religious Orders in Late Medieval Bologna* (Cambridge, Cambridge University Press, 2014), 10–11, 47–50; Christiane Ulrike Kurz, *"Ubi et est habitatio sororum et mansio fratrum": Doppelklöster und ähnliche Klostergemeinschaften im mittelalterlichen Österreich* (*Diözese Passau in den Ausdehnungen des 13. Jahrhunderts*) (Kiel: Solivagus Verlag, 2015), 1–19; Charles de Miramon, *Les "donnés" au Moyen Âge: une forme de vie religieuse laïque, v. 1180–v. 1500* (Paris: Cerf, 1999), 128–145.

89 Letter of Clement IV, 22 April 1265, Ut Per Litteras Apostolicas: https://clio.columbia.edu/catalog/4346120, last accessed November 22, 2021. Printed in Édouard Jordan, ed., *Les Registres De Clement IV, 1265–1268* (Paris: Thorin et Fils, 1894), Nr. 1554.

90 Ut Per Litteras Apostolicas: https://clio.columbia.edu/catalog/4346120, last accessed November 22, 2021. The letters of Benedict are printed in Charles Grandjean, ed., *Le Registre de Benoît XI* (Paris: Thorin et Fils, 1883), Nr. 1181, Nr. 1188.

91 See, for example, A. T. Bannister, ed. *The Register of Adam de Orleton, Bishop of Hereford* (*A.D. 1317–1327*) (Hereford: Wilson and Phillips, 1907), 11; José Luis Martin, *Documentación medieval*

The distinctive role of *leprosaria* did not make them legally separate from multipurpose hospitals and other religious houses. Nicholas III, in enjoining penance on a count in 1280, included the stipulation that he should make a donation "for the uses of the poor, to the houses of God, hospitals, *leprosaria*, religious and other pious places" in Paris.[92] The profusion of labels is indicative of the flexibility—even ambiguity—of hospitals' institutional form, but also of the fact that they were seen as coming within the remit of canon law. In sending a mandate to restore "ancient conventions" between the hospitals of Harbledown and Northgates and the archbishop of Canterbury, Nicholas IV made no distinction between the leper house and the multipurpose institution.[93] In clarifying what the King of France is permitted to take from ecclesiastical and religious persons, Boniface VIII lists "masters, preceptors, or priors, or prelates, by whatever name they are known, of houses of god, leper hospitals, and hospitals of the poor."[94]

The majority of papal letters from the latter half of the thirteenth century deal with hospitals' privileges as religious institutions to be exempt from tithes. No single form letter was used for this purpose, but from the 1270s, a set formula for the exemptions themselves came to dominate: "*De reditibus et proventibus leprosarium, domorum Dei, et hospitalium pauperum, qui in usus infirmorum et pauperum convertuntur, decima non solvetur.*" This formula was taken directly from the Council of Paris concerning the rights of religious persons. First appearing in a letter of Gregory X confirming that council, it appears frequently in letters to tithe collectors and bishops.[95] Such letters were issued fairly regularly throughout the thirteenth century, dropping off abruptly in the first decade of the fourteenth. This suggests that the 1311 Council of Vienne was perceived as providing a set of guidelines

de la iglesia catedral de Coria, Acta Salmanticensia 12 (Salamanca: Universidad de Salamanca, 1989), 147–148, in an episcopal letter of 1322.

92 Nicholas III, 27 March 1280. The relevant Latin reads: "in usus pauperum, domorum Dei hospitalium, leprosariarum, religiosorum ac aliorum piorum locorum." Ut Per Litteras Apostolicas: https://clio.columbia.edu/catalog/4346120, last accessed November 22, 2021. Printed in Jules Gay, ed., *Les Registres de Nicolas III* (Paris: Thorin et Fils, 1898), Nr. 621.

93 Nicholas IV, 3 February 1290, Ut Per Litteras Apostolicas: https://clio.columbia.edu/catalog/4346120, last accessed November 22, 2021.

94 The relevant Latin reads: "...magistros, preceptores seu priores sive prelates, quocumque nomine censeantur, domorum dei, leprosariarum, hospitalium pauperum." Boniface VIII, 28 January 1299, Ut Per Litteras Apostolicas: https://clio.columbia.edu/catalog/4346120, last accessed November 22, 2021.

95 Letters of Gregory X, 23 October 1274 and 13 February 1277; Letters of Nicholas III, 9 February 1278, 13 November 1278, 9 August 1278, 22 September 1278, 25 September 1278; Letter of Honorius IV, 17 June 1285, 7 July 1289, 23 June 1289, 20 September 1290; Boniface VIII, 29 September 1301. Ut Per Litteras Apostolicas: https://clio.columbia.edu/catalog/4346120, last accessed November 22, 2021.

concerning the rights and obligations of hospitals that could be used instead of the reactive letters of preceding decades.

There are only nine letters in the papal registers relevant to hospitals within the province or archdiocese of Mainz. Most of these, moreover, are concerned with the interests of the papacy or of the powerful Hospitallers, rather than local conditions or events.[96] In 1224, almost certainly in response to a petition, Honorius III took the rector and brothers of the hospital of St. Martin in Erfurt under his protection, confirming them in all the privileges granted by the archbishop of Mainz.[97] The fact that the hospital community sought out such privileges from ecclesiastical authorities suggests that they were aware both of the desirability of legal privileges as a religious institution, and of the potentially ambiguous criteria for obtaining them. A letter of Nicholas IV to Archbishop Gerhard II and his suffragans demonstrates that claims of hospital identity could be contentious. In 1290, the pope wrote to the ecclesiastical leaders of Mainz condemning in strong language those who falsely asserted that they belonged to the Templars, the Hospitallers, or other "diverse orders of hospitals," and obtained alms and donations under these pretenses. The problem was not limited to Mainz, but the pope did want the condemnation of such practices publicly condemned in the cities and churches of that territory.[98] Notably, Nicholas IV specifies in the conclusion of this letter that legitimate members of hospital communities are by no means to be restricted from the preaching and gathering of alms.[99] The question of how proper and improper claims to hospital status were to be distinguished is left up to local authorities. It is, then, to the practical negotiation of hospitals' religious status, and the

96 Letter of Honorius III, 7 April 1223; letter of Urban IV, 9 November 1261; letter of Gregory X, 23 March 1275; letter of Boniface VIII, 23 March 1299. Boniface includes the abbot of St. Alban in Mainz among the addressees of a letter concerning the molestation of Hospitallers. Ut Per Litteras Apostolicas: https://clio.columbia.edu/catalog/4346120, last accessed November 22, 2021.

97 Letter of Honorius III, 7 March 1224: "Rectori et fratribus Hospitalis sancti Martini in Erphordia Eos et locum in quo divino obsequio sunt mancipati, sub protectione recipit nec non possessiones et libertates a Maguntino archiepiscopo de capituli sui assensu pia liberalitate eisdem concessas confirmat." Ut Per Litteras Apostolicas: https://clio.columbia.edu/catalog/4346120, last accessed November 22, 2021. Printed in Pietro Pressutti, *Regesta Honorii papae III, 1216–1227* (Hildesheim: Georg Olms Verlag, 1978).

98 Letter of Nicholas IV, 11 October 1290. Ut Per Litteras Apostolicas: https://clio.columbia.edu/catalog/4346120, last accessed November 22, 2021.

99 Letter of Nicholas IV, 11 October 1290. "Per hoc autem fratres militie Templi, Hospitalis Sancti Johannis et domorum ac hospitalium predictorum a questu licito nolumus prohiberi." Ut Per Litteras Apostolicas: https://clio.columbia.edu/catalog/4346120, last accessed November 22, 2021.

effects of that status on hospitals in the archdiocese of Mainz, that the following chapters turn.

Conclusion: Canon Law and the Hospitals of Mainz

The first record of care for the sick-poor in Mainz dates to the tenure of the influential Archbishop Willigis (r. 975–1011). The late tenth and early eleventh centuries also saw the creation of numerous religious foundations in and around Mainz, and the city's great cathedral was constructed under Willigis' leadership.[100] A note in a tenth-century gospel book records Archbishop Willigis' gift of alms in the form of food and drink to the sick-poor. These alms were regularly distributed, possibly to a regular clientele, in Mainz's cathedral close. This distribution was done both for the good of Willigis' soul and in memory of his sister Mathilda, who had been an abbess. The language of the memorial does not allow a conclusive answer to the question of whether the *pauperes* receiving Willigis' alms were already defined by residence in a hospital, or selected at the archbishop's or provost's discretion.[101] As noted above, the duties of a hospital to provide care were defined as providing for the comforts of the poor. This central duty clarified and confirmed hospitals' social functions and legal responsibilities.[102]

100 Ludwig Falck, "Die Erzbischöfliche Metropole, 1011–1244," in *Mainz: Die Geschichte der Stadt*, edited by Franz Dumont, Friedrich Schütz, and Ferdinand Scherf, (Mainz: Philipp von Zabern, 1998), 113–114. The foundations first recorded under Willigis include St. Stephan, St. Victor, St. Alban, and Altmünster.

101 Stiftsbibliothek Aschaffenburg MS Perg 37 146r. The relevant passage reads: "Sancta intencione hoc | extituit memoriale quatinus quot annis in festivitate omnum sanctorum ex parte archiepiscopi detur una livra denariorum pauperibus eroganda | et ex parte proposite totidem pauperum pascio in potu et cibo et ut | eodem die sancta clericorum congregacio tale convivium habeat | unde se honeste reficere valeat."

102 Bodleian MS Laud Misc 430, fols. 54r–55r, in a life of St. Elisabeth of Hungary, treats the regular distribution of alms as part of the function of a hospital; Odo Rigaldus, *Registers of Eudes of Rouen*, trans. Sydney M. Brown, ed. J. F. Sullivan (New York: Columbia University Press, 1964), 614–615, describes the visitation of a leper hospital (Salle-aux-Puelles) near Rouen where alms were distributed thrice weekly. For secondary literature on the later Middle Ages, see Davis, "Hospitals, Charity, and the Culture of Compassion," 41; John Henderson, *Piety and Charity in Late Medieval Florence* (Oxford: Clarendon Press, 1994), 242, noting parallels between hospitals and other religious institutions; Daniel Le Blévec, *La Part du Pauvre: l'assistance dans les pays du Bas-Rhône du XIIe siècle au milieu du XVe siècle,* vol. 1 (Rome: École française de Rome, 2000), 92, 113; Orme and Webster, *The English Hospital,* 56–64, assert that alms might be distributed ritually to both transient and permanent populations. Miri Rubin, *Charity and Community in Medieval Cambridge* (Cambridge: Cambridge University Press, 1988), 245–250.

The later eleventh and early twelfth centuries saw an expansion of the hospital landscape, along with the growth of Mainz itself into a powerful urban center.[103] The prosperous canonry of Liebfrauen, that supervised the St. Barbara hospital, dates from the late eleventh century; this period, too, contains the first mentions of a community in the location where the lepers of Heilig Kreuz would later gather.[104] Several twelfth-century archbishops—notably Adalbert I and Marcolf—took an active interest in the religious institutions of the city and its environs, providing patronage or intervening in administration.[105] It was probably under the latter that the city's oldest hospital received its first independent buildings; his successor, Heinrich, placed the hospital under the administration of a house of canons. The mid-twelfth century also saw increasing political tensions between the burghers of Mainz and the archbishops. Dietrich Demandt calls the resulting constellation of power "tripolar," with the cathedral chapter, the burghers of Mainz, and the archbishop fighting for influence over ecclesiastical and civic control.[106] In the latter half of the twelfth century, the archbishops were conspicuously caught up in the power struggles between pope and emperor; their engagement in the administration of Mainz and its archdiocese is less visible.[107] During this period, the religious houses of Mainz were primarily aristocratic in their composition and their patronage; Benedictine houses and canonries dominated the religious landscape.

The consent of the chapter to archiepiscopal decrees was a novel requirement in the early thirteenth century. Dependent on this consent were *inter alia* sale or lease of church property, rents, and church subsidies; the fact that this consent is explicitly affirmed in hospital statutes indicates that hospitals were seen as religious houses.[108] The 1230s–1250s would see a

103 Michael Kläger, "Das Stadtbild im Wandel," in *Beiträge zur Mainzer Geschichte* 28 (1988), 24.

104 Falck, "Die Erzbischöfliche Metropole," 114. Kläger, "Das Stadtbild im Wandel," 17–18.

105 Josef Semmler, "Vita Religiosa und Bischof bis gegen 1200," in *Handbuch der Mainzer Kirchengeschichte: Christliche Antike und Mittelalter*, ed. Friedhelm Jürgensmeier, vol. 2 (Würzburg: Echter Verlag, 2000), 631–640.

106 Dietrich Demandt, *Stadtherrschaft und Stadtfreiheit im Spannungsfeld von Geistlichkeit und Bürgerschaft in Mainz (11-15. Jahrhundert)* (Wiesbaden: Franz Steiner Verlag 1977), 50–68; see also Semmler, "Vita Religiosa und Bischof," 644–645, and StAM U/8 September 1260. StAM U/1 February 1275 resolves a dispute between the archbishop and the burghers, the archbishop having been "freventlich gestoert."

107 Semmler, "Vita Religiosa und Bischof," 644669, esp. 667–669; Falck, "Die Erzbischöfliche Metropole," 123–128: while archiepiscopal and civic factions were rivals for power, religious leaders and institutions often pursued independent policies.

108 Irmtraud Liebeherr, *Der Besitz des Mainzer Domkapitels im Spätmittelalter* (Mainz: Gesellschaft für Mittelrheinische Kirchengeschichte, 1971), 12–14.

wave of centralization efforts by powerful archbishops. Nonnenmünster and Altmünster, in Worms and Mainz, respectively, were but two of the houses in the archdiocese brought into the Cistercian Order through the joint intervention of pope and archbishop.[109] The language of the papal letter on Altmünster, leaving scarcely a legal term unelaborated, suggests an audience (or at least an imagined audience) for whom religious identity was not easily denoted by a set vocabulary.[110] The same decades saw the creation of a new rule for Mainz's oldest hospital, and the creation of a new community of hospital sisters. New trends in the religious life of city and archdiocese took shape at the same time that the legal boundaries between civic and ecclesiastical privileges remained under dispute. Over the course of the next two centuries, when Mainz enjoyed its golden age, hospitals appear alongside other religious houses of the archdiocese in waves of reform, and as agents and prizes in often turbulent ecclesiastical politics. The subsequent chapters examine the activities of these diverse hospitals, and their commitment to their distinctive institutional vocation, as well as the protection of their legal rights.

109 On Nonnenmünster, see Christine Kleinjung, *Frauenklöster als Kommunikationszentren und soziale Räume. Das Beispiel Worms vom 13. bis zum Beginn des 15. Jahrhunderts* (Korb: Didymos Verlag, 2008) 45–52. This house's incorporation was a process of several decades from 1236–1252, with the bishop of Worms aggressively involved following a letter from Gregory IX to the archbishop. The official letter of incorporation dates to 1244 and was reaffirmed in the 1290s.

110 StAM U / 7 February 1235 is the remarkably beautiful papal charter concerning Altmünster, described as a correction and reform of the monastery "in its head and in its members," a "suitable reform of orders and of regular observance." The hand is regular and the ruling generous; this and the elegantly embellished capitals suggests that the charter was made to impress those who were to live in a manner befitting "religious and honest persons."

2 Civic Hospitals in the City and Archdiocese of Mainz

Abstract
This chapter discusses the establishment of an archiepiscopal rule for Mainz's hospital, and the hospital's subsequent transfer to civic oversight. Studying how the hospital's inclusion in the 1244 charter of civic liberties affected its claim to the privileges of religious status sheds new light on the transfer's effects. I pursue the hospital's late medieval history through 1462, when the archbishops of Mainz reasserted their political control over the city, and their rights over the administration of the hospital. I compare the civic hospitals of Worms and Speyer, and their relationships with civic and episcopal authority. Over the course of the later Middle Ages, civic hospitals in the Rhineland used their claims to religious status to carve out institutional independence.

Keywords: urban history, medieval hospitals, Worms, Mainz, Speyer

On 1 August 1236, Archbishop Siegfried III authorized the move of Mainz's hospital to new buildings on the edge of the city.[1] In the elaborate prologue to the statutes issued on this occasion, the archbishop described his role in high-flown terms:

> "We know that it is only fitting for us to eagerly assist, maintain, and guide all places where the sick and pilgrims find welcome, the weary rest, the hungry food, the thirsty drink, and all, whether rich or poor,

1 This has, on occasion, mistakenly been interpreted as the foundation document of the hospital: Erich Hinkel, *Das Gau-Algesheimer Hospital. Beiträge zur Geschichte des Gau-Algesheimer Raumes,* (Carl-Brilmayer-Gesellschaft: Gau-Algesheim, 1987), 1; Karl W. Heyden, "Die Hospitäler in Oppenheim," *Oppenheimer Hefte* 1 (1990), 16.

Barnhouse, Lucy C. *Hospitals in Communities of the Late Medieval Rhineland. Houses of God, Places for the Sick.* Taylor & Francis Group, 2023
DOI: 10.5117/9789463720243_CH02

find solace. We also know that their special care is incumbent upon us [as a duty.]"[2]

In invoking provision for the sick as the key reason for the hospital's move, the document echoes early thirteenth-century councils that defined hospitals' religious identity in terms of their provision of such necessities.[3]

In the first half of the thirteenth century, many of the urban hospitals of Europe emerged from the aegis of episcopal patrons, establishing themselves as independent institutions. This process was in part a response to the changing requirements of canon law, and itself raised new questions about hospitals' religious status. The early thirteenth-century history of Mainz's oldest hospital is representative of this process in the hospital's acquisition of a written rule, its move away from the cathedral close, and its oversight by the city council.[4] The hospital is not consistently named until the thirteenth century; for the institution's early history, therefore, I avoid the designation "Heilig Geist Spital." Within the span of a few decades—from the 1230s to the 1250s—Mainz's hospital moved from the cathedral close to the city walls, acquired statutes proclaiming its conformity to the canonical requirements for religious status, was transferred from archiepiscopal to civic oversight, and dismissed its vowed female staff. Each of these processes had legal catalysts and consequences, affecting the hospital's position in the religious networks of Mainz. These changes can be better understood through the lens of canon law than through an analysis focused primarily on the variables of civic politics. Municipal elites could use hospitals' religious status to their own financial and social advantage, but were more interested in maintaining hospitals separate from direct ecclesiastical control than with administering the hospitals themselves.

Analysis of hospitals' thirteenth-century development has often resulted in simplified narratives of lay elites asserting their newfound social power against ecclesiastical control.[5] Assumptions that disputes over hospital

2 StAM 6/40 (3). Printed in Valentin Ferdinand Gudenus, *Codex diplomaticus: exhibens anectoda ab anno DCCCLXXXI ad MCCC Moguntiaca, ius Germanicum, et S.R.I. historiam illustrantia* I, (Göttingen: Sumptu Regiae Officinae Librar. Academ., 1743), 637.

3 See Joseph Alberigo, Joseph A. Dossetti, Pericles Joannou, Claude Leonardi, and Paul Prodi, eds., *Conciliorum Oecumenicorum Decreta*, 3rd ed., (Bologna: Istituto per le scienze religiose, 1973), 322. Cf. Giovan Domenico Mansi, *Sacrorum conciliorum nova et amplissima collectio*, vol. 22 (Florence: Antonio Zatta, 1759), col. 826–827.

4 See Ludwig Falck, "Mainzer Hospitäler im Mittelalter," in *Moguntia Medica: Das medizinische Mainz von Mittelalter bis ins 20. Jahrhundert*, ed. Franz Dumont (Wiesbaden: B. Wylicil, 2002), 409–411.

5 Thomas Just and Herwig Weigl, "Spitäler im südöstlichen Deutschland und in den österreichischen Ländern im Mittelalter," in *Europäisches Spitalwesen. Institutionelle Fürsorge in*

administration were inevitable, however, neglect the agency of hospital communities themselves, as well as one of their signal characteristics, disturbing to ecclesiastical and civic authorities alike: the ability to escape definite compartmentalization.[6] I contest the conventional narrative about such urban institutions which holds that hospitals passed from archiepiscopal into civic control as pawns of the dominant political interests. In many interpretations, regionalism is seen as trumping characteristics unique to hospitals, with site-specific conflicts between civic and ecclesiastical authorities driving events.[7] Analyzing institutional uses of canon law enables supra-regional comparison. This is not meant to replace one monocausal explanation with another. Rather, it is intended to shed light on the ways in which civic hospitals developed as independent institutions. From the thirteenth century onwards, Mainz's oldest hospital used its claim to religious status to negotiate a substantially independent course, both before and after it passed from archiepiscopal to civic oversight. In Speyer and

Mittelalter und Früher Neuzeit, eds. Martin Scheutz, Andrea Sommerlechner, Herwig Weigl, and Alfred Stefan Weiß (Munich: R. Oldenbourg Verlag, 2008), 158–159, have pointed this out. For examples, see Siegfried Reicke, *Das Deutsche Spital und sein Recht im Mittelalter*, vol. 1 (Stuttgart: Enke, 1932), 111–127; Wolfgang W. Schürle, *Das Hospital zum Heiligen Geist in Konstanz; ein Beitrag zur Rechtsgeschichte des Hospitals im Mittelalter* (Sigmaringen: Jan Thorbecke Verlag, 1970), 29–37; Ulrich Knefelkamp, "Stadt und Spital," in *Städtisches Gesundheits- und Fürsorgewesen vor 1800*, ed. Peter Johanek (Köln: Böhlau Verlag, 2000), 30–40, asserts that hospitals were not only both economically important and socially significant, but functioned as "prestige buildings" symbolizing burghers' priorities.

6 See for example Benjamin Laqua, *Bruderschaften und Hospitäler während des hohen Mittelalters: Kölner Befunde im westeuropäisch-vergleichende Perspektive* (Stuttgart: Hiersemann, 2011), 99–108, on the hospital of Lüttich. Michel Pauly, *Peregrinorum, pauperum ac aliorum transeuntium receptaculum: Hospitäler zwischen Maas und Rhein im Mittelalter* (Stuttgart: Franz Steiner Verlag, 2007), 167–171, 179–180, 208–212, points out that conflicts over hospital administration could arise from rivalries among different urban interest groups, rather than between municipal and ecclesiastical authorities imagined as monolithic, but still characterizes hospitals primarily as objects rather than agents of change.

7 See Franz Meffert, *Caritas und Krankenwesen bis zum Ausgang des Mittelalters* (Freiburg im Breisgau: Caritas Verlag, 1927), 312–313; Jesko von Steynitz, *Mittelalterliche Hospitäler der Orden und Städte als Einrichtungen der Sozialen Sicherung* (Berlin: Duncker und Humblot, 1970), 103–105; Ernst-Adolf Meinert, *Die Hospitäler Holsteins im Mittelalter: Ein Beitrag zur mittelalterlichen Stadtgeschichte* (Neumünster, Wachholtz Verlag, 1997), 17–23; Mathias Kälble, "Sozialfürsorge und kommunale Bewegung. Zur Bedeutung von Hospitälern für die politische Gruppenbildung in der Stadt," in *Sozialgeschichte Mittelalterlicher Hospitäler*, 237–242; Knefelkamp, "Stadt und Spital," in *Städtisches Gesundheits- und Fürsorgewesen vor 1800*, ed. Peter Johanek (Köln: Böhlau Verlag, 2000), 30–40. Sheila Sweetinburgh, "Royal Patrons and Local Benefactors: The Experience of the Hospitals of St. Mary at Ospringe and Dover in the Thirteenth Century," in *Religious and Laity in Western Europe 1000–1400: Interaction, Negotiation, and Power*, ed. Emilia Jamroziak and Janet Burton (Turnhout: Brepols, 2006), 122–126.

Worms, too, hospitals were both supported by civic elites, and assiduous in asserting their legitimacy as religious institutions.

When Mainz's first hospital enters the documentary record in 1145, archiepiscopal involvement in its administration is simultaneously commemorated and affirmed. Invoking his predecessors, Archbishop Heinrich I placed the hospital under the supervision of a house of canons in order to regularize its religious observance.[8] In 1236, the hospital received its first statutes, reinforcing its identity as a religious institution, and the privileges and obligations thereby conferred on its staff. Amid shifting dynamics of power in the growing city of Mainz, the hospital and its residents maneuvered to maintain both the privileges of their religious status, and their independence from external control.[9]

The winning of privileges by civic authorities has often been touted as a form of administrative control over the institution, and typical of thirteenth-century developments in urban hospitals.[10] The council's acquisition of rights over appointing the hospital priest as a civic liberty in 1244 was not, however, followed by an exercise of civic control over the affairs of the hospital. The

8 Gudenus, *Codex diplomaticus*, 167–169. Yvonne Monsees, *Das Zisterzienserinnenkloster Gottesthal im Rheingau* (Wiesbaden: Selbstverlag der Historischen Kommission für Nassau, 1986), 15–17, rebuts the supposition that the 1145 charter was a forgery. She presumes that the hospital must have been relocated in connection with this transfer of administration. I see no evidence to support this theory.

9 On the relationships between Mainz's civic and ecclesiastical authorities in the first half of the thirteenth century, see Friedhelm Jürgensmeier, "Pro und Contra: Die Stellung der Erzbischöfe (1160–1249) im Reichsgeschehen," in *Handbuch der Mainzer Kirchengeschichte: Christliche Antike und Mittelalter*, edited by Friedhelm Jürgensmeier, vol. 1 (Würzburg: Echter Verlag, 2000), 338–346; Dietrich Demandt, *Stadtherrschaft und Stadtfreiheit im Spannungsfeld von Geistlichkeit und Bürgerschaft in Mainz (11–15. Jahrhundert)* (Wiesbaden: Franz Steiner Verlag, 1977), 50–74; Falck, *Geschichte der Stadt Mainz*, vol. 2, 138–160; Ernst-Dieter Hehl, "Goldenes Mainz und Heiliger Stuhl," in *Mainz: die Geschichte der Stadt*, eds. Franz Dumont, Friedrich Schütz, and Ferdinand Scherf (Mainz: Phillip von Zabern, 1998), 838–857.

10 See, for example, Paul Bonenfant, "Les premiers 'hospitia' de Bruxelles au XIIe siècle," *Annales de la Société belge d'histoire des hôpitaux* 11 (1973), 9–13; Thomas Coomans, "Belfries, Cloth Halls, Hospitals, and Mendicant Churches: A New Urban Architecture in the Low Countries around 1300," in *The Year 1300 and the Creation of a New European Architecture*, ed. Alexandra Gajewski (Turnhout: Brepols, 2007), 185–202; James W. Brodman, *Charity and Welfare: Hospitals and the Poor in Medieval Catalonia* (Philadelphia: University of Pennsylvania Press, 1998) 19–27. On tensions between civic and ecclesiastical authorities concerning hospitals more generally, see Reicke, *Das deutsche Spital und sein Recht*, vol. 2, 56–72; also Uhrmacher, *Lepra und Leprosorien*, 26–28, 56–70; Bettina Toson, *Mittelalterliche Hospitäler in Hessen zwischen Schwalm, Eder, und Fulda* (Darmstadt: Hessiche Historische Kommission, 2012), 39–45, 161; Riegel, *Lepra, Pest, und andere Seuchen*, 36–46; Wilhelm Frohn, *Der Aussatz im Rheinland: sein Vorkommen und seine Bekämpfung* (Jena: G. Fischer, 1933), 205–213; Hans Liermann, *Handbuch des Stiftungsrechts. Vol. 1: Geschichte des Stiftungsrechts* (Tübingen: J.C.B. Mohr, 1963), 96–100.

municipal elites who managed the hospital did so in ways consistent with a view of the hospital as a religious institution integrated in the economic and charitable networks of the city. Their desire to remove the hospital from archiepiscopal control was not tantamount to a desire for its secularization. Rather, the council worked to protect the privileges of the hospital as a religious institution. The unusually well-documented thirteenth-century history of Mainz's oldest hospital has been frequently invoked but never analyzed in depth.[11] This chapter compares its institutional trajectory to those of similar hospitals elsewhere in the archdiocese.

Urban Hospitals

The increasing prominence of hospitals in the burgeoning European cities of the twelfth and thirteenth centuries has been widely noted. Hospitals were integrated with their neighborhoods, and with wider urban environments. They were connected to their communities by the habit and pledge of mutual assistance with the surrounding population, not just the most poor and vulnerable. Hospitals, identified over a century ago as one of the characteristic institutions of the European Middle Ages, were focal points of civic life, and functioned as instruments of social integration for the vulnerable persons they served.[12] The question of whom they were to serve, however, was a fraught one.

While medieval burghers' concern about the eternal implications of almsgiving should not be discounted, invocations of piety in the historiography of hospitals can verge on the ahistorical.[13] Demonstrating that the

11 Kälble, "Sozialfürsorge und kommunale Bewegung," 242–246; Michel Pauly und Martin Uhrmacher, "Die Koblenzer Hospitäler in zentralörtlicher Perspektive," in *Zwischen Maas und Rhein: Beziehungen, Begegnungen und Konflikte in einem europäischen Kernraum von der Spätantike bis zum 19. Jahrhundert*, ed. Franz Irsigler (Trier: Universität Trier, 2006), 340–342; Michel Pauly, "Hospitäler im Mittelalter-wann und wo gehörte das Hospital zur Stadt?" in *Was machte im Mittelalter zur Stadt? Selbstverständnis, Außensicht und Erscheinungsbilder mittelalterlicher Städte*, eds. Kurt-Ulrich Jeschke and Christhard Schrenk (Heilbronn: Stadtarchiv Heilbronn, 2007), 251; Demandt, *Stadtherrschaft und Stadtfreiheit*, 76–82.

12 Rotha Mary Clay, *The Medieval Hospitals of England* (London: Methuen, 1909), xvii-xviii, 15–16; cf. Pauly, "Für eine raumbezogene Hospitalgeschichte," 13–14; Christianne Jéhanno, "L'emplacement de l'Hotel Dieu de Paris," in *Hôpitaux et maladreries au moyen âge: espace et environnement: actes du colloque international d'Amiens-Beauvais, 22, 23 et 24 novembre 2002*, ed. Pascal Montaubin (Rouen: CAHMER, 2004), 35–49. Pauly, *Peregrinorum, Pauperum ac aliorum transeuntium receptaculum*, 16.

13 Sharon Farmer, "The Beggar's Body," in *Monks and Nuns, Saints and Outcasts: Religion in Medieval Society*, eds. Sharon Farmer and Barbara Rosenwein (Ithaca: Cornell University Press,

recipients of hospital care were deserving was advantageous to hospitals themselves, as it proved that they were providing the service that gave them, in canon law, their *raison d'être*.[14] Hospitals' legal status can help explain several developments hitherto viewed either in particularist terms, or as part of teleological narratives. Religious status, even as late as the thirteenth century, was defined not necessarily by the following of a particular rule or the adoption of clothing, but by a way of life stricter and less indulgent than that of the laity, geared towards spiritual purification.[15] The late medieval drive to provide clearer definitions of the sick-poor could bolster or undermine the assertions of legitimacy by the institutions designed for their support and care.

The popularity of hospitals with the laity—as founders, benefactors, and staff—has often been described as a manifestation of lay piety paralleling the rise of new religious movements.[16] While the phenomena are unquestionably connected, lay hospital foundations and entrance into hospital service were not merely the result of devotion.[17] Historiographic judgments on the success or failure of hospitals' "true" charitable purpose have sometimes been made according to anachronistic views of the relative worthiness of different groups—the poor versus the aged, for example—to receive care.[18] For many

2000), 162–164. Cf. Frank Rexroth, "Zweierlei Bedürftigkeit. Armenhäuser und selektive caritas im England des 14. bis 16. Jh.," in *Sozialgeschichte Mittelalterlicher Hospitäler*, eds. Neithard Bulst and Karl-Heinz Spiess (Ostfildern: Jan Thorbecke Verlag, 2007), 14.

14 Alberigo et al, eds. *Conciliorum Oecumenicorum Decreta*, 322; Mansi, *Sacrorum conciliorum*, vol. 22, col. 906.

15 Nicole Bériou, "La predication au beguinage de Paris pendant l'annee liturgique 1272–1273," *Recherches augustiniennes* 13 (1978), 129, cites canonist Heinrich de Susa on this point.

16 Michel Mollat, *The Poor in the Middle Ages: An Essay in Social History*, trans. Arthur Goldhammer (New Haven: Yale University Press, 1986), 98–102.

17 Reicke, *Das deutsche Spital*, vol. 1, 13–25, esp. 20–21; Gabriel Cros-Mayrevieille, *Les frères donnés à la léproserie du bourg de Narbonne* (Toulouse: Privat, 1930), 1–3; Liermann, *Handbuch des Stiftungsrechts*, 160–162; Heyden, "Die Hospitäler in Oppenheim," 15; Luke Demaitre, *Leprosy in Premodern Medicine: A Malady of the Whole Body* (Baltimore: Johns Hopkins University Press, 2007), 81; Jennifer Stemmle, "From Cure to Care: Indignation, Assistance, and Leprosy in the High Middle Ages," in *Experiences of Charity, 1250–1650*, ed. Anne M. Scott (Farnham: Ashgate, 2015), 45. This tendency and its dangers were noticed in Rudolf Virchow, "Der Hospititaliter-Orden des Heiligen Geist, zumal in Deutschland," in *Monatsberichte der Königlich Preussischen Akademie der Wissenschaften zu Berlin* 43 (1878), 342–343. Bonenfant, "Les premiers 'hospitia' de Bruxelles," 9–13, notes that piety by itself does not found hospitals. On hospital service, particularly, see for example Gunther Risse, *Mending Bodies, Saving Souls: A History of Hospitals* (Oxford: Oxford University Press, 1999), 143–148.

18 On corrodians, see Liermann, *Handbuch des Stiftungsrechts*, 71–77; Knefelkamp, *Das Gesundheits- und Fürsorgewesen der Stadt Freiburg*, 41; Schürle, *Das Hospital zum Heiligen Geist in Konstanz*, 70–80. Ute Mayer and Rudolf Steffens, *Die spätmittelalterliche Urbare des*

medieval thinkers, though, the concept of *infirmitas* extended to the weak and aged, thus making those unable to earn their own living worthy objects of hospital care.[19] The claim that hospitals were staffed by religious men and women because hospitals "closely followed the patterns of monastic life" ignores the fact that those who took permanent vows as hospital staff became religious men and women by virtue of hospital service.[20] Religious houses, including hospitals, were seen as places in which to live a holy life in imitation of Christ and his apostles.[21]

The enthusiasm of men and women for joining religious communities outstripped the ability of ecclesiastical legislation and infrastructure to keep pace with them.[22] Narratives of spiritual motivation in the texts of religious

Heiliggeist-Spitals in Mainz (Stuttgart: Franz Steiner Verlag, 1992), 25, claim without substantiation that Mainz's hospital was chiefly a place of recourse for corrodians by the turn of the fourteenth century. Laqua, *Bruderschaften und Hospitäler*, 33–43, is unusually cautious in his assessment.

19 On this notion, see C.H. Talbot, *Medicine in Medieval England* (London: Oldbourne, 1955), 172–173; Joel Agrimi and Chiara Crisciani, "Charity and Aid in Medieval Christian Civilization," in *Western Medical Thought from Antiquity to the Middle Ages*, ed. Mirko D. Grmek (Cambridge, MA: Harvard University Press, 1998), 170–176; Marilyn Oliva, *The Convent and the Community in Late Medieval England: Female Monasteries in the Diocese of Norwich, 1350–1540* (Woodbridge: Boydell, 1998), 111–113; Adam J. Davis, *The Medieval Economy of Salvation: Charity, Commerce, and the Rise of the Hospital* (Ithaca: Cornell University Press, 2019), 208.

20 Charlotte A. Stanford, *Commemorating the Dead in Late Medieval Strasbourg: The Cathedral's Book of Donors and its Use (1320–1521)* (Farnham: Ashgate, 2011), 268–269. Cf. Jessalynn Lea Bird, "Medicine for Body and Soul: Jacques de Vitry's Sermons to Hospitallers and their Charges," in *Religion and Medicine in the Middle Ages*, eds. Peter Biller and Joseph Ziegler (Rochester, NY: York Medieval Press, 2001), 99, for the claim that "bishops and hospital officials [in the early thirteenth century] drew upon recent conciliar work, the customs of houses successfully adapted to local conditions, and rules imported from famous institutions."

21 The creation of hospitals for twelve staff members like the apostles is one tangible example of this emulation; see Franz Staab, "Reform und Reformgruppen im Erzbistum Mainz. Vom 'Libellus de Willigisi consuetudinibus' zur 'Vita domnae Juttae inclusae,'" in *Reformidee und Reformpolitik im Spätsalisch-Frühstaufischen Reich: Vorträge der Tagung der Gesellschaft für Mittelrheinische Kirchengeschichte vom 11. bis 13. September 1991 in Trier* (Trier: Gesellschaft Mittelrheinische Kirchengeschichte, 1992), 90–92; Touati, "Places of Conversion," 28–29.

22 Michael D. Bailey, "Religious Poverty, Mendicancy, and Reform in the Late Middle Ages," *Church History* 72 (2003), 457–483; Constance Hoffman Berman, *The Cistercian Evolution: The Invention of a Religious Order in Twelfth-Century Europe* (Philadelphia: University of Pennsylvania Press, 2000), 9–12, 36–41 et passim; Herbert Grundmann, *Religious Movements in the Middle Ages: The Historical Links Between Heresy, the Mendicant Orders, and the Women's Religious Movement in the Twelfth and Thirteenth Century, with the Historical Foundations of German Mysticism*, trans. Steven Rowan (Notre Dame, IN: University of Notre Dame Press, 1995); Lutz Kaelber, *Schools of Asceticism: Ideology and Organization in Medieval Religious Communities* (University Park, PA: Pennsylvania State University Press, 1998); Malcolm Lambert, *Medieval Heresy: Popular Movements from the Gregorian Reform to the Reformation* (Oxford: Blackwell Publishers, 2002);

orders have justly been given critical analysis in recent decades, but similar attention has not yet been given to the pious rhetoric concerning hospital staff.[23] Similarly, while the concrete impact of reforming rhetoric on religious communities has been productively questioned, applying such analysis to hospital development remains a desideratum.[24] An illustration is found in the changing language used for the residents of both leprosaria and multipurpose hospitals. Statutes and charters of the eleventh and twelfth centuries use vocabulary that conflates the sick and hospital staff.[25] By the thirteenth century, as is illustrated by the 1236 statutes of Mainz's oldest hospital, clearer distinctions were being drawn between those who received care from hospitals, and those responsible for giving that care.[26] This trend arose in response to the development of canon law governing religious institutions and persons in the late twelfth and early thirteenth centuries.[27] Stricter and

Patricia Ranft, "An Overturned Victory: Clare of Assisi and the Thirteenth-Century Church," *Journal of Medieval History* 17 (1991), 123–134.

23 On lay piety and its intersections with the religious life, see, still foundationally, André Vauchez, *The Laity in the Middle Ages: Religious Beliefs and Devotional Practices,* ed. Daniel E. Bornstein, trans. Margery J. Schneider (Notre Dame, IN: University of Notre Dame Press, 1993); Jörg Oberste, "Donaten zwischen Kloster und Welt. Das Donatenwesen der religiösen Ritterorden in Südfrankreich und die Entwicklung der städtischen Frömmigkeitspraxis im 13. Jahrhundert," *Zeitschrift für historische Forschung: Halbjahresschrift für die Erforschung des Spätmittelalters und der frühen Neuzeit* 29 (2002), 1–37. On the religious observance of hospital staff see: Françoise Bériac, "Les fraternités de lépreux et lépreuses," in *Doppelklöster und andere Formen der Symbiose männlicher und weiblicher Religiosen im Mittelalter,* ed. Kaspar Elm and Michel Parisse (Berlin: Duncker und Humblot, 1980), 209–211; James Brodman, "Shelter and Segregation: Lepers in Medieval Catalonia," in *On the Social Origins of Medieval Institutions: Essays in Honor of Joseph F. O'Callaghan,* ed. Donald J. Kagay and Theresa M. Vann (Leiden: Brill, 1998), 44; idem, *Charity and Welfare,* 52–53; Angers, "La bourgeoisie de Falaise," 237; Thomas Frank, "Spätmittelalterliche Hospitalreformen und Kanonistik," *Reti Medievali Rivista* 11 (2010), 10–11, on liturgical observance as legal privilege.

24 See for example Elizabeth M. Makowski, *A Pernicious Sort of Woman: Quasi-Religious Women and Canon Lawyers in the Later Middle Ages* (Washington, DC: Catholic University of America Press, 2005), 1–13 et passim; Franz Josef Felten. "Die Zisterzienserorden und die Frauen," in *Vita religiosa sanctimonialium: Norm und Praxis des weiblichen religiösen Lebens vom 6. bis zum 13. Jahrhundert,* ed. Christine Kleinjung (Korb: Didymos-Verlag, 2011), 199–205; Alan Forey, "Women and the Military Orders in the Twelfth and Thirteenth Centuries," in *Military Orders and Crusades* (Aldershot: Variorum, 1994), 67–71, 89–92, points out the differences between the statutory exclusion of women and de facto relations they had as donors, assistants, and consorores with the Templars.

25 Sommerlechner, "Spitäler in Nord- und Mittelitalien," 108–118.

26 Touati, "Places of Conversion," 63–70; Risse, *Mending Bodies, Saving Souls,* 144–147.

27 Robert Génestal, *Le Privilegium fori en France: du Décret de Gratian à la fin du XIVe siècle* (Paris: Éditions Ernest Leroux, 1921), 14–20; James A. Brundage, *Medieval Canon Law* (New York: Longman, 1995), 55–69; Wilfried Hartmann and Kenneth Pennington, eds., *The History of Medieval Canon Law in the Classical Period, 1140–1234: From Gratian to the Decretals of Pope*

clearer legal criteria for religious status rendered it both possible and desirable for vowed hospital staff to be differentiated from the sick-poor whom they served. This ongoing process was not unique to hospital communities. Rather, the parameters of religious status for individuals, no less than for institutions, remained the subject of active debate throughout the thirteenth century.[28] While hospital staff have sometimes been identified as lay religious persons, surviving statutes governing their communal life, and charters confirming their privileges, do not place qualifiers on their religious status.[29] The directive of the Council of Rouen (1270) that both secular persons and vowed religious should be active in the care of the sick and the giving of alms is characteristic. Certainly, this performance of the works of mercy could express individual charitable impulses. But it also took place within hospitals, and helped to define hospitals as religious institutions.[30] The policies of hospital staff and administrators were shaped by the desire to maintain both the legal privileges of religious status, and their institutional independence.[31]

Care for Mainz's Sick-poor: Episcopal Charity

The origins of Mainz's hospital can be putatively linked to the activities of Willigis, the city's first archbishop (975–1011).[32] Willigis made a substantial

Gregory IX (Washington, DC: Catholic University of America Press, 2008), esp. Kenneth Pennington, "The Decretalists 1190 to 1234," in *The History of Medieval Canon Law in the Classical Period, 1140-1234: From Gratian to the Decretals of Pope Gregory IX,* eds. Wilfried Hartmann and Kenneth Pennington (Washington, DC: Catholic University of America Press, 2008), 211–245.

28 Charles de Miramon, *Les 'donnés' au Moyen Âge: une forme de vie religieuse laïque, v. 1180–v. 1500* (Paris: Cerf, 1999), 128–145, esp. 142–145; Sherri Franks Johnson, "The Lateran Canons and their Predecessors: Shifting Monastic Networks in Medieval Italy," AHA annual meeting, 6 January 2022.

29 Cf. Miramon, *Les donnés au Moyen Âge*, 28–58, on the vows and charters typical of lay oblation.

30 Mansi, *Sacrorum conciliorum*, vol. 22, col. 826–827. On the works of mercy, see for example Miri Rubin, *Charity and Community in Medieval Cambridge* (Cambridge: Cambridge University Press, 1988), 54–74; Agrimi and Crisciani, "Charity and Aid in Medieval Christian Civilization," 170–176; Carole Rawcliffe, *The Hospitals of Medieval Norwich* (Woodbridge: Boydell, 1995), 16–17; Carl Johann Heinrich Villinger, "Wormser Hospitäler. Ein Beitrag zur Geschichte der Wormser Caritas im Mittelalter," *Jahrbuch für das Bistum Mainz* 2 (1947), 185.

31 Mansi, *Sacrorum conciliorum*, vol. 22, col. 826–827. See Bodleian MS Laud Misc 430, f51–82, for the use of the works of mercy to structure and legitimate a hagiographical narrative, in this case that of St. Elizabeth of Thüringen.

32 Martin Uhrmacher, *Leprosorien in Mittelalter und früher Neuzeit* (Köln: Rheinland-Verlag, 2000), 1–4; Laqua, *Bruderschaften und Hospitäler*, 48–49. On Mainz see Ludwig Falck, *Mainz im frühen und hohen Mittelalter* (Düsseldorf: Richter Verlag, 1972), 53, 71–77; Irmtraud Liebeherr,

gift for regular alms to the sick-poor. The fact that the archbishop intended this as a permanent memorial for himself suggests that this donation formed part of a regularized system of care.[33] The proprietary language of later archbishops would be consistent with such a scheme. Although no mention of purpose-built accommodation for the sick-poor survives from Willigis' tenure as archbishop, their care formed an integral part of publicly administered charity under his administration. The role of *pater pauperum*, father of the poor, was enjoined upon bishops by conciliar law, and the legal obligations of bishops to the most vulnerable among their flock are raised repeatedly in early medieval ecclesiastical legislation.[34] Early medieval European hospitals were concentrated in cathedral cities, suggesting that the episcopal duty of care was taken seriously.[35]

In addition to endowing regular alms, Archbishop Willigis also took initiative in the unusual dedication of Mainz's cathedral to St. Martin, helping to create a topography of charity with the care of the sick-poor at its heart.[36] The centrality of charity in Martin's *vita* had implications for the public image of Mainz's archbishops and citizens alike. Donations to Mainz's hospitals—of bread and chickens, clothing, coins, and candles—designated for Martin's feast day indicate that charity was seen as central to the saint's veneration, and support of the city's hospitals as a worthy way of honoring

Der Besitz des Mainzer Domkapitels im Spätmittelalter (Mainz: Gesellschaft für Mittelrheinische Kirchengeschichte, 1971), 12.

33 Stiftsbibliothek Aschaffenburg MS Perg 37 146r.

34 Elke Weingärtner, *Das Medizinal- und Fürsorgewesen der Stadt Trier im Mittelalter und der frühen Neuzeit* (Trier: Porta Alba Verlag, 1981), 24–25; see also Joseph P. Huffman, "Potens et pauper: charity and authority in jurisdictional disputes over the poor in medieval Cologne," in *Plenitude of Power: The Doctrines and Exercise of Authority in the Middle Ages. Essays in Honor of Robert Louis Benson* (Aldershot: Ashgate, 2006), 107–108.

35 Karl Baas, *Mittelalterliche Gesundheitsfürsorge im Gebiet des heutigen Rheinhessens*, Veröffentlichungen aus dem Gebiete der Medizinalverwaltung (Berlin: Richard Schoetz, 1931), 11; Franz Irsigler, "Matriculae, xenodochia, hospitalia und Leprosenhäuser im Frühmittelalter," in *Einrichtungen der sozialen Sicherung im mittelalterlichen Lotharingien. Actes des 13es Journées Lotharingiennes (12–15 Oct. 2004.)*, ed. Michel Pauly (Linden: Section Historie de l'Institut Grand-Ducal, 2008), 322–326. Falck, *Mainz im frühen und hohen Mittelalter*, 53–71; Sally Mayall Brasher, *Hospitals and Charity: Religious Culture and Civic Life in Medieval Northern Italy* (Manchester: Manchester University Press, 2017), 14. See also Cornel Dora, "Der soziale heilige St. Gallens," in *Vater für die Armen: Otmar und die Anfänge des Klosters St. Gallen* (Basel: Schwabe Verlag, 2019), 46–47.

36 Fritz Viktor Arens, "St. Martin, der Mainzer Dom, und das Erzstift," *Neues Jahrbuch für das Bistum Mainz* (1982), 9–12. The St. Johanniskirche probably served as the cathedral until the early tenth century; work on the cathedral in its present location was started by Willigis shortly after his assumption of the archiepiscopal dignity in 975, and finished in 1036 (after a fire in 1009 had destroyed much of the work to that point.)

the saint. The location of the hospital adjacent to—and later, opposite—the cathedral of St. Martin made it part of a topography of devotion and charity under the aegis of Mainz's archbishops.[37] Hospitals were often built as an expansion of regular care without dedicated buildings but within the cathedral close, and this was likely the case in Mainz.[38] The hospital itself is not mentioned until the mid-twelfth century; in this it is typical of high medieval foundations. The hospital by Trier's cathedral is first mentioned in 1136; before the twelfth century, only prescriptive evidence for hospitals attached to religious houses survives. Reicke posited that the hospitals of Mainz, Worms, and Speyer were among the earliest in Germany.[39] When Mainz's oldest hospital enters the written record, it is as an established institution, both an object of episcopal patronage, and a house with legal rights and privileges of its own.

Twelfth-Century Reforms

The 1145 charter containing the earliest evidence of the hospital as an independent institution was preserved by the hospital in multiple copies.[40] In it, Archbishop Heinrich I speaks of "our hospital," indicating that the hospital was under archiepiscopal patronage.[41] The primary purpose of the charter was to transfer the administration of the hospital from the cathedral

37 Reicke, *Das deutsche Spital und sein Recht*, vol. 1, 32–33. Stiftsbibliothek Aschaffenburg MS Perg 37 146r; StAM 30/4.

38 For Mainz's cathedral close in the central Middle Ages, see Arens, "St. Martin, der Mainzer Dom, und das Erzstift," 9–12; for this pattern, see Peregrine Horden, "Religion as Medicine: Music in Medieval Hospitals," in *Religion and Medicine in the Middle Ages*, ed. Peter Biller and Joseph Ziegler (Rochester, NY: York Medieval Press, 2001), 135–140, and Frederick S. Paxton, "Anointing the Sick and Dying in Christian Antiquity and the Early Medieval West," in *Health, Disease, and Healing in Medieval Culture*, eds. Sheila Campbell, Bert Hall, and David Klausner (New York: St. Martin's Press, 1992), 93–102.

39 Monika Eschner-Apsner, "Geistliche Institutionen und Hospitäler," in *Caritas im Bistum Trier: Eine Geschichte des Helfens und Heilens*, ed. Roland Ries and Werner Marzi (Trier: Kliomedia Verlag, 2006), 78–77; Reicke, *Das deutsche Spital*, vol. 1, 32–38.

40 The original no longer survives. The transcriptions of eighteenth-century antiquarian L. S., however, reveal that three slightly different versions survived in the archives of the hospital. StAM 6/40; Wolfgang Wann, "Die alten Mainzer Archive," *Archivalische Zeitschrift* 60 (1964), 101.

41 StAM 6/40 (3). Printed in Gudenus, *Codex diplomaticus I*, 167. On the role of Mainz's archbishops in shaping the direction of Mainz's religious foundations during the eleventh and twelfth centuries, cf. Staab, "Reform und Reformgruppen im Erzbistum Mainz," 172–196. Cf. James Brodman, *Charity and Religion in Medieval Europe* (Washington, DC: Catholic University of America Press, 2009), 58.

chapter to a house of Augustinian canons, in Gottesthal; it also provides the hospital with territory on an island in the Rhine from which to draw revenue. The ongoing prayer of the sick-poor in the hospital for those whom the archbishop nominates, for his predecessors, and in honor of Heinrich's own anniversary of ordination, is listed as the sole condition of the gift. These prayers are referred to as a way of meditating (presumably in gratitude) on alms already received.[42] In making this grant, Heinrich refers to rights and properties granted to the hospital by Marcolf and his other predecessors. The hospital probably received its first buildings during Marcolf's brief tenure as archbishop (1141–1142). This would be consistent with Marcolf's known policies regarding religious institutions, and with known histories of similar hospitals.[43] The posited centrality of archiepiscopal patronage to the hospital's identity was more than a rhetorical flourish on Heinrich's part. The charter's testimony to such patronage strengthened the hospital's claim to the legal exemptions enjoyed by religious institutions.[44] In a similar case two years before, the hospital of Strasbourg, also in the province of Mainz, had its privileges confirmed by the bishop, along with a gift of property.[45]

Such privileges would have been particularly valuable to the hospital of Mainz in the face of the tensions suggested by the transfer of hospital

42 StAM 6/40 (3). On Heinrich's policies towards religious houses more generally, see Ludwig Falck, "Klosterfreiheit und Klosterschutz. Die Klosterpolitik der Mainzer Erzbischöfe von Adalbert I. bis Heinrich I (1100–1153)," in *Archiv für Mittelrheinische Kirchengeschichte* 8 (1958), 68–75. Cf. Oliver Auge, "'Ne pauperes et debiles in…domo degentes divinis careant.' Sakral-religiöse Askpete der mittelalterlichen Hospitalgeschichte," in *Sozialgeschichte mittelalterlicher Hospitäler*, eds. Neithard Bulst and Karl-Heinz Spiess (Ostfildern: Jan Thorbecke Verlag, 2007), 92–95, on twelfth-century attitudes towards the prayers of the poor.

43 Pauly, "Hospitäler im Mittelalter," 246–250, provides evidence for episcopal care of the sick and building of hospitals in the late tenth through early twelfth centuries. Josef Semmler, "Vita Religiosa und Bischof bis gegen 1200," in *Handbuch der Mainzer Kirchengeschichte: Christliche Antike und Mittelalter*, ed. Friedhelm Jürgensmeier, vol. 2 (Würzburg: Echter Verlag, 2000), 633, states that it was Marcolf, and not Heinrich, who was responsible for handing over the administration of Mainz's hospital to Erenfridus, citing the letter as printed in Peter Acht, ed., *Mainzer Urkundenbuch*, vol 2 (Darmstadt: Selbstverlag der Hessischen Historischen Kommission Darmstadt, 1971), 149 Nr. 75. J.F. Böhmer and Cornelius Will, eds., *Regesta archiepiscoporum Maguntinensium. Register zur Geschichte der Mainzer Erzbischöfe von Bonifatius bis Heinrich II.*, vol. 1 (Innsbruck: Wagner, 1886), 317–318, nr. 9, shows Marcolf giving the cloister of Gottesthal an island in the Rhine near Eltville for an annual memorial.

44 Frank, "Spätmittelalterliche Hospitalreformen und Kanonistik," 10–11; on the predominance and importance of episcopal foundations cf. Irsigler, "Matriculae, xenodochia, hospitalia und Leprosenhäuser im Frühmittelalter," 331–334; Pauly, *Peregrinorum, pauperum ac aliorum transeuntium receptaculum*, 160–161, identifies Mainz's hospital as an episcopal foundation.

45 Wilhelm Wiegand, ed., *Urkundenbuch der Stadt Strassburg* (Strasbourg: Trübner, 1888), 70–72.

administration to a house of canons, and by the unusually elaborate preamble of the charter recording it. Placing the hospital temporarily under the authority of Gottesthal may have been an attempt to resolve tensions between the archbishop and cathedral chapter, although the transfer is presented as a work of charity, providing for the needs of Christ's poor and for the financial security of the canons of Gottesthal through the use of the hospital's resources.[46] Archbishop Heinrich's desire to have the religious status of the hospital and its staff confirmed is further indicated by a letter he issued in 1151, granting property rights to the community. The eighteenth-century copyist of this letter interpreted it as referring to an Augustinian house in Winckel, but the "brothers and sisters sharing the common life under the rule of St. Augustine" should rather be interpreted as identical with the hospital community.[47] This hypothesis is supported by the fact that the property concerned is found in the hospital's unambiguous possession a century later.[48] Furthermore, as in the charter of 1145, the favor of Archbishop Marcolf is identified as a precedent for Heinrich's patronage.[49] The gift is made in exchange for the prayers not only of the brothers and sisters, but of the poor to whom they will regularly give alms.[50]

The expression "naked following the naked Christ" makes clear that the hospital staff embraced voluntary poverty.[51] Heinrich writes of wishing to preserve the community from oblivion and neglect, indicating that the archbishop wished to ensure that the hospital and its staff were recognized

46 StAM 6/40 (3). The anathemas against those daring to violate the terms of the agreement were standard for this period; cf. Brigitte Miriam Bedos-Rezak, "Medieval Identity: A Sign and a Concept," *The American Historical Review* 105 (2000), 1507–1508. Reicke, *Das deutsche Spital*, vol. 1, 20–21, attributes the engagement of bishops in putting hospitals under cloister management in the eleventh and twelfth centuries to a desire not to see hospitals mismanaged.

47 StAM 6/40 (4). Moreover, Carl Julius Böttcher, ed., *Germania Sacra Abt. 2: Kirchenprovinz Mainz* (Berlin: De Gruyter, 1929), 559, on Winkel, makes no mention of an Augustinian house or a hospital in that place.

48 StAWü MBVI 17, f 122. Relevant documents are printed in Böhmer and Will, eds., *Regesta archiepiscoporum Maguntinensium*, 317–318, nr. 9: Marcolf (1141–1142) gives the cloister of Gottesthal an island in the Rhine near Eltville for an annual memoria ["known" only from Heinrich's charter of 1145]; 328–329, nr. 46: Regest of Heinrich's 1145 confirmation of the island and transfer of HGS admin; 346, nr. 142: Heinrich (1151 before September 1) confirms possession of island on request of "Abbot" Robert.

49 StAM 6/40 (4).

50 StAM 6/40 (3).

51 StAM 6/40 (4). See Giles Constable, "Nudus Nudum Christum Sequi and Parallel Formulas in the Twelfth Century: A Supplementary Dossier," in *Continuity and Discontinuity in Church History: Essays Presented to George Hunston Williams*, eds. F. Forrester Church and Timothy George (Leiden: Brill, 1979), 83–91.

as having religious status.[52] In this document, the brothers and sisters of the hospital are surrounded by too many idealizing tropes for their communal goals to be clear. But for the men and women who took up this service, behind the rhetoric of carrying Christ in their bodies lay a reality of demanding physical and emotional labor in ministering to the needs of the sick, as well as liturgical observance.[53]

Mainz's hospital does not appear again in the records of Gottesthal in the second half of the twelfth century. Parallel instances of short-lived transfer suggest that the involvement of the canons was used as a temporary reform measure, or as a way of asserting archiepiscopal control over the hospital. In Lüttich, for example, mixed hospital administration was accompanied by debate throughout the late twelfth century concerning the authority of ecclesiastical and civic authorities over the hospital.[54] The catalyst for the return of the hospital to the aegis of the cathedral chapter may have been the conversion of Gottesthal itself into a house of canonesses, or, later, into a Cistercian house.[55] Reinhold Rörig has suggested that the cathedral chapter administered the hospital under the official supervision of the archbishops. Although the surviving records of the chapter hold no direct indication of such ties, the hospital's location in the cathedral close would certainly have rendered such a connection convenient.[56] The

52 StAM 6/40 (4).

53 Andrew T. Crislip, *From Monastery to Hospital: Christian Monasticism and the Transformation of Health Care in Late Antiquity* (Ann Arbor: University of Michigan Press, 2005), 9–38; Bird, "Medicine for Body and Soul," 103–104.

54 Reicke, *Das deutsche Spital*, vol. 1, 33–35. Cf. Laqua, *Bruderschaften und Hospitäler*, 99–108.

55 Wolfgang Seibrich, "Monastisches Leben von ca. 1200 bis zur Reformation," in *Handbuch der Mainzer Kirchengeschichte: Christliche Antike und Mittelalter*, ed. Friedhelm Jürgensmeier, vol. 2 (Würzburg: Echter Verlag, 2000), 694, places the transfer of the house to canonesses at the turn of the thirteenth century. Böhmer-Will, *Regesta archiepiscoporum Maguntinensium*, 312 nr. 44: a charter of Christian II's refers to the nuns of Gottesthal as "those who have gone over to the Cistercians," suggesting that this affiliation was a recent development. The stability of this new identity is uncertain, however; in 329 nr. 119, Gerhart, Gottesthal appears alongside another Augustinian house. In 364 nr. 122, Gottesthal appears as a Cistercian cloister, which Wernher transfers to the supervision of Eberbach along with Dalheim, Oppenheim, and Syon, incorporating it formally into the order. Cf. Franz Joseph Bodmann, *Rheingauische Alterthümer oder Landes und Regimentsverfassung des westlichen oder Niederrheingaues im Mittlern Zeitalter*, (Mainz: Florian Kupferberg, 1819), 227–233. For a similar case, see Kay Peter Jankrift, "Hospitäler und Leprosorien im Nordwesten des mittelalterlichen Regnum Teutonicum unter besonderer Berücksichtigung rheinisch-westfälischer Städte," in *Europäisches Spitalwesen. Institutionelle Fürsorge in Mittelalter und Früher Neuzeit*, eds. Martin Scheutz, Andrea Sommerlechner, Herwig Weigl, and Alfred Stefan Weiß (Munich: R. Oldenbourg Verlag, 2008), 298.

56 Reinhold Rörig, *Die Mainzer Spitäler und Krankenhäuser: Ein Rückblick auf 2000 Jahre Krankenhausgeschichte* (Mainz: Schmidt, 1989), 20. Liebeherr, *Der Besitz des Mainzer Domkapitels*

hospital's next appearance in the documentary record, however, explicitly presents it as an independent institution. Cathedral canons served as hospital administrators after its transfer to a new location, but as the twelfth-century history of the institution shows, this was not a post which they held exclusively.

That Mainz's hospital was integrated within the city's religious networks is indicated by the fact that its administrators were also affiliated with other religious institutions of Mainz. The Erenfridus named as *prepositus* of the hospital in 1145 may be the same Erenfridus who appears in an 1151 charter of Gottesthal as a candidate for a disputed benefice; he is there referred to as a canon of St. Maria ad Gradus in Mainz.[57] The same document identifies a certain Fridericus, provost of the chapter of St. Maria ad Gradus as Erenfridus' successor (but not in the benefice). If this Erenfridus and the one of 1145 are the same man, it seems probable that Fridericus succeeded him as overseer of the hospital.[58] The preservation of the records naming these men suggests that the hospital staff saw the involvement of the canons as bolstering the legitimacy of the hospital's religious status. The brothers and sisters of the hospital appear to have remained substantially autonomous, as was not uncommon among twelfth-century hospitals.[59] Neither the records of the hospital, nor those of the canonries from which its twelfth-century overseers came, contain the evidence of dispute or agreement that might be expected, had other foundations overseen the hospital's administration. The statutes of 1236 suggest that Mainz's oldest hospital developed its own customs and robust internal organization.

im Spätmittelalter, 44–45, points out that much of the chapter's property was concentrated just north of the city, often in localities where the hospital also held property.

57 HHStAW Abt. 29 U 3.

58 HHStAW Abt. 29 U 3.

59 On twelfth-century hospitals see, for example, Anne E. Lester, "Cares Beyond the Walls: Cistercian Nuns and the Care of Lepers in Twelfth- and Thirteenth-Century Northern France," in *Religious and Laity in Western Europe 1000–1400: Interaction, Negotiation, and Power,* ed. Emilia Jamroziak and Janet Burton (Turnhout: Brepols, 2006), 197–208; Pauly, "Von der Fremdenherberge zum Seniorenheim: Funktionswandel in mittelalterlichen Hospitälern an ausgewählten Beispielen aus dem Maas-Mosel-Rhein-Raum," in *Funktions– und Strukturwandel spätmittelalterlicher Hospitäler,* 104–105; idem, *Peregrinorum, pauperum ac aliorum transeuntium receptaculum,* 74–76; Sheila Sweetinburgh, *The Role of the Hospital in Medieval England: Gift-Giving and the Spiritual Economy* (Portland, OR: Four Courts Press, 2004), 54–60; François-Olivier Touati, "Les Léproseries aux XIIème et XIIIème siècles: Lieux de Conversion?" in *Voluntate Dei Leprosus: les lépreux entre conversion et exclusion aux XIIème et XIIIème siècles,* Nicole Bériou and François-Olivier Touati (Spoleto: Centro Italiano di studi Sull'altro Medioevo, 1991), 72–73.

The Comforts of the Poor and the Rights of the Hospital: 1236–1244

The statutes issued for Mainz's hospital in 1236 draw a distinction between the sick and the vowed hospital staff, a trend noticeable throughout Europe in the first half of the thirteenth century. Increasingly, entrance into hospital service was defined as a way of entering the religious life, as detailed by numerous hospital rules across Europe.[60] For Mainz's oldest hospital, its statutes marked an important step in its institutional development. Issued shortly after the promulgation of the *Liber Extra* in 1234, they echoed its formulations of the criteria for religious status.[61] They asserted the conformity of its staff with the requirements of canon law—stability, the profession of a rule, the wearing of a habit—and their entitlement to its privileges, including exemptions from taxes. Although it has been posited that the statutes of 1236 replaced earlier rules, it seems more likely that they were created in response to the evolving legal requirements governing the religious status of hospitals and their staff.[62]

The staff of Mainz's hospital was composed of both clerical and lay brothers, and women as well as men. The vocabulary is more refined than that of the twelfth century, but ongoing cooperation between men and

60 For examples of hospital rules defining hospital service as a way of taking up the religious life, see Léon Le Grand, *Statuts d'hôtels-Dieu et de léproseries: recueil de textes du XIIe au XIVe siècle* (Paris: Alphonse Picard et Fils, 1901), passim. On Mainz, see Staab, "Reform und Reformgruppen im Erzbistum Mainz," 172–196. Laqua, *Bruderschaften und Hospitäler*, 43–49, sees early confirmation for vowed staff in glosses of the early thirteenth century.

61 Lotte Kéry, "Verbrechen und Strafen im kanonischen Recht des Mittelalters," in *Kriminalität in Mittelalter und früher Neuzeit: Soziale, Rechtliche, Philosophische und Literarische Aspekte*, eds. Sylvia Kesper-Biermann and Diethelm Klippel (Wiesbaden: Harrassowitz Verlag, 2007), 13–14; Johannes Helmrath, "Partikularsynoden und Synodalstatuten des späteren Mittelalters im europäischen Vergleich: Vorüberlegungen zu einem möglichen Projekt," in *Das europäische Mittelalter im Spannungsbogen des Vergleichs. Zwanzig internationale Beiträge zu Praxis, Problemen und Perspektiven der historischen Komparatistik*, ed. Michael Borgolte (Berlin: Akademie Verlag, 2001), 139–140, on the standardization of the synodal form. On the similarity between hospital statutes and monastic customs, see Edward J. Kealey, *Medieval Medicus: Physicians and Health Care in England, 1100–1154* (Baltimore: Johns Hopkins University Press, 1981), 107–117.

62 Falck, "Mainzer Spitäler," 52–54. For descriptions of the document as "statutes," see Reicke, *Das deutsche Spital und sein Recht*, vol. 2, 32–34, 76–77; Monsees, *Das Zisterzienserinnenkloster Gottesthal im Rheingau*, 15–17; Böhmer and Will, *Regesta archiepiscoporum Maguntinensium*, 243–244, describes them as "merkwürdige Statuten." Gisela Drossbach, *Christliche caritas als Rechtsinstitut: Hospital und Orden von Santo Spirito in Sassia 1198–1378* (Paderborn: Ferdinand Schöningh, 2005), 55, notes that charters of privilege could be retrospectively identified as statutes.

women, clergy and laypersons, is accepted as normative.[63] The rule makes no distinction between male and female staff in enjoining customs and duties.[64] The brothers and sisters of Mainz's hospital are explicitly exhorted to serve the sick, "ministering to them in food and drink, and other things suited to their needs, humbly and devoutly."[65] The service of the sick is often identified in hospital statutes of this period as a hallmark of the apostolic life, with the sick often paralleling saints in the founding documents of religious communities.[66] Mainz's comprehensive welcome to the sick and pilgrims, to weary travelers, the hungry and thirsty (who may have included beggars), and to rich and poor alike, is unusual in its scope.[67] This inclusive language was not merely formulaic. Contemporaneous hospital rules often included lists of those requiring specialized care that the hospital could or would not provide.[68]

Archbishop Siegfried III is recorded as issuing the statutes at the insistence of the citizens of Mainz, with the consent and counsel of the city's clergy and the cathedral chapter.[69] Although the collaborative nature of the decision is reiterated several times, the move suggests that the hospital staff may have sought increased autonomy, as well as more space for their community. There is much rhetoric emphasizing the archbishop's generosity, but the economic and legal concessions made to the hospital community suggest that they had the upper hand in negotiations. The hospital, its

63 Laqua, *Bruderschaften und Hospitäler*, 238–239, suggests that such arrangements were fairly common, and reflected in the daily life of hospitals as well as in their prescriptive statutes.

64 See Le Grand, *Statuts d'hôtels-Dieu*, 18–21, 29, 36–38, 55, 119–121.

65 Gudenus, *Codex Diplomaticus* I, 637–638. The section concerning the hospital's religious status as an institution concludes with the command "fratres vero et sorores, infirmis cibum et potum, et alia ipsorum necessitati conveniencia ministrent humiliter et devote."

66 Just and Weigl, "Spitäler im südöstlichen Deutschland und in den österreichischen Ländern im Mittelalter," 168. For more on hospital statutes, see Le Grand, *Statuts d'hotels-dieu*, 18–22, 25–26; Brodman, *Charity and Welfare*, 142–143; Hubert Kolling, "Die Sorge für die Kranken," in *Der Dienst am Kranken: Krankenversorgung zwischen Caritas, Medizin und Ökonomie vom Mittelalter bis zur Neuzeit*, Gerhard Aumüller, Kornelia Grundmann, and Christina Vanja, eds. (Marburg: Elwert, 2007), 65–86.

67 StAM 6/30 (4): "Venerabilia Deo dicata loca, in quibus egentes et peregrini gratum receptaculum, fatigati quietem, refectionem esurientes, potum sicientes, et alii, tam divites quam pauperes gratum et acceptum solacium semper inveniunt…"

68 Le Grand, *Statuts d'hotels-Dieu*, 25–26, 115. Cf. Stanford, *Commemorating the Dead in Late Medieval Strasbourg*, 268–269.

69 Gudenus, *Codex Diplomaticus* I, 640. Ludwig Falck, "Die Erzbischöfliche Metropole, 1011–1244," 129–136, observes that more political activity under Siegfried II and Siegfried III brought more influence to Mainz but also more conflict within the city, and more demands on the part of civic leadership for independence from the potentially polarizing policies of the archbishops.

staff, and their belongings, are all declared "free and immune" from all taxes (*angariis et perangariis*) owed to the archbishop as the temporal lord. The lack of any reference to such rights as traditional suggests that they reflect contemporary legal preoccupations.[70] As indicated by papal letters, concerns about the question of which institutions and properties were entitled to such exemptions due to ecclesiastical status peaked during the 1230s–1240s. Two references to *angariis* in the 1220s, during the papacy of Honorius III, are succeeded by no fewer than thirteen in the 1230s, under Gregory IX, three of which respond specifically to the petitions of religious institutions for confirmations of their legal rights.[71] The specification that the brothers and sisters of Mainz are to go "with their property to this new location," indicates some ambiguity over their property rights.[72] At the Council of Rouen, in 1213, ecclesiastical authorities expressed anxiety that the implementation of canon law concerning moveable and immoveable property, and religious vows, might be impeded by the laity.[73] The language of Mainz's hospital statutes suggests similar concerns, and further supports the hypothesis that the hospital staff were influential in shaping the terms of the hospital charter.

The episcopally-issued statutes also bolster the claim of Mainz's hospital to religious status by specifying which types of donation the hospital was allowed to accept, along with the right of the hospital clergy to celebrate Mass, hear confessions, and administer the other sacraments of the church.[74] Notably, the hospital rector is given final say over how often, and by whom, these sacraments are to be procured. The archbishop reserved his right to appoint this priest in charge; but the quotidian administration of the hospital was left in the hands of the brothers and sisters themselves. The

70 Drossbach, *Christliche caritas als Rechtsinstitut*, 80–83, offers a useful discussion of the developing concept of "ordo" and attempts through decrees and councils to organize religious life from the second half of the twelfth century through Lateran IV.

71 *Ut per litteras apostolicas*, https://clio.columbia.edu/databases/4346120. Last accessed March 25, 2022.

72 StAM 6/30 (4). On hospital property, and ambiguities concerning the same, cf. Jean Imbert, *Histoire des hôpitaux français: contribution à l'étude des rapports de l'église et de l'état dans le domaine de l'Assistance Publique: les hôpitaux en droit canonique du décret de Gratien à la sécularisation de l'administration de l'Hôtel-Dieu de Paris en 1505* (Paris: J. Vrin, 1947), 18–26; Timothy S. Miller, *The Birth of the Hospital in the Byzantine Empire* (Baltimore: Johns Hopkins University Press, 1985), 104–110; *Regesten der Bischöfe von Strassburg*, 326–327. Drossbach, "Liber Regulae," 32–34, records that the rule devised by Pope Innocence III for the hospital of Santo Spirito in Rome in 1204 specified that the hospital staff were not entitled to private property, moveable or immoveable.

73 Mansi, *Sacrorum conciliorum*, col. 922, XXXII.

74 StAM 6(40), 3, printed in Gudenus, *Codex Diplomaticus* I, 638.

specification that clergy and laypersons who wished to enter the religious life might do so through undertaking service in the hospital is unusually explicit. Lateran IV is echoed in the statement that vowed staff are thereby exempted from the authority of a secular tribunal, and barred from leaving hospital service unless to enter a canonically stricter order. Siegfried II, the previous archbishop of Mainz, was an active participant at the Fourth Lateran Council, and may have been tasked with bringing copies of its canons to the archdiocese.[75]

Considerable evidence argues against the hypothesis that Mainz's hospital belonged to the order of the Holy Spirit, founded by Guido of Montpellier and given its first rule by Innocent III.[76] Although early modern editors glossed twelfth- and thirteenth-century letters as belonging "to the hospital of the Holy Spirit," the earliest use of this name for Mainz's oldest hospital appears in its fourteenth-century account books.[77] The Order is not mentioned in connection with the hospital's transfer to the supervision of the council, or the separation of the male and female staff in 1259. Had Mainz's hospital been a daughter house of Santo Spirito, undertaking these actions without communicating with Rome would have contravened canon law.[78]

One of the distinctive characteristics of the Order of the Holy Spirit was its centralization. The papal rule for the house in Rome lays out the

75 StAM 6(40), 3, printed in Gudenus, *Codex Diplomaticus* I, 638. Paul B. Pixton, *The German Episcopacy and the Implementation of the Decrees of the Fourth Lateran Council 1216–1245: Watchmen on the Tower* (Leiden: Brill, 1995), 50–51; Adam J. Davis, *The Holy Bureaucrat: Eudes Rigaud and Religious Reform in Thirteenth-Century Normandy* (Ithaca: Cornell University Press, 2006), 6–68; Jane Lang, "The Reform Work of the Episcopate on the Lines Laid Down by the Lateran Council of 1215," in Marion Gibbs and Jane Lang, *Bishops and Reform, 1215–1272: With Special Reference to the Lateran Council of 1215*, (Oxford: Oxford University Press, 1934), 94–99, 105–113; Werner Maleczek, "Der Mittelpunkt Europas im frühen 13. Jahrhundert: Chronisten, Fürsten, und Bischöfe an der Kurie our Zeit Papst Innocenz' III," *Römische Historische Mitteilungen* 49 (2007), 89–97.

76 Susanne Schlösser, "Armen– und Krankenfürsorge im Gebiet des heutigen Rheinhessen," *Archiv für hessische Geschichte und Altertumskunde* 49 (1991), 61–84; Ulrich Craemer, *Das Hospital als Bautyp des Mittelalters* (Köln: W. Kohlhammer Verlag, 1963), 55. Other scholars, while noting the lack of direct evidence for such a connection, present it as a probability. Reicke, *Das Deutsche Spital*, vol. 1, 166–182; Von Steynitz, *Mittelalterliche Hospitäler der Orden und Städte*, 74–102; Klaus Militzer, "Die Hospitaltätigkeit des Deutschen Ordens," in *Einrichtungen der Sozialen Sicherung*, 421–436. For an early chronology of the foundation in Rome, see Drossbach, *Christliche caritas als Rechtsinstitut*, 72–80.

77 StAM 6/30 (4); StAM 33/1; Gudenus, *Codex Diplomaticus* I, 167–169, 537–541.

78 Drossbach, *Christliche Caritas als Rechtsinstitut*, 60–61, 80–83. Given the scanty survival of the thirteenth-century records of Mainz's hospital, the absence of an affiliation letter would not in itself be surprising, but the lack of any documented contact with Rome is striking.

obligations of daughter institutions in no uncertain terms.[79] If Mainz's hospital belonged to the Order, the mother house in Rome would have had authority to intervene not only in the move to the banks of the Rhine, but the transfer of rights of appointment in 1244 as well.[80] Not only is there no mention of this rule in documents issued in Mainz, but no records survive of complaints from Rome about the independent path taken by Mainz's hospital.[81] The statutes of the hospital themselves were designed to serve, potentially, a regional network of hospitals formed with Mainz's hospital as the mother house: "If (by the aid of divine mercy) the above house is amplified to such an extent that it begins to have other hospitals, those shall be governed by the same law and grace in all things."[82] The dove of the Holy Spirit appeared on the hospital's seal (first surviving on a charter of 1260), but the text on the seal makes no reference to an order; furthermore, the Order of the Holy Spirit itself is not known to have had a seal before 1383.[83]

Despite all the evidence against Mainz's hospital having been formally affiliated with the Order of the Holy Spirit, the staff entering the hospital were required to profess "regulariter Santo Spirito." The invocation of a hospital's patron saint in the vows taken by its members was common throughout the twelfth and thirteenth centuries. The specification that the men and women of Mainz were to profess *regulariter* points to the importance of *a* hospital rule to the religious life, not to the use of an external rule.[84] The statutes do not borrow vocabulary or structure from the Rule

79 Drossbach, *Christliche Caritas als Rechtsinstitut*, 76–77, 86–89. Drossbach sees parallels between Innocent's patronage and control over the strongly centralized Order of the Holy Spirit and Hugolino of Ostia's efforts in creating (organized, centralized) houses for religious women.

80 This has been justly pointed out by Eva Gertrud Neumann, *Rheinisches Beginen- und Beghardenwesen: Ein Mainzer Beitrag zur religiösen Bewegung am Rhein* (Meisenheim am Glan: Hein, 1960), 24.

81 This is so although Alexander IV and his predecessor show awareness of the religious communities of Mainz and concern about the reform of hospital communities. Potthast, *RPR*, Gregory IX: vol. 1, nr. 1017 (594–595; Alexander IV, nrs. 1171, 1338, 1701–1702.

82 StAM 6/30 (4). Tiffany A. Ziegler, *Medieval Healthcare and the Rise of Charitable Institutions: The History of the Municipal Hospital* (London: Palgrave Macmillan, 2018), 85–99, analyzes the hospital of St. John in Brussels as a similar regional model.

83 Drossbach, *Caritas als Rechtsinstitut*, 174. HStAD A2 168/30 preserves only a partial seal; Gudenus, I, 640, reproduces a clearly identical seal as it appeared on a 1283 confirmation of the hospital statutes.

84 Le Grand, *Statuts d'hotels-Dieu*, 142–143, 189, 234; Davis, *The Holy Bureaucrat*, 163; Imbert, *Histoire des hôpitaux français*, 100–101; Pauly, "Für eine raumbezogene Hospitalgeschichte," 12–13; Clay, *The Medieval Hospitals of England*, 245–259; Frohn, *Aussatz im Rheinland*, 151. Pauly, *Peregrinorum, pauperum ac aliorum transeuntium receptaculum*, 304–318. Cf. Meffert, *Caritas und Krankenwesen*, 214f, 236–238; Craemer, *Das Hospital als Bautyp*, 54–69.

of Santo Spirito; nor do they mention papal authority. The rule created for the Roman hospital in 1204 was devised by Innocent III. Its papal approval made it a valuable badge of appropriate religious observance, which would almost certainly have been invoked, had there been a connection between Mainz's hospital and the order.[85] Invocation of the service of the sick as the justification for the form as well as the fact of the hospital's institutional life is increasingly standardized as a legal trope, and not distinctive to the Rule of Santo Spirito.[86] The staff of Mainz's hospital made sure to assert their conformity with the criteria for religious status, in order to secure their claim to the privileges of that status. Similar patterns are visible in the history of St. Agnes, examined in the next chapter. For the men and women taking vows in Mainz's oldest hospital, the rule that gave them their corporate identity as religious persons also ensured their independence from affiliation.

Space, Identity, and Liturgy: The Locations of Civic Hospitals

Hospitals functioned as central points for personal interactions, for the concentration and circulation of intentions, goods, and money. They thus reinforced the centrality of cities in the surrounding landscapes, not only providing services to those in the city, but contributing to the function of cities as centers for travelers, traders, and pilgrims.[87] The growth and multiplication of hospitals as independent institutions was, however, a gradual process. The independent hospitals of the twelfth century usually had scattered territory in locations determined by hospital need, and by

85 Drossbach, *Caritas als Rechtsinstitut*, 55–63.

86 Archives de Strasbourg, 1AH 215; Adam J. Davis, "Hospitals, Charity, and the Culture of Compassion in the Twelfth and Thirteenth Centuries," in *Approaches to Poverty in Medieval Europe: Complexities, Contradictions, Transformations, c. 1100–1500*, ed. Sharon Farmer (Turnhout: Brepols, 2016), 30–35; Kenneth Baxter Wolf, *The Life and Afterlife of St. Elizabeth of Hungary* (Oxford: Oxford University Press, 2011), 67–74. Rubin, *Charity and Community*, 89–94. On the rule and order of Santo Spirito, see Drossbach, *Christliche Caritas als Rechtsinstitut*, 91–102; Gisela Drossbach, "Bild und Text im *Liber Regulae* des römischen Hospitals von Santo Spirito in Sassia," in *Sozialgeschichte Mittelalterlicher Hospitäler*, ed. Neithard Bulst and Karl-Heinz Spiess (Ostfildern: Jan Thorbecke Verlag, 2007), 146–148.

87 Jean-Luc Fray, "Institutions hospitalières médiévales et problématique historienne de la centralité…" in *Zwischen Maas und Rhein*, 352–354, 361; Pauly and Uhrmacher, "Die Koblenzer Hospitäler in zentralörtlicher Perspektive," 346–347; Nicole Brocard, *Soins, secours, et exclusion: Etablissements hospitaliers et assistance dans le diocèse de Besançon, XIVe et XVe siècles* (Paris: Presses Universitaires Franc-Comtoises, 1998), 19–38.

topography (e.g. the location of vineyards), as well as by proximity to the institution itself.[88] In considering the thirteenth century, Anne E. Lester has written of a charitable landscape in which intramural and extra-mural hospitals—multipurpose institutions and *leprosaria* alike—participated alongside other religious houses.[89]

Hospitals also functioned as points of orientation in the symbolic topographies of late medieval cities. From the thirteenth century onwards, hospitals were increasingly seen as an essential element of urban landscapes and neighborhoods, part of how the ideal city was imagined.[90] Through the twelfth century, many such hospitals were located in or near the cathedral close, and thus associated with the sacred authority of the bishop. In the course of twelfth- and thirteenth-century urban development, episcopal buildings, including hospitals, became sites of increasingly contested power. Not infrequently, the location of these buildings shifted to reflect this.[91] The late medieval development of towns and town neighborhoods, with the movement and construction of buildings, inevitably altered the symbolic community; the perception of Mainz's hospital changed with its thirteenth-century move from the cathedral close to the new walls of the city.[92]

In the early decades of the thirteenth century, many civic hospitals found new sites, changing the symbolic as well as the physical topographies of their cities.[93] Even as urban expansion made central spaces increasingly

88 Pauly and Uhrmacher, ""Die Koblenzer Hospitäler in zentralörtlicher Perspektive," 334–340.

89 Anne E. Lester, "Crafting a Charitable Landscape: Urban Topographies in Charters and Testaments from Medieval Champagne," in *Cities, Texts, and Social Networks, 400–1500: Experiences and Perceptions of Medieval Urban Space,* edited by Caroline Goodson, Anne E. Lester, and Carol Symes (Farnham: Ashgate, 2010), 141.

90 Keith Lilley, *City and Cosmos: The Medieval World in Urban Form* (London: Reaktion Books, 2009), 15–37, 65–73.

91 Maureen C. Miller, *The Bishop's Palace: Architecture and Authority in Medieval Italy* (Ithaca: Cornell University Press, 2000), 125–169. See also Katerina Hornickova, "To Be Seen: The Visual Aspect in Urban Symbolic Communication," in *Faces of Community in Central European Towns: Images, Symbols, and Performances, 1400–1700*, ed. Katerina Hornickova (Lanham, MD: Rowman and Littlefield, 2018), ix-xviii, esp. xii.

92 Faber, "Geschichtslandschaft," 20–23. See also Robert Simunek, "The Bohemian Town as a Space for Symbolic Communication," in *Faces of Community in Central European Towns*, 20–21, 31–33.

93 Pauly and Uhrmacher, "Koblenzer Hospitäler," 340–341; Pascal Montaubin, "Hôtel-Dieu d'Amiens au XIIIe siècles: un hôpital dans les enjeux urbanistiques," in *Hôpitaux et maladreries au moyen âge*, 71–75; Dieter Staerk, "Gutleuthäuser und Kotten im südwestdeutschen Raum. Ein Beitrag zur Erforschung der städtischen Wohlfahrtspflege in Mittelalter und Frühneuzeit," in *Die Stadt in der europäischen Geschichte: Festschrift Edith Ennen*, eds. W. Besch and F. Irsigler (Bonn: n.p., 1972), 551–553, points out that this could be true for l*eprosaria* as well as multipurpose hospitals.

crowded, a growing and increasingly mobile population placed more demands on hospitals than ever before.[94] These multifunctional institutions were, increasingly, both economically important and socially significant as "prestige buildings."[95] The association of these developments with a chronology of "communalization" and increasing civic control has proved durable in the historiography on hospitals.[96] Such a narrative, however, obscures not only tensions between civic and ecclesiastical authorities, but the agency of hospitals themselves. An illuminating case is found in Košice, in the kingdom of Hungary. The hospital was, in fact, under the parish's jurisdiction, and its earliest written source, dating to 1283, says that it had been so for some time. The governing body of the town, however, viewed Košice itself "as the founder and patron of the hospital and jealously protected [their] rights in this capacity."[97] The relationship of hospitals to civic authorities and civic identity could become still more complex in cities boasting multiple hospitals.

Like Mainz, the cathedral city of Speyer had a decentralized hospital landscape in the thirteenth and fourteenth centuries. The old hospital of St. Stephan, traditionally under episcopal control, was transferred to the Teutonic Knights in 1220 by Bishop Conrad III, a move which formed part of the pan-European attempts to regulate religious communities in the wake of Lateran IV. It also aligned with the efforts of Archbishop Siegfried II to bring prosperous houses under stricter forms of religious observance.[98] Thus connected to interests independent of those of the city, the hospital appears to have been comparatively neglected by Speyer's burghers, although it does sometimes appear in charters where multiple hospitals are recipients. The emergence of multiple hospitals as independent institutions of record in subsequent decades suggests a pattern of established communities seeking new forms of legitimacy, rather than diversification in Speyer's hospital landscape. This process is most clearly indicated in the case of the

94 Uhrmacher, *Leprosorien in Mittelalter und früher Neuzeit*, 23–25; Jankrift, "Hospitäler und Leprosorien," 302–305, strikes a more skeptical note on the demands posed by population pressure alone. Knefelkamp, *Stadt und Spital*, 30, discusses urban topography and the architectural complexes of hospitals, using Mainz as an example.

95 Ulrich Knefelkamp, *Das Heilig-Geist-Spital in Nürnberg vom 14–17. Jahrhundert: Geschichte, Struktur, Alltag* (Nürnberg: Verein für Geschichte der Stadt Nürnberg, 1989), 32–38.

96 Pauly and Uhrmacher, "Koblenzer Hospitäler," 340–342. Although civic rectors are only visible from the 1350s, council witnesses appear in hospital charters in the late 1280s.

97 Tim Juckes, *The Parish and Pilgrimage Church of St. Elizabeth in Košice: Town, Court, and Architecture in Late Medieval Hungary* (Turnhout: Brepols, 2011), 31.

98 Böhmer and Will, eds., *Regesta archiepiscoporum Maguntinensium*, I, 192, nr. 505. Cf. Bodmann, *Rheingauische Alterthümer* I, 200.

St. Nicolaus hospital. The first extant reference to this institution comes from 1239, when Pope Gregory IX, in response to a petition from the hospital, confirmed its property rights and its freedom from taxes, suggesting that St. Nicolaus' religious privileges were under dispute.[99]

The new location of Mainz's hospital led to the development of new relationships with neighbors, with visitors to the city, and with civic and ecclesiastical authorities. Built into the walls near a gate, the hospital was both one of the first landmarks of the city to be seen by outsiders, and a point of orientation for citizens. The move to the periphery of the city, far from removing the hospital from spaces of social or economic activity, placed it in close contact with travelers and traders on the Rhine, as well as with the butchers and fishmongers of neighboring streets.[100] The city walls were constructed so that the hospital formed a reinforcing corner; its new location was thus one of responsibility as well as privilege.[101] The construction of the walkway on the city walls leading through the upper level of the hospital may have been designed to offer the guards a few minutes' respite from the elements, possibly with the provision of fire and refreshment by the hospital.[102] Mainz's hospital is somewhat unusual in its literally liminal placement.[103] Its position on the periphery of the city facilitated the collection of rents from its extra-urban properties, and, still more importantly, the direct reception of belated travelers and those seeking aid.[104]

99 Meffert, *Caritas und Krankenwesen*, 191–194.

100 That it was so is suggested by the Maskopp'chen Stadtplan, StaWü Mainz Risse und Plane Nr. 17. For parallel instances see e.g. Lester, "Crafting a Charitable Landscape," 125–129; François-Olivier Touati, "La géographie hospitalière médiévale," in *Hôpitaux et maladreries*, 7–20; Jéhanno, "L'emplacement de l'Hotel Dieu de Paris," 35–49; Andreas Rehberg, "Die Römer und ihre Hospitäler: Beobachtungen zu den Trägergruppen der Spitalsgründungen in Rom (13.–15. Jahrhundert)," in *Hospitäler im Mittelalter*, esp. 242–250.

101 Rörig, *Mainzer Spitäler*, 27–28. Ernst Neeb, "Zur Baugeschichte des Hospitals zum Heiligen Geist und der mittelalterlichen Stadtmauer der Rheinseite zu Mainz," *Mainzer Zeitschrift* 15/16 (1920/1921), 56–61. The portal of the hospital is now in Mainz's cathedral, at the entrance of the St. Gotthard chapel. For another move of a hospital to the city walls, in Montpellier, see Reyerson, "Urban Development vs. Defense," 101–107.

102 Meyer and Steffens, *Die spätmittelalterliche Urbare des Heiliggeist-Spitals*, 22–25.

103 On gatehouses and the delimitation of religious spaces, see Nicolas Reveyron, "Lieux d'accueil et limites régulières dans l'organisation de l'espace monastique au Moyen Âge en Occident," 31–45, though this proposes a strict typology based largely on prescriptive texts.

104 On the reception of pilgrims and travelers see Rörig, "Mainzer Spitäler," 27–28; Neeb, "Zur Baugeschichte des Hospitals zum Heiligen Geist," 56–57; Huffman, "Potens et pauper," 118; Pauly, "Pilgerverkehr und Hospize," 229–239; Susanne Schlösser, *Den Armen und Elenden zu Troste und Frommen...600 Jahre Hospital zu Alzey* (Alzey: Altertumsverein, 1987), 55; Fray, "Institutions hospitalières médiévales," 352–354, argues that hospitals contributed to the function of cities as centers for travelers and pilgrims. On city walls and city identity see also Heinz Stoob, "Die

Wolfgang Schürle has observed that the hospital of Konstanz was constructed at what he terms "a hotspot of economic activity" in the growing city, surrounded by (other) buildings—market, Rathaus—displaying civic pride.[105] In the case of Mainz, the hospital appears to have drawn significant buildings and activities to it, rather than the other way around. The Rathaus was constructed near the hospital some years after its relocation.[106] The scale of the hospital's new buildings, and the speed of its strategic acquisitions, indicate both the prosperity of the community and its commitment to providing the universal welcome celebrated in its statutes. The hospital staff quickly acquired properties surrounding the main building, including a chapel, a cemetery, and a small auxiliary building which may have been used for the care of lepers. They were diligent, moreover, in asserting their rights to perform liturgy and administer the sacraments in their new parish.[107]

The new hospital itself was a spacious, two-story construction. Its interior has been frequently remodeled, meaning that theories concerning how the space was used must be tentatively drawn, based on textual evidence and comparison to better architectural survivals. The chapel was probably at the eastern end, allowing for maximum visibility by all the patients. Side altars may also have been used, as in the tiny hospital of San Jacopo in Florence.[108] A tantalizing reference in a fourteenth-century charter suggests that, at that period, the seriously ill were grouped together at one end of the hospital, where a fire was kept burning for their comfort and for the purification of

Stadtbefestigung. Vergleichende Überlegungen zur bürgerlichen Siedlungs- und Baugeschichte, besonders der frühen Neuzeit," in *Europäische Städte im Zeitalter des Barock: Gestalt, Kultur, Sozialgefüge*, ed. Kersten Krüger. Cologne: Böhlau Verlag, 1988), 25–43.

105 Schürle, *Das Hospital zum Heiligen Geist in Konstanz*, 29–37.

106 Wolfgang Dobras, "Verfassung, Gesellschaft und Wirtschaft in Mainz im 14. Jahrhundert," in Mittelalterliche Kaufhäuser im europäischen Vergleich," ed. Franz Josef Felten (Stuttgart: Franz Steiner Verlag, 2015), 31–54.

107 Meyer and Steffens, *Die spätmittelalterliche Urbare des Heilig Geist Spitals*, 27–35. Such a division is known for other hospitals in the region; StAM 33/1, f61. On hospital cemeteries, cf. Imbert, *Histoire des hôpitaux français*, 67–71; Roberta Gilchrist, *Requiem: The Medieval Monastic Cemetery in Britain* (London: Museum of London Archaeology Service Monograph, 2005), 103–104, 205–207. HStAD A2 168/14 makes clear that St. Gereon had no connection with the hospital before the latter's transfer. This charter, from 1210, ends a dispute between St. Maria ad Gradus and the former chaplain of St. Gereon. StAM 6/30 contains a summary heading of the transfer letter that includes the identification of the new hospital location as "juxta capellam Sancta Gereonis."

108 John Henderson, "Caring for the Poor: Commessi and commesse in the Hospitals of Renaissance Florence," in *Hospitäler in Mittelalter und früher Neuzeit: Frankreich, Deutschland und Italien. Eine Vergleichende Geschichte*, ed. Gisela Drossbach (Munich: Oldenbourg, 2007), 163–172.

the air.[109] The hospital conferred on the sick in residence there a communal identity that endured across generations. Like many other medieval urban hospitals, it also served as a focal point for the regular distribution of alms to the less seriously ill.[110] Some rivalry with the cathedral chapter may have been involved here; there are indications that the chapter distributed alms in bread on feast days, particularly during the Easter season.[111]

The male and female staff of Mainz's hospital inhabited the first and second floors of the new complex, respectively.[112] In all probability, they cooperated closely in hospital administration. For the brothers and sisters of Mainz's hospital, the most significant characteristic of their location appears to have been its proximity to the chapel of St. Gereon, owned by the cathedral chapter. The statutes of 1236 identify the plot for the new buildings as adjacent to the chapel, suggesting that the preexistence of a consecrated building provided one reason for the choice of site.[113] The chapel, although not directly controlled by the hospital, could have provided a space for the performance of liturgical functions during the construction

109 Richard Dertsch, ed., *Die Urkunden des Stadtarchivs Mainz: Regesten*, vol. 3 (Mainz: Stadtarchiv, 1963), Nr. 1377, from a priest's will: "ligna cremabilia pro foco ignis egenis peregrines et in dicta hospitali degentibus." On the use of fire as a method of air purification see Johann Peter Schunk, ed. *Beyträge zur Mainzer Geschichte, mit Urkunden*, vol. 1 (Frankfurt: Fleischer, 1788), 346–348; Stiftsbibliothek Aschaffenburg MS Pap 16, f152v; Miller, *The Birth of the Hospital*, 141–166.

110 StAM U 9 September 1385, a testament, contains evidence of alms distributed regularly on Mondays (the bequest is "zu hulfe den almosen die man wochclichen uff den mandag gibt in dem vorgenanten spiedale zum heiligen geiste"). A summary of the record is printed in Dertsch, *Die Urkunden des Stadtarchivs Mainz*, Nr. 2260. When this custom began is uncertain, although Ernst Vogt, ed., *Regesten der Erzbischöfe von Mainz* (Leipzig: Veit & Co., 1913), 275–277, contains evidence for active alms-collectors in the early fourteenth century, and François-Olivier Touati, *Archives de la lèpre: Atlas des léproseries entre Loire et Marne au moyen âge* (Paris: Comité des Travaux historiques et scientifiques, 1996), 29, points out that records relating to almsgiving were often created or compiled considerably after the practice's date of origin. On the practice of almsgiving in hospitals more generally, see Bernd Fuhrmann, "Einleitung," in *Norm und Praxis in der Armenfürsorge in Spätmittelalter und früher Neuzeit*, Sebastian Schmidt and Jens Aspelmeier, eds.(Stuttgart, Steiner, 2006), 15; Gerhard Oexle, "Armut, Armutsbegriff, und Armenfürsorge," in *Soziale Sicherheit und soziale Disziplinierung: Beiträge zu einer historischen Theorie der Sozialpolitik*, Christoph Sachse und Florian Tennstedt, eds. (Frankfurt am Main: Suhrkamp, 1986), 79–80.

111 Martinus-Bibliothek HS 3, f56–62.

112 Neeb, "Zur Baugeschichte des Hospitals zum Heiligen Geist," 59; Meyer and Steffens, *Die spätmittelalterliche Urbare des Heilig Geist Spitals*, 227. There is no basis for the assertion of Craemer, *Das Hospital als Bautyp des Mittelalters*, 38, that this two-story design provided a template for houses of the Order of Santo Spirito elsewhere in Germany.

113 StAM 6/30; Meyer and Steffens, *Die spätmittelalterliche Urbare des Heilig Geist Spitals*, 227–228, identify the chapel as having stood at the northeast corner of the hospital buildings.

of the new buildings. The Fourth Lateran Council made explicit that any religious institution—including any hospital—needed its own priest, and the capability of administering the Sacraments to the sick.[114] The importance of St. Gereon is confirmed in a charter of November 1252, detailing the terms of the chapel's sale to the brothers and sisters of the hospital by the cathedral chapter. The terms of the agreement suggest that the sale and its conditions were fiercely fought for by the hospital community.[115] Conspicuous by its absence is any reference to the hospital by name; at this stage, it is still simply the hospital of Mainz.

A donation charter of 1257 hints at tensions between the hospital and the parish of St. Quintin, in which the new buildings were situated, over the provision of the sacraments and other elements of pastoral care.[116] The gift, from a prosperous matron and her son, arranged for both the chapel of St. Gereon and St. Quintin to receive monies for memorial lights, but with the stipulation that St. Gereon was required to pay the parish church a measure of oil.[117] The brothers and sisters of the hospital are collectively identified as issuers of the charter, together with the rector, the only member of the hospital staff with a named role. By contrast, all of the officials of the cathedral chapter are mentioned; the claim that they gave the chapel "charitably and freely (*pie et liberaliter*)" is more likely a rhetorical flourish than a reflection of reality.[118] Whether the phrasing was chosen by the canons or the hospital staff, it served to reinforce the hospital's rights as a religious institution at a moment when its position in the city's religious and ecclesiastical networks was contested. The chapel may have become an inconvenience to the hospital, either because of its location or its size. The hospital obtained explicit permission to "dispose of the chapel through building, through destroying, or by any means whatsoever, as it may appear most healthy and convenient for us and for our house."[119]

114 Alberigo et al, eds., *Conciliorum Oecumenicorum Decreta*, 263.

115 StAM U/1252. Copied in the records of the cathedral chapter, StaWü MBVI 17, CXXII, with the superscription "Centenario olei quod dat hospitale." Printed in Gudenus, *Codex Diplomatica* I, 627 Nr. 261. StAM 33/1 f 61, 71, the latter entry with a marginal note on an increased rent, indicating careful management; StAM 33/4 f 37. Cf. Meyer and Steffens, *Die Urbare des Heilig Geist Spitals von Mainz*, 227–228.

116 Juckes, *The Parish and Pilgrimage Church of St. Elizabeth in Košice*, 31, describes a possibly parallel case. The hospital of Košice boasted a church (*ecclesia*) independent from the parish from at least 1366.

117 HStAD C1 A Nr. 78, pg. 37.

118 StAM U / 15 November 1252. On the limitations of gifts to hospitals, see Mansi, *Sacrorum conciliorum*, vol. 22, col. 835–836.

119 StAM U / 15 November 1252.

Whether the hospital staff wished to tear down the chapel in order to expand the accommodations for the sick or to expand the chapel itself for the communal performance of liturgy, or whether these and other possibilities were still under debate, is unclear. In any case, the value the hospital placed on the chapel was considerable, as indicated by the pledge of a *centenarium* of oil to be paid to the chapter annually on St. Martin's Day. Still conforming to the terms of canon law, the oil is described as a "free gift" to the cathedral chapter, but the circumstances indicate that the terms of the sale were contested. That the brothers and sisters were unanimous in pledging the rent on behalf of themselves and their successors is an impressive testimony to the community's rapid expansion, and to their already-attained prosperity.[120] The hospital's rights over the property, and obligation to the cathedral chapter, are reiterated in the records of both institutions into the early fourteenth century.[121]

Civic Administration, Religious Status: The Hospitals of Mainz, Worms, and Speyer

A parallel case to that of Mainz's hospital is found in Speyer, also around the midpoint of the thirteenth century. Speyer's hospital of St. Georg, or "new hospital," as it was frequently known, has been referred to as a foundation of the mid-thirteenth century.[122] Its first extant records, however, from 1259 and 1261, suggest that the crucial procedure was a clarification of rights, not the establishment of an entirely new community. Moreover, as illustrated in Mainz, the label of a "new hospital" could endure for decades for the sake of distinguishing between multiple urban foundations. In 1259, the burgher Ulrich Klüpfel made an extensive gift to Speyer's "new hospital," endowing it with properties in two nearby villages and the rights of appointment over a priest in one of them.[123] Several of the witnesses to this charter are clerics, indicating that negotiations may have been necessary to ensure that the activities of the hospital priest were not seen as infringing upon parochial rights, as in the case of Mainz's Heilig Geist Spital and St. Quintin. When

120 StAM U / 15 November 1252.

121 StAWü MBVI XVII, f122r; HStAD A2 168/14; StAM 33/4 f61; StAM 33/1 f71; Gudenus I, 627 Nr. 261.

122 Wolfgang Eger, "Beispiel europäischer Hospitalgeschichte: vom St. Georgen-Spital zum Stiftungskrankenhaus," *Speyer: Vierteljahreshefte des Verkehrsvereins* 32 (1992), 3–4.

123 Alfred Hilgard, ed., *Urkunden zur Geschichte der Stadt Speyer* (Strassburg: Trübner, 1885), Nr. 92.

Speyer's St. Georg received its administrative statutes from the council two years later, its properties were explicitly exempted from taxation.[124]

Following the refining of criteria for religious status in the early thirteenth century, changes in hospital administration became increasingly frequent. For example, lay founders might sign over administration to the bishops in order that the hospital might retain the legal privileges of a religious institution. The existence of such transfers alongside those from ecclesiastical to civic authorities provides a salutary caution against assuming the primacy of local politics and municipal identity in transfers which did move hospitals, their staff and property, into the hands of city councils.[125] The variety in such changes, and in the negotiations between civic and ecclesiastical authorities, has caused confusion among those who have tried to sketch a chronology for the so-called secularization of the medieval hospital.[126] The increasing influence of lay elites—like Ulrich Klüpfel—over hospital administration has often been interpreted as a reflection of spiritual decline. Indeed, such decline and lax administration have been the "chief historiographical villains" in studies of late medieval hospitals.[127] Such interpretations echo the language of prescriptive sources, and parallel trends in the historiography of monastic houses.[128] They neglect, however, the complexity of the social questions that arose as a consequence of hospitals' contested legal status. In evaluating council involvement in the governance of Rhineland hospitals, I

124 Hilgard, ed., *Urkunden zur Geschichte der Stadt Speyer*, Nr. 98.

125 See Pauly, *Peregrinorum, pauperum ac aliorum transeuntium receptaculum*, 113, 179–180, 208–212.

126 Bettina Toson, *Mittelalterliche Hospitäler in Hessen zwischen Schwalm, Eder, und Fulda* (Darmstadt: Hessiche Historische Kommission, 2012), 25–26; Christopher Bonfield, Therapeutic Regimens," in *Hospital Life*, 21–48, offers a useful study of continuities in attitudes and practices in English hospitals from the fourteenth to thesixteenth centuries.

127 Sethina Watson, *Fundatio, Ordinatio, and Statuta: The Statutes and Constitutional Documents of English Hospitals to 1300* (Oxford: D.Phil., 2003), 222–223. Falck, "Mainzer Hospitäler im Mittelalter," 410; Reicke, *Das deutsche Spital und sein Recht*, vol. 1, 86–92; Margaret A. Seymour, "The Organization, Personnel, and Functions of the Hospital in the later Middle Ages," *The Bulletin of the Institute for Historical Research* 21 (1948), 249–250; Marie-Louise Windemuth, *Das Hospital als Träger der Armenfürsorge im Mittelalter* (Stuttgart: Franz Steiner Verlag, 1995), 75–87.

128 See Glenn Warren Olsen, *The Legal Definition of the Ecclesiastical Benefice During the Period of the Appearance of Papal Provisioning* (Ph.D. Diss., University of Wisconsin, 1965), 239–244; Gert Melville, "Nuove Tendenze della storiografia monastica di area tedesca," in *Dove va la storiografia monastica in Europa?: temi e metodi di ricerca per lo studio della vita monastica e regolare in età medievale alle soglie del terzo millennio : atti del convegno internazionale Brescia-Rodengo, 23–25 marzo 2000*, ed. Giancarlo Andenna (Milan: Vita e Pensiero, 2001), 35–39, for a review of the paradigms of renewal and decline in the historiography.

attempt to reframe debates about alleged secularization, and the concrete importance of administrative control.[129]

Mainz's hospital obtained its statutes as an independent religious house at a time when tensions among different interest groups ran high. The hospital itself was of no small social and economic importance, and the implications of its legal status were considerable.[130] The burghers of Mainz, after over a decade of challenges and concessions, gained political freedom from the archbishop in 1244.[131] The charter of civic emancipation included rights of administration over the hospital. Although the hospital's relationships with lay and religious authorities changed appreciably with this agreement, the institution did not lose its religious status. Under the rules of 1236, those who worked there took permanent vows as religious persons, and both they and their property were exempted from secular taxes. These privileges were retained after its administrative transfer. In gaining rights over the hospital, the city council gained a say in the management of its valuable—and tax-exempt—properties. Before examining the terms of this transfer in detail, it is worth considering the political and religious context in which it took place.

Archbishop Siegfried von Eppstein succeeded his uncle as archbishop in 1230. He would be followed by Wernher von Eppstein, whose tenure was hardly less turbulent.[132] The two decades of Siegfried's tenure as political and spiritual lord of Mainz were characterized by tension with the clergy of the diocese and the laity alike, especially in the prosperous city of Mainz.[133] His zeal for the regularization of religious institutions is particularly visible in the city itself.[134] A chronicle penned by a cathedral canon describes the

129 This strategy is recommended by Pauly and Uhrmacher, "Die Koblenzer Hospitäler in zentralörtlicher Perspektive," 340–341.

130 Cf. Fray, "Institutions hospitalières médiévales," 352–354. Rubin, *Charity and Community*, 202–235.

131 Demandt, *Stadtherrschaft und Stadtfreiheit*, 76–82; Friedhelm Jürgensmeier, "Siegfried III," in *Handbuch der Mainzer Kirchengeschichte: Christliche Antike und Mittelalter*, ed. Friedhelm Jürgensmeier, vol. 1 (Würzburg: Echter Verlag, 2000), 342–346; Christian Eckert, "Der Mainzer Rat vom 13. Nov 1244 bis 28 Oct 1462," *Archiv für Hessische Geschichte und Altertumskund* 2 (1899), 321–357.

132 Friedhelm Jürgensmeier, "Das Erzbistum Mainz," in *Die Bistümer des Heiligen Römischen Reiches von ihren Anfängen bis zur Säkularisation*, ed. Erwin Gatz (Freiburg im Breisgau: Herder, 2003), 412–414.

133 Jürgensmeier, "Siegfried III," 342.

134 Pixton, *The German Episcopacy*, 225–282. On the archbishop's involvement at Lateran IV, see Stephan Kuttner and Antonio Garcia y Garcia, "A New Eyewitness Account of the Fourth Lateran Council," *Traditio* 20 (1964), 147–148, 158–159, and Maleczek, "Der Mittelpunkt Europas," 89–97.

archbishop as "raised up in heart, and of great pride.... Assuming the face and spirit of a lion," writes the outraged chronicler, "he became a lion indeed; and he began to make orphans and widows, to burn towns, to destroy cities, to consume men, and turn the earth into a desert."[135] Though this jeremiad ought not to be taken at face value, the patterns of administration it describes align with scholarly analysis.[136] Siegfried was an adept political strategist, and the charter by which he granted Mainz its civic freedom may have been calculated to pacify a chronically restive—and increasingly powerful—municipal elite.

The charter, issued on 15 November 1244, marked a sea-change in Mainz's administration: a council was created to assume political leadership of the city.[137] The privileges enshrined in the charter were to be repeatedly confirmed in subsequent decades by both the cathedral chapter and Mainz's archbishops. When Siegfried III himself confirmed these privileges, the rights over the hospital were singled out.[138] The prescriptions concerning taxes, tolls, and armed retinues are of a specificity suggesting long and rancorous debate. Although ancient customs are alluded to, such issues as the exemption of expanding housing from taxation were a consequence of recent urban growth.[139] After demarcating the economic and political rights of the archbishop and the citizens of Mainz, the charter turns to the hospital.[140] In contrast with the other provisions of the charter, rights over the hospital are granted to a named man, Arnelm, suggesting that the council negotiated for such rights specifically.

The newly formed city council is granted power over presenting the hospital priest, and, more unusually, of deposing him "if his fault shall

135 "Christiani chronicon Moguntinum," in Jaffé, ed., *Monumenta Moguntina,* 697.

136 Jürgensmeier, "Siegfried III,", 342–346. Siegfried III was elected without significant opposition, and initially followed the policies of his predecessor, which were in line with the interests of the cathedral chapter. However, Siegfried was excommunicated in 1240 as a result of his imperial politics; when he turned against the Staufer, however, the cathedral chapter of Mainz turned against him.

137 StAM U 1244. Jürgensmeier, as above, interprets Siegfried's grant of civic freedoms as a gesture intended to win Mainz for the archbishop's anti-Staufer policies, removing it from the line of pro-imperial Rhenish cities.

138 HStAD A2 168/250; StAWü MBVI 75, f. 13r–13v. Further confirmations by the cathedral chapter and successive archbishops are found on folia 14r–15v, 17r–18r, 28r-v.

139 StAM U 1244.

140 Keith Lilley, *City and Cosmos: The Medieval World in Urban Form* (Chicago: University of Chicago Press, 2009), 143–146, suggests that such charters containing urban statutes reflected the priorities of social order. Such an analysis would place the hospital low among the concerns of Mainz's lay elites.

require it."[141] Both processes are to be mediated by archiepiscopal authority. The fact that the power to make such a concession lay in Siegfried's power indicates that the oversight of the house of Augustinian canons had been a temporary measure. A similar case is known in Trier; further records on the late twelfth-century leadership of Mainz's hospital are not extant.[142] The delegation of authority of the council is not tantamount to secularization. The decretals of Gregory IX, and their commentaries, demonstrate that laypersons were legally capable of choosing priests.[143] Administration of the hospital's temporal possessions was granted to "citizens who are seen to be suitable." These administrators, however, never became dependent on the council; nor did Mainz's hospital have the statutes affirming its religious status—and that of the persons who resided there as vowed staff—rescinded or superseded. The change in administration did, however, mean the migration of a substantial source of income from the archbishop to the city's nascent political elite. Once the hospital was removed from the control of the archbishop and chapter, the council appeared content to intervene only rarely. The hospital's presence in the charter granting civic privileges suggests that it held a place of symbolic and practical importance in the minds of Mainz's burghers. Still, the council wanted the hospital to remain a religious institution, with continued exemption from taxation.[144]

Like the archiepiscopal letter of 1236, the charter of 1244 uses labile vocabulary to designate the members of the laity involved. "All the citizens of Mainz" reportedly petitioned the archbishop for the first transfer.[145] Resent-

141 StAM U 1244.

142 Gregory IX, in a bull of 29 April 1227, reiterates the mid-thirteenth-century concern with unlawful impositions "not only on men of the church, but churches themselves, and other ecclesiastical persons." L. Auvray (éd.), *Les registres de Grégoire IX (1227–1241)*, Paris, 1890–1955, 4 vols. (BEFAR), https://clio.columbia.edu/databases/4346120. Accessed October 15, 2020. The language of StAM U 1244 makes clear that the hospital's religious status was preserved in its transition to civic oversight. Cf. Hostiensis, *Summa Aurea, Liber I* (Venice: Senneton, 1574), col. 90–96, on the nomination of priests. See also Mayer and Steffens, *Die spätmittelalterliche Urbare des Heiliggeist-Spitals*, 25–29; Reicke, *Das deutsche Spital*, 32–33.

143 Hostiensis, *Summa Aurea*, (Venice: n.p., 1574), col. 99–104, 133–137 on the powers of election and confirmation.

144 Joachim Wollasch, "Anmerkungen zur Gemeinschaft des Heiliggeistspitals zu Freiburg i.Br. im Spätmittelalter," in *Civitatum communitas: Studien zum europäischen Städtewesen. Festschrift Heinz Stoob zum 65. Geburtstag*, ed. (Köln: Böhlau Verlag, 1984), 607–609, finds a parallel instance in Freiburg. On hospitals and civic power and identity more generally, see Pauly, *Peregrinorum, pauperum ac aliorum transeuntem receptaculum*, 167–180, 208–212. For more detail on the council's role in dividing the mixed-gender staff of the hospital, see Chapter 3.

145 StAM 6(40), 3, printed in Gudenus, *Codex Diplomaticus* I, 638.

ment of urban property being held by ecclesiastical institutions—including hospitals—was widespread throughout the thirteenth and fourteenth centuries, and Mainz appears to have been no exception.[146] Such resentment may have been a catalyst for the first move of the hospital, away from the city's central market and public space by the cathedral. The transfer to civic control preceded the development of the area near the hospital into a second locus of power. The town hall, the mint, and a commercial building (Kaufhaus) were all constructed adjacent to the hospital, in the thirteenth and fourteenth centuries, making the locality a political and economic center.[147] In the aftermath of Mainz's obtaining civic freedoms in 1244, it has been argued, the hospital helped to constitute a sort of civic forum.[148] Although the hospital was connected to Mainz's merchant elites in the later thirteenth and fourteenth centuries, such links are not readily visible in either the statutes of 1236 or the charter of 1244. Arnelm is granted rights over the hospital *ex officio* as a council member, rather than based on any relationship with the institution.[149] The hospital statutes' focus on individual and collective property exemptions suggests the possibility of staff members prosperous enough to have a pragmatic concern for their possessions, as well as for the rights afforded them by canon law, including the right to accept bequests and *inter vivos* donations.[150]

In thirteenth-century Worms, the council intervened still less in hospital affairs. They contributed to hospital upkeep in the 1280s, but little is known about their collective involvement.[151] Unusually, cathedral canons and a council member appear as joint administrators of the city's hospital in 1299.[152] The same document provides a partial inventory of the hospital's property at the time of its former procurator's death. That the hospital

146 Franz-Josef Arlinghaus, "The Myth of Urban Unity: Religion and Social Performance in Late Medieval Braunschweig," in *Cities, Texts, and Social Networks, 400–1500: Experiences and Perceptions of Medieval Urban Space*, eds. Caroline Goodson, Anne E. Lester, and Carol Symes (Farnham: Ashgate, 2010), 215–224.

147 Rita Heuser, *Namen der Mainzer Straßen und Örtlichkeiten. Sammlung, Deutung, sprach- und motivgeschichtliche Auswertung* (Stuttgart: Franz Steiner Verlag, 2008), 573.

148 Andreas Puth, "'Our and the Empire's Free City on the Rhine': Visualizing the Empire in the Mainz Kaufhaus Reliefs," in *Mainz and the Middle Rhine Valley*, eds. Ute Engel and Alexandra Gajewski (Leeds: British Archaeological Association, 2007), 89–90.

149 StAM U / 1244. Cf. Dertsch, *Die Urkunden des Stadtarchivs Mainz*, vol. 1, 183–197.

150 StAM 6(40), 3, printed in Gudenus, *Codex Diplomaticus* I, 638. On *inter vivos* donations, see Le Grand, *Statuts d'hôtels-dieu*, 36–38; Imbert, *Histoire des hôpitaux français*, 18–24.

151 Ludwig Baur, *Hessische Urkunden: Die Provinz Rheinhessen von 963–1325*, vol. 2 (Darmstadt: Der historische Verein für das Grossherzogthum Hessen, 1862), 365–366.

152 StAW U / 1299 Mai.

held, as the year's produce, over 450 measures of flour, eighty measures of wheat, thirty pigs, and six sheep testifies to the scale on which it could and did provide food to those in need.[153] The charter's language of committing all these things "and the care of the sick" to the new procurator suggests that it was intended to legitimate the hospital's claim to religious status by demonstrating that its plentiful resources were being used in accordance with the prescriptions of canon law.

The statutes of Speyer's St. Georg hospital, issued by the city council in 1261, provide another example of how civic authorities invoked canon law in establishing hospital privileges. The statutes affirm the house's legal privileges, relying on the vocabulary of Christian charity. The judges and council members of Speyer do not identify themselves by name in the opening formulae of the charter, but rather *ex officio* as the creators of the document "together with all the citizens of Speyer." They then turn to a long excursus on the saving work of Christ for his "sick sheep," which inspires them to "mercifully perform the works of charity."[154] Three citizens are established as administrators of the hospital, with the provision that no rents, properties, or other possessions may be alienated without the consent of the whole council. The comfort of the sick may indeed have been a priority for hospital administrators; but it would be naive to ignore the legal and economic privileges that the charter secured for the hospital as an institution. Both the specification that the hospital should provide for the sick of Speyer and the association of temporal assistance with mindfulness of eternal welfare are typical of trends observed by historians of German hospitals in the later Middle Ages.[155] The hospital of Kiel, for instance, staffed by a mixed-gender community, is on record as having their privileges confirmed multiple times from the mid-thirteenth to the mid-fourteenth centuries, having first been given statutes (probably some time after the hospital's origin) by the bishop in the 1250s.[156]

The careful negotiation of religious status in the development of civic hospitals demonstrates that, for late medieval burghers, the realization of political power and social identity could come through religious institutions, rather than in opposition to them. The multiplication of urban hospitals in

153 StAW U / 1299 Mai.

154 Hilgard, ed., *Urkunden zur Geschichte der Stadt Speyer*, Nr. 98.

155 See for example Laqua, *Bruderschaften und Hospitäler*, 109–113, 168–169, 207–209, 238–239, 383.

156 Meinert, *Die Hospitäler Holsteins im Mittelalter*, 59–67. Cf. Rawcliffe, *Hospitals*, 69–77, on the membership of Norwich's hospitals, and 77–85, on financial records that provide evidence of high expenses and struggles to meet them, but also of conscientious management.

the written records of the twelfth and thirteenth centuries is not necessarily indicative of a commensurate multiplication in the number of such institutions.[157] The types of documents created by and for these hospitals indicate a concern with their recognition as independent religious institutions. As the criteria for religious status changed, hospital statutes—whether sought, imposed, or granted—reflected the evolving responsibilities and privileges associated with that status.[158] The physical and symbolic hospital landscapes of the major cities of the Rhineland differed from each other, as did the chronologies of hospital development in each city. Similar patterns are visible, however, in the thirteenth-century negotiation over hospitals' property rights, and over their relationships to civic and ecclesiastical authorities. In the often tense relationships between the region's powerful bishops and archbishops, and increasingly prosperous urban elites, hospitals appear as places fraught with significance, but not as mere pawns. Rather, hospital staff and administrators were tenacious in asserting and preserving their individual and collective rights to religious status.

157 Le Grand, *Statuts d'hôtels-Dieu*, 96–100; Meinert, *Die Hospitäler Holsteins im Mittelalter*, 14–15, offers an unusually sensitive treatment of the emergence of hospitals into the written record in the twelfth century and external reforms in the latter half of the thirteenth century.
158 Cf. Brasher, *Hospitals and Charity*, 93–107.

3 Mainz's Hospital Sisters and the Rights of Religious Women

Abstract

This chapter analyzes how Mainz's hospital sisters, and similar communities, can be understood as part of the history of women's religious houses. The late medieval history of the independent hospital formed by the hospital sisters has hitherto been virtually unexamined, and its administration has been misattributed to the cathedral chapter. This seriously distorts, I argue, the image of Mainz's decentralized hospital landscape. Although civic authorities and male religious leaders in Mainz sought to have the women incorporated into one of the city's Cistercian houses, the women themselves saw hospital service as central to their religious identity. That the management of their hospital was a communal priority for the women of St. Agnes is suggested by the fact that they funneled resources towards it and concentrated properties around it.

Keywords: medieval hospitals, religious women, canon law, Cistercians

On 14 August 1260, Hildeborg, elaborately identified as "the magistra of the convent of nuns of the hospital in Mainz," on behalf of the community, made over to the hospital the house which the sisters owned "in the courtyard of the hospital, next to the cookhouse."[1] Temporary residence on hospital property could have been an attempt to satisfy civic and ecclesiastical authorities, without suddenly depriving the hospital of a significant number of its staff; or, indeed, a concession to the women as they sought a new place of residence. In the charter of 1260, the sisters still appear closely connected with the hospital. Six members of the community witness the charter: Godesman, the provisor, two hospital priests, and three lay brothers.[2] This

1 HStAD A2 168/30.
2 HStAD A2 168/30.

Barnhouse, Lucy C. *Hospitals in Communities of the Late Medieval Rhineland. Houses of God, Places for the Sick.* Taylor & Francis Group, 2023
DOI: 10.5117/9789463720243_CH03

degree of specification concerning the roles of the men within the hospital is itself unusual; in documents of practice, the status of healthy and sick, staff and patients, are usually less distinct than in regulations. Despite the *de jure* separation, Hildeborg refers to the image of the Dove of the Holy Spirit, pressed into red wax, as "our seal," used to affirm that the sale is permanent, and that the rights of the brothers must be undisputed.[3] The division of Mainz's hospital staff along gendered lines was a response to increasing suspicion of mixed-gender religious communities, and marked the beginning of the sisters' efforts to form a new community, managing a new hospital.

Religious Status and Women's Communities: The Case of Hospitals

The vowed sisters of Mainz's oldest hospital, who, after their enforced departure from it, formed the community of St. Agnes, saw their identity as hospital sisters as central to their status as religious women. After leaving the civic hospital in 1259, the most fraught question for the women was that of their institutional identity. The women's attempts to establish a convent in Mainz's burgeoning urban center in the 1260s–1270s met with initial hostility from the laity. The archbishops of Mainz sought to place their community under increasingly strict regulation. In order to preserve their autonomy, the sisters of St. Agnes deployed the rhetoric of religious status knowledgeably. The development of St. Agnes demonstrates that religious identity in the later Middle Ages could be fluid, negotiable, and—perhaps above all—situational.[4] A credulous reading of the extant sources led early historians of Mainz to conclude that these women joined the Cistercian Order, following the plan of the city council and religious

3 HStAD A2 168/30.

4 Herbert Grundmann, *Religious Movements in the Middle Ages: The Historical Links Between Heresy, the Mendicant Orders, and the Women's Religious Movement in the Twelfth and Thirteenth Century, with the Historical Foundations of German Mysticism*, trans. Steven Rowan (Notre Dame, IN: University of Notre Dame Press, 1995), 75–153; Jo Ann Kay McNamara, *Sisters in Arms: Catholic Nuns Through Two Millennia* (Cambridge, MA: Harvard University Press, 1996), 252–259. Cf. Venarde, *Women's Monasticism and Medieval Society*, 133–186; Anne E. Lester, *Creating Cistercian Nuns: The Women's Religious Movement and Its Reform in Thirteenth-Century Champagne* (Ithaca: Cornell University Press, 2011), 78–116 et passim; Heidi L. Febert, "The Poor Sisters of Söflingen: Religious Corporations as Property Litigants, 1310–1317," *Traditio* 68 (2013), 327–340; Gertrude Jaron Lewis, *By Women, for Women, about Women: The Sister-Books of Fourteenth-Century Germany* (Toronto: Pontifical Institute of Medieval Studies, 1996), 3–9, 176–199.

men of Mainz, as outlined in the charter formally separating the sisters and brothers of Mainz's oldest hospital.[5] In forming their community of St. Agnes, the hospital sisters of Mainz evaded affiliation with the Cistercians, choosing rather to pursue their vocation independently. This policy led to tensions with both the laity and the ecclesiastical leaders of Mainz in the latter half of the thirteenth century. The sisters of St. Agnes ensured their community's survival by appealing to bishops and archbishops across Europe for letters of indulgence, which provided them both with religious legitimacy and, indirectly, with additional financial support.[6] For the women of St. Agnes, their role as hospital sisters was central to their sense of communal purpose; and they recognized religious status as crucial to their communal survival.

For the women of St. Agnes, forging an institutional identity required that they negotiate relationships with the laity of Mainz as their neighbors and donors, and with ecclesiastical elites in Mainz and beyond. In the latter decades of the thirteenth century, the understandings of the religious identity of St. Agnes and of its hospital were attentively managed by the women. This is revealed through the regulation—and patronage—of the community by ecclesiastical authorities, and through St. Agnes' relationships with members of the laity. The sisters were heavily invested in the hospital's management, cultivating diverse properties for its support. Their administration of the hospital, however, was not without controversy; multiple charters testify to archiepiscopal efforts to bring it under a stricter religious observance. By the mid-fourteenth century, the laity of Mainz had accepted the community of St. Agnes as part of the city's religious landscape, while the archbishops persisted in attempts to regulate the religious observance both of St. Agnes and of its hospital more strictly. The

5 Karl Schaab, *Die Geschichte der Stadt Mainz* (Mainz: F. Kupferberg, 1841), 361, 367–368; Franz Joseph Bodmann, *Rheingauische Alterthümer oder Landes und Regimentsverfassung des westlichen oder Niederrheingaues im Mittlern Zeitalter*, (Mainz: Florian Kupferberg, 1819), 242; Ute Mayer and Rudolf Steffens, *Die spätmittelalterliche Urbare des Heiliggeist-Spitals in Mainz* (Stuttgart: Franz Steiner Verlag, 1992), 24–25. The women themselves invoked Cistercian identity, while remaining free from visitation.

6 On indulgences and hospitals, see Carla Keyvanian, *Hospitals and Urbanism in Rome, 1200–1500* (Leiden: Brill, 2015), 295–296; Miri Rubin, *Charity and Community in Medieval Cambridge* (Cambridge: Cambridge University Press, 1987), 264–269; Gerhard Fouquet, "Zwölf-Brüder-Häuser und die Vorstellung vom verdienten Ruhestand im Spätmittelalter," in *Sozialgeschichte mittelalterlicher Hospitäler*, 45; Beate Sophie Gros, *Das Hohe Hospital in Soest (ca. 1178 –1600). Eine prosopographische und sozialgeschichtliche Untersuchung* (Münster: Aschendorff, 1999), 64; Franz Meffert, *Caritas und Krankenwesen bis zum Ausgang des Mittelalters* (Freiburg im Breisgau: Caritas Verlag, 1927), 287–312.

identity of hospital sisters was that which was most actively pursued and cultivated by the sisters themselves.[7]

Sisters and Brothers: The Division of Mainz's Hospital Staff

In 1259, the men and women who, having vowed themselves to the religious life, had jointly issued charters and cared for the sick in Mainz's hospital were divided. The hospital property was divided likewise, in order to enable the hospital sisters to support themselves. Research on the separation of Mainz's hospital staff has been marked by confusion about both chronology and institutional identity.[8] This confusion has been exacerbated by the fragmentary nature of extant sources, and also by the tensions between official rhetoric, which claimed the existence of near-schism within the hospital community, and the evidence for ongoing relationships between the hospital brothers and sisters. Although the archivist Joseph Bodmann dated the division of the hospital staff to 1254, the first record of the staff's separation is a charter issued by Mainz's council in May 1259. I believe that this charter marked the legal finalization of a recent process.[9]

In an 8 March agreement with the Cistercian house of Eberbach, the hospital provisor identifies himself as speaking on behalf of all the brothers of the hospital, without mentioning the sisters, but this may have been a diplomatic omission in response to external pressure.[10] The transaction with Eberbach shortly before the sisters' putative transfer to its supervision might seem suggestive of concealed motives. The property transferred, however, was sold for the tidy sum of four and a half silver marks, and no mention of other connections—even to disclaim their relevance—is made. Moreover, there is no evidence to support the presumption that St. Agnes came under Eberbach's supervision before the fifteenth century. The separation of the brothers and sisters was one of many such processes legally finalized

7 For more on the vocabulary used to describe the women, by themselves and others, see Lucy C. Barnhouse, "Disordered Women? The Hospital Sisters of Mainz and Their Late Medieval Identities," *Medieval Feminist Forum* 55:2 (2020), 60–97.

8 Bodmann, *Rheingauische Alterthümer*, II, 900–903, identifies the charter of 1259 as formalizing the separation which he earlier describes as taking place ca. 1250. His assessment of the situation in 1260 is that some sisters must have remained in the hospital, and some sisters have separated, but still lived next to the hospital as nuns. Ludwig Falck, *Mainz in seiner Blütezeit als Freie Stadt (1244–1328)*, Geschichte der Stadt Mainz III (Düsseldorf: Verlag Rau, 1973), 54.

9 HStAD A2 115/1. Bodmann, *Rheingauische Alterthümer*, I, 202. Bodmann attributes his decision to "an ancient and unprinted document," not further identified.

10 HStAD A2 208/5. A duplicate copy of the record survives under HStAD A2 208/6.

around the midpoint of the thirteenth century.[11] Traditional explanations of religious or charitable zeal, echoing contemporary claims, provide inadequate explanation for such a pattern.[12] Thirteenth-century divisions of hospital communities along gendered lines can be better understood as attempts, initiated by administrators, to safeguard the religious status of hospitals as institutions.

The formal division of the hospital's male and female staff marks the first instance of Mainz's council exercising control over the hospital since their acquisition of rights in 1244. Their intervention demonstrates that, contradicting popular historiographical narratives, the council wanted the hospital they administered to retain its status as a religious institution.[13] The council wrote that they made their decision after taking conference with the Dominicans, the cathedral chapter, and other religious men of Mainz, signaling larger issues at stake in the religious and social landscape of the city.[14] Internal dissent alone would have been unlikely to attract such extensive involvement from groups outside the hospital. The "religious men" of Mainz may have been consulted in order to find an affiliation for the women that would satisfy the demands of canon law—which dictated that vowed persons could not leave their community unless joining a stricter observance—while not upsetting the balance of power among the city's numerous monastic houses.

The process of dividing the hospital property between the brothers and sisters was monitored by a carefully chosen committee. The council placed hospital brothers on the committee because of their intimate knowledge of the property. Under conditions of internal strife in the hospital, this arrangement might have been expected to result in protest,

11 Wolfgang Seibrich, "Monastisches Leben von ca. 1200 bis zur Reformation," in *Handbuch der Mainzer Kirchengeschichte: Christliche Antike und Mittelalter*, ed. Friedhelm Jürgensmeier, vol. 2 (Würzburg: Echter Verlag, 2000), 685–688.

12 Hans Liermann, *Handbuch des Stiftungsrechts, vol. 1: Geschichte des Stiftungsrechts* (Tübingen: J. C. B. Mohr, 1963), 101–123; Andrea Sommerlechner, "Spitäler in Nord- und Mittelitalien vom 11. bis zum Beginn des 14. Jahrhunderts," in *Europäisches Spitalwesen. Institutionelle Fürsorge in Mittelalter und Früher Neuzeit*, eds. M. Scheutz, A. Sommerlechner, H. Weigl, and A. S. Weiß (Vienna: Oldenbourg, 2008), 116f. Sommerlechner, noting that such arrangements increased in frequency from the 1230s onwards, has interpreted them as a response to the *Liber Extra*'s sharpened emphasis on the criteria for religious identity, both for individuals and institutions.

13 The process of late medieval hospital secularization is treated as typical and sometimes as inevitable: Falck, *Mainz in seiner Blütezeit*, 54; idem, "Mainzer Hospitäler im Mittelalter," in *Moguntia Medica*, 410–411. Otto Winckelmann, *Das Fürsorgewesen der Stadt Strassburg vor und nach der Reformation bis zum Ausgang des sechzehnten Jahrhunderts: ein Beitrag zur deutschen Kultur- und Wirtschaftsgeschichte* (Leipzig: Heinsius, 1922), 1–26.

14 HStAD A2 115/1.

or at least in rigid identifications of the property divisions eventually made, but neither occurred.[15] The sharply drawn battle-lines of the charter's preamble are revealed as a rhetorical fiction distant from reality.[16] The council represents the brothers and the sick as on one side of an ostensibly ongoing dispute, the sisters—here described as the *magistra* and nuns (*monialium*) of the hospital—on the other. The categorization of the sick as a homogenous group echoes the language of early thirteenth-century councils that framed the legal status of hospitals in terms of their care for the sick.[17]

The opportunity afforded by hospitals for men and women to serve side by side was increasingly scarce in religious communities of the high Middle Ages.[18] When hospital rules limited interaction between men and women, it was almost always between the healthy and sick, limiting the intimacies of care to those of the same gender as their patients.[19] In the mid-thirteenth century, mandated limitations on the contact of male and female staff became increasingly common in episcopally-issued statutes.[20] Mixed-gender religious communities were obvious targets for ecclesiastical and municipal officials seeking to make complex realities align with the

15 HStAD A2 115/1: "We, by the will and with the consent of the above nuns and monks and poor persons elect for this purpose: Ulrich de Rosebaum [and] Arnold Eckenkeller, lawyers of Kostheim; and Beowulf of Eisenhof, our fellow citizens, that they might conclude a separation and division discreetly and faithfully. Of these, Arnold and Henry were brothers of the hospital, and thus all of the properties were known to them. They divided the goods that the convent possessed in two parts and by lots yielded to the aforesaid nuns the goods enumerated below."

16 HStAD A2 115/1.

17 HStAD A2 115/1. For the Councils of Paris and Rouen, which were held in 1212 and 1213, respectively, see Giovan Domenico Mansi, *Sacrorum conciliorum nova et amplissima collectio*, vol. 22 (Florence: Antonio Zatta, 1759), col. 827, 906.

18 For examples of hospitals with mixed-gender staff, see, inter alia, Gabriel Cros-Mayrevieille, *Les frères donnés à la léproserie du bourg de Narbonne* (Toulouse: Privat, 1930), 12–15; Jennifer Kolpacoff Deane, "Geistliche Schwestern: the pastoral care of lay religious women in medieval Würzburg," in: *Partners in Spirit: Women, Men, and Religious Life in Germany, 1100–1500*, eds. Fiona J. Griffiths and Julie Hotchin (Turnhout: Brepols, 2014), 248–250; Frank G. Hirschmann, "Frauenklöster und Beginenhöfe im Maas-Mosel-Raum des 12. und 13. Jh.," in *Landschaft(en): Begriffe, Formen, Implikationen*, eds. Franz Josef Felten, Harald Müller, and Heidrun Ochs (Stuttgart: Franz Steiner Verlag, 2012), 245, 251–260; De Keyser, "Le 'dépistage' de la lèpre," 100–101; Meinert, *Die Hospitäler Holsteins*, 59–67.

19 The hospital rule of Santo Spirito provides an example of this. Gisela Drossbach, *Christliche caritas als Rechtsinstitut: Hospital und Orden von Santo Spirito in Sassia 1198–1378* (Paderborn: Ferdinand Schöningh, 2005), 34–35 et passim. See also Angers, "La Bourgeoisie de Falaise," 228–231; Brodman, *Charity and Welfare*, 52–53.

20 Léon Le Grand, *Statuts d'hôtels-Dieu et de léproseries: recueil de textes du XIIe au XIVe siècle* (Paris: Alphonse Picard et Fils, 1901), 22, 36–38, 46, 55, 61.

categories of law.[21] Mainz's hospital had its privileges as a *locus religiosus* affirmed in the statutes of 1236. By the 1250s, however, the standards for such institutions had been further sharpened. Moreover, the hospital's transfer to civic administration had paved the way for a potential reopening of debate over its status as a religious institution. Despite the council's acquisition of administrative rights in 1244, the hospital continued to be administered by an ecclesiastical provisor, who appears to have been traditionally chosen from among the canons of St. Stephan. This complexity has been a source of scholarly puzzlement, and may have resulted in contemporary ambivalence as well.[22]

That civic and religious authorities in Mainz intended the hospital sisters to join the Cistercian Order provides further evidence that the statutes of 1236, discussed in the previous chapter, were still in force. In contrast to the legal separation of the hospital staff, their practical separation was neither immediate nor unambiguous. The sisters faced a transitional period of several decades. The location of their community remained uncertain, and sometimes beleaguered; the vocabulary used for the women was labile; and support from the laity of Mainz remained elusive. Such uncertainties might seem to support a view of hospitals' thirteenth-century legal development "as migratory, even rudderless."[23] The women's pursuit of support for their community, however, and their vision for its future, were both linked to their sense of religious identity as hospital sisters.

21 For the concerns of legislators, see Bodleian MS Laud Misc 307, f15v; Brigitte Flug, "Mainz, Dalen," in *Die Männer- und Frauenklöster der Benediktiner in Rheinland-Pfalz und Saarland,* ed. Friedhelm Jürgensmeier, *Germania Benedictina,* vol. 9 (St. Ottilien: EOS Verlag, 1999), 428–433; UCLA Digital Library Program. *Corpus Juris Canonici (1582)* <http://digital.library.ucla.edu/canonlaw> Last accessed April 14, 2020. As the thirteenth century drew on, commentaries on the decrees of the *Liber Extra* laid increased emphasis on the difference between *loca religiosa*, with all the privileges of religious identity, and *loca sacra*, dedicated to pious purposes, but not entitled to the exemptions conferred on regular institutions. Oliver Auge, "'Ne pauperes et debiles in…domo degentes divinis careant.' Sakral-religiöse Askpete der mittelalterlichen Hospitalgeschichte," in *Sozialgeschichte mittelalterlicher Hospitäler,* eds. Neithard Bulst and Karl-Heinz Spiess (Ostfildern: Jan Thorbecke Verlag, 2007), 77, 98–102.

22 Falck, *Die Geschichte der Stadt Mainz*, 52f.; Bodmann, *Rheingauische Altertümer*, vol. 1, 202.

23 Sethina Watson, *Fundatio, Ordinatio, and Statuta: The Statutes and Constitutional Documents of English Hospitals to 1300* (Oxford: D.Phil., 2003), 213, critiquing this common historiographical view. Cf. Christian-Frederik Felskau, "Von Brabant bis Böhmen und darüber hinaus. Zu Einheit und Vielfalt der 'religiösen Frauenbewegung' des 12. und des 13. Jahrhunderts," in *Fromme Frauen-unbequeme Frauen? Weibliches Religiosentum im Mittelalter*, ed. Edeltraud Klueting (Hildesheim: Georg Olms Verlag, 2006), 72–74.

The Sisters of St. Agnes: Building a New Religious Community

When Hildeborg and the other women issuing the charter of 1260 moved—away from the banks of the Rhine, into the center of town—they had to cope with financial difficulties, lay protests, and the problem of insufficient space. Still, they remained determined to pursue the formation of their own institutional identity, identifying themselves as "the nuns of St. Agnes at the hospital, in Mainz."[24] Either the women were still associating themselves with the hospital they had left, or associating themselves with service in a hospital that had not yet been built. Based on the charter of 1260, Bodmann has posited an intermediate step in the migrations of the sisters, suggesting that they stayed for some time in the house adjacent to the hospital.[25] The fact that the charter refers to the brothers and sisters of the hospital jointly has led some historians of Mainz to the hypothesis that it was but a few women, animated by desire for a more demanding form of the religious life, who left the hospital in 1259, and that their uncomfortable fervor caused the "long discord" to which the charter issued by the council refers.[26] A number of factors undermine this hypothesis. Firstly, charters issued by the civic hospital after the separation identify the hospital staff, collectively and individually, as male. There is one woman who is a named exception at the end of the fourteenth century, but it may be taken that she is a lay nurse; parallel instances are known.[27] A complete list of hospital residents from the end of the fifteenth century lists a married couple among its corrodians, but

24 Ludwig Baur, *Hessische Urkunden: Die Provinz Rheinhessen von 963–1325*, vol. 2 (Darmstadt: Der historische Verein für das Grossherzogthum Hessen, 1862), 204 (nr. 223.)

25 Bodmann, *Rheingauische Alterthümer*, vol 1, 298. and vol. 2, 900–902. Bodmann suggests that some of the sisters remained in the hospital, while some lived next to it "as nuns." The charter in question is HStAD 168/30, and is dated 14 August 1260. The house in question is described by the magistra and her sisters as "domum nostram sitam in foribus hospitali ad vicinam coquine fraternitatis."

26 Falck, *Mainz in seiner Blütezeit als freie Stadt*, 54; Bodmann, *Rheingauische Alterthümer* II, 900–902; Schaab, *Geschichte der Stadt Mainz*, vol. 2, 328–329, hypothesizes that some of the hospital sisters of St. Agnes, perhaps the older ones, stayed behind at the separation to continue work as nurses, and notes that the brothers and sisters must have still had some goods in common despite official separation by the council.

27 Sharon Strocchia, "Caring for the 'Incurable' in Renaissance Pox Hospitals," in *Hospital Life: Theory and Practice from the Medieval to the Modern*, eds. Laurinda Abreu and Sally Sheard (Oxford: Peter Lang, 2013), 82–91; Siegfried Reicke, *Das deutsche Spital und sein Recht im Mittelalter*, vol. 2 (Stuttgart: Enke, 1932), 95–116. Reicke, somewhat problematically, goes from the evidence for the presence of laywomen as nursing staff to interpreting all female hospital staff as nurses or assistants.

women appear only as lay staff.[28] The sisters referred to in the charter of 1260 might have been either lay staff housed elsewhere, or sick persons acknowledged as members of the community. It is difficult to see what purpose the division would have served, and why Mainz's civic leadership and religious elites would have been involved in it, had it left the civic hospital as a mixed-gender community.[29]

The next local record concerning St. Agnes is a letter of 1275, issued by Archbishop Wernher von Eppstein in response to the sisters' request to move to a new location in response to lay protests.[30] The choice of the new location, the curia "ad testam," on the bustling Dietmarkt, appears to have been the women's own.[31] Notable for its inclusion in the efficient letter is the archiepiscopal permission granted to the women of St. Agnes to exhume and relocate the bodies of their dead.[32] In 1279, the Cistercian convent of Altmünster gave the women of St. Agnes the use of a house adjoining their new buildings, which had been previously occupied by a community of quasi-religious women. The numbers of the *inclusae* of St. Walpurgis were probably small, but it is worth noting that the combination of their community with that of St. Agnes seemed reasonable to all parties involved.[33] Ambiguous though it may be on some points, the charter is scrupulously detailed regarding the legal privileges and obligations of all parties involved.

The house of Altmünster is obliged to provide the *inclusae* with priests, and to provide them with legitimacy as a religious community: clad in the gray habit of the Cistercians, supplied with the sacraments, and permanently

28 StAM 33/9: Fragmentary account book of 1487–1488, written by Heinrich Schopp in Latin and German. On an inserted sheet of paper (78a) is a list of hospital community members, 23 in all. There are only three women: one chief maid and two nurses: "Item dye hochmaget Lise / Item Anne die siechen maget / Item Else auch eyn siechen maget."

29 Maria Pia Alberzoni, "Norditalienische Pilgerhospize im 12. und 13. Jahrhundert," in *Wege zum Heil: Pilger und Heilige Orte an Mosel und Rhein*, eds. Thomas Frank, Michael Matheus, and Sabine Reichert (Stuttgart: Franz Steiner Verlag, 2009), 280–281, has called attention to the problem that the cooperation of men and women has often been ignored because it had been phased out of existence by the time a hospital came to be more thoroughly documented or to its "final" institutional form.

30 HStAD A2 115/5. For more detail on this charter, see Barnhouse, "Disordered Women," 69–70. Cf. Katherine Gill, "Scandala: Controversies Concerning Clausura and Women's Religious Communities in Late Medieval Italy," in *Christendom and its Discontents: Exclusion, Persecution, and Rebellion, 1000–1500*, eds. Peter D. Diehl and Scott L. Waugh (Cambridge: Cambridge University Press, 1996), 192.

31 HStAD A2 168/30.

32 HStAD A2 115/5.

33 HStAD A2 118/4. For the chronology given by Bodmann, *Rheingauische Alterthümer* II, 902–903, there is no solid basis in the surviving evidence.

enclosed, subject to the abbess of Altmünster. Any rebellion against these terms is to be punished by the abbot of Eberbach, referred to reverently by the abbess and nuns of Altmünster as *visitator noster*.[34] Given the emphasis on the supposed eagerness of the *inclusae* to enter a new community on these terms, the detailed descriptions of the methods to ensure obedience and punish rebellion are surprising.[35] Whose initiative is seen here, and whose concern? The subsequent history of the community of St. Agnes makes clear that the sisters were not strictly enclosed. They continued to interact with laypersons through liturgy and alms, as well as caring for the sick; nor are the women ever referred to as *inclusae* again.[36] Furthermore, there is no evidence that they were submitted to the supervision of Altmünster.[37] One possibility is that a subset of the women who left the hospital splintered off in order to follow a different form of the religious life. Another is that this charter represents a failed attempt by external authorities—perhaps the influential abbot of Eberbach—to bring the hospital sisters under the governance of an established rule, and an established order. Charters issued by the women of St. Agnes attest their continued independence. In the latter decades of the thirteenth century, they engaged in ambitious endeavors to ensure the viability of their existence as a self-supporting community.

Once installed on the Dietmarkt, the women of St. Agnes sought out support in the form of episcopal indulgences. They did not seek such support from Archbishop Wernher. Although surviving charters suggest that Wernher may have wished to support—as well as regulate—the community, he was in no position to do so without alienating municipal elites. In the rapidly transforming cities of late medieval Europe, open conflict could be provoked if one group sought power outside a customary sphere, either of authority or of geography.[38] Wernher's archiepiscopate was characterized by tensions with the civic leaders of Mainz; the struggle of St. Agnes to

34 HStAD A2 118/4. It is specified that the abbess of Altmünster will have one of two keys to the dwelling of the *inclusae*, and the senior among these women will keep the second.

35 HStAD A2 118/4.

36 For more on *inclusae* as a designation, and its ambiguity, see Jennifer Kolpacoff Deane, "From Case Studies to Comparative Models: Würzburg Beguines and the Vienne Decrees," in *Labels and Libels: Naming Beguines in Northern Medieval Europe*, ed. Letha Böhringer (Turnhout: Brepols, 2014), 56–61.

37 For more on St. Agnes' ambivalent relationship with the Cistercian Order, see Barnhouse, "Disordered Women," 60–74.

38 Franz-Josef Arlinghaus, "The Myth of Urban Unity: Religion and Social Performance in Late Medieval Braunschweig," in *Cities, Texts, and Social Networks, 400–1500: Experiences and Perceptions of Medieval Urban Space*, eds. Caroline Goodson, Anne E. Lester, and Carol Symes (Farnham: Ashgate, 2010), 215–224.

establish itself in a new location became a focal point of such tension. The fact that Wernher belonged to the Von Eppstein dynasty was not immaterial. Wernher was the third of that line to hold the archiepiscopate, and he exercised his considerable power autocratically in the face of the rising political self-assertion of the burghers of Mainz.[39] Lay resentment of the hospital sisters' move may have been provoked either by the creation of a new ecclesiastical space, or by the loss of staff from the old hospital, the one religious institution in Mainz that was also under the administration of civic authorities.[40] In Bologna, Sherri Franks Johnson has also found that the location of religious houses could reflect changes in the social relationships of these communities. The women of St. Agnes, once established on the market, seemed determined to stay, and to make themselves useful to the laity through the provision of liturgical and sacramental services. In order to strengthen their position within the city, they appealed far beyond its borders, obtaining numerous episcopal indulgence letters from the 1270s to the 1290s.[41]

The fact that the women of St. Agnes had their letters of privilege, once issued by obliging prelates, confirmed by the judges of Mainz, suggests that they felt the need of asserting their position of privilege as a religious institution relative to municipal as well as ecclesiastical authorities. In 1304, the women sought confirmation of episcopal privileges multiple times. In January, they received from the court confirmation of a letter apparently jointly issued by prelates across Europe and beyond.[42] Amid so much effort at establishing a secure legal identity, the women of St. Agnes never appealed or referred to Eberbach, the great monastery that was responsible for the supervision of all the Cistercian houses of Mainz. Despite the uncertainties

39 For Wernher's relationship with the council and the laity, see Paul-Joachim Heinig, "Die Mainzer Kirche am Ende des Hochmittelalters (1249–1305)," in *Handbuch der Mainzer Kirchengeschichte: Christliche Antike und Mittelalter*, ed. Friedhelm Jürgensmeier, vol. 1 (Würzburg: Echter Verlag, 2000), 351–356. In the time of Peter von Aspelt, Wernher was referred to as having admirably respected the privileges of the laity: StAWü MBVI 75, f1r.

40 On the concentration of religious houses in certain urban and periurban districts, see Lester, "Crafting a Charitable Landscape," passim, and Sherri Franks Johnson, *Monastic Women and Religious Orders in Late Medieval Bologna* (Cambridge: Cambridge University Press, 2014), 24–26. On the significance of religious houses in the topography—literal and symbolic—of cities and regions, see Felten, "Klosterlandschaften," in *Landschaft(en): Begriffe, Formen, Implikationen*, 157–176, and Gert Melville, "'Klosterlandschaft': Kritische Bemerkungen zum wissenschaftlichen Wert einer Wortschöpfung," ibid, 195–196.

41 For more detail, see Barnhouse, "Disordered Women," 74–77.

42 HStAD A2 115/29 is unusually elaborate, and specifies that the judges have added the letters to a register.

surrounding their communal future, they deliberately maintained distance from the Cistercian Order which civic and religious authorities in Mainz had intended them to join in the 1250s.

Women, Sisters…Nuns? The Legal Status of St. Agnes

For those pursuing the religious life in the thirteenth century, and for those who sought their prayers, the perception of religious status appears to have been determined by social as well as legal realities.[43] Such lability was not viewed with equanimity by Mainz's thirteenth-century archbishops. Siegfried III, especially, worked closely with Pope Gregory IX to bring religious houses to stricter forms of obedience.[44] A 1241 papal letter on women illicitly claiming religious status was deemed important enough by the ecclesiastical authorities of Mainz that the copy sent to Siegfried III was preserved. The pope claims to have received word of numerous women (*non nulle mulieres*) wandering through cities and dioceses, falsely claiming religious status, and wearing habits to which they have no right. Their presence, according to Gregory, is the cause of "confusion, discredit and… scandal" to religious orders.[45] Bishops and archbishops are commanded to make clear that such women are the targets of apostolic and ecclesiastical censure. The letter makes clear both the variety of ways in which the religious life could be pursued, and the desire to more clearly delimit and define them. This copy of the papal letter, less elaborate than the charter issued to Altmünster, would almost certainly have

43 On women's religious identity and the difficulty of imposing firm categories upon it, at least for the twelfth and thirteenth centuries, see Felskau, "Von Brabant bis Böhmen und darüber hinaus," 90–92; Heidi Febert, *Between the Law and the World: Defining Women's Religious Identity in the Later Middle Ages*, (Ph.D. Diss., Fordham University, 2012), 10–27.

44 Werner Maleczek, "Der Mittelpunkt Europas im frühen 13. Jahrhundert: Chronisten, Fürsten, und Bischöfe an der Kurie our Zeit Papst Innocenz' III," *Römische Historische Mitteilungen* 49 (2007), 89–97; Winfried Wilhelmy, "Ein unbekanntes Krönungsrelief der Mainzer Erzbischöfe: Bonifatius und die Bildpropaganda der sedes Moguntiae im Zeitalter der Goldenen Bulle," *Mainzer Zeitschrift* 99 (2004), 28–29; Karl von Hegel, *Die Chroniken der mittelrheinischen Städte: Mainz* (Leipzig: Hirzel, 1881), 3–17; Friedhelm Jürgensmeier, "Das Erzbistum Mainz," in *Die Bistümer des Heiligen Römischen Reiches von ihren Anfängen bis zur Säkularisation*, hrsg. Erwin Gatz (Freiburg im Breisgau: Herder, 2003), 413; Karl W. Heyden, "Die Hospitäler in Oppenheim," *Oppenheimer Hefte* 1 (1990), 16; Paul B. Pixton, *The German Episcopacy and the Implementation of the Decrees of the Fourth Lateran Council 1216–1245: Watchmen on the Tower* (Leiden: Brill, 1995), 279–280; Mathias Kälble, "Sozialfürsorge und kommunale Bewegung. Zur Bedeutung von Hospitälern fur die politische Gruppenbildung in der Stadt," in *Sozialgeschichte Mittelalterlicher Hospitäler*, 251.

45 StAM U / 21 February 1241.

been displayed and read aloud in Mainz. The groups named in the charter as discredited by imposture were not prominent in the archdiocese of Mainz. That the papal letter was nonetheless preserved and referenced in synodal legislation indicates that concerns about religious identity were pervasive, though what regional emphasis they took is incompletely known.[46] Further regulation was not imposed on St. Agnes itself before the end of the fifteenth century, when visitation by Eberbach is recorded for the first time.[47]

Apart from the letter of Altmünster referring to the women as *inclusae*, there is no evidence suggesting that the community became more strictly cloistered after the letter of 1275. When limiting the number of the community to thirty, in 1290, Archbishop Gerhard uses the term *sanctimoniales,* but makes no mention of a cloister or claustration. No one is forced to leave, he specifies, but no new postulants are to be admitted until the number of nuns is decreased by death. Unusually, the archbishop adds a proviso: "We wish," he writes, "to see these terms observed in your monastery in perpetuity unless, by the Lord's favor, your resources grow in such measure that superior authority may allow your numbers to be increased."[48] Neither the Pope nor the abbot of Eberbach is on record as raising the quota; this double silence is further suggestive of the continuation of St. Agnes' communal life without reliance on formal affiliation to an order.

In Mainz, quasi-religious women cultivated relationships with more strictly regulated communities to an unusual degree, a practice that appears to have influenced lay perceptions; late medieval testaments list beguines, unaffiliated houses, and hospitals alongside houses belonging to established orders.[49] These diverse and complex relationships have contributed to the historiographical confusion surrounding the status of St. Agnes. Eva Gertrud Neumann, in her study of beguines and beghards in the Rhineland, referred to the sisters of St. Agnes as a "beguine-like group."[50] Although charters spanning the fourteenth century attest to ties between St. Agnes and individual beguines, there is nothing to suggest that the women of St. Agnes regarded themselves as "beguine-like," or were regarded so by others.[51]

46 StAM 013/001, f14, for reference to the charter.

47 HHStAW Abt. 22 Nr. 550.

48 HStAD A2 115/24.

49 StAM 13/370, 3, 21; StAM 13/330, 8–9; HStAD A2 168/273 ; HStAD C1 A Nr. 89 22r–22v; HStAD A2 168/474 (19 January 1373); HStAD A2 168/83.

50 Neumann, *Rheinisches Beginen- und Begardenwesen*, 23–24. On the variable status of beguines in canonical legislation, see Makowski, *A Pernicious Sort of Woman*, 23–50.

51 StAM U 1302 März; HStAD A2 168/83 (23 September 1293); HStAD A2 168/133 (1306); HStAD A2 168/350 (1345); HStAD C1 A Nr. 89, f. 22r–22v.

The women of St. Agnes, although not hierarchically tied to the Cistercian Order, did enter into a confraternity with Cistercian convents in and near Mainz (Altmünster, Weißfrauen, and Dalen) and shared staff with them, at least from the second half of the 1300s.[52] Although evidence for Eberbach's exercise of rights of visitation, hearing confessions, and confirming abbesses exists for these other houses, no such evidence survives for St. Agnes. In the case of St. Agnes, the earliest record of such privileges in Eberbach's possession is an eighteenth-century copy of a 1509 confirmation of them.[53] In 1310, Eberbach paid a debt of twenty marks owed to the archbishop of Mainz to St. Agnes instead. The initiative in the arrangement appears to have lain with Archbishop Peter von Aspelt; no mention is made of any obligations connecting the two religious communities. The archbishop, who took a particular interest in medical care, may have sought this method of shoring up the beleaguered women's finances.[54] Under a multitude of names, the women of St. Agnes appear to have evaded direct control by either prelates or Order. Assiduous in defending their religious status, the women remained primarily dedicated to their identity as hospital sisters. It is to the evidence for St. Agnes' continued provision of care for the sick, and connections to Mainz's "new hospital," that I now turn.

Sisters of the Hospital: St. Agnes and the "neues Spital"

In the case of the "new hospital" of Mainz, as so often in medieval hospital history, the community's self-sufficiency works against the creation of an ample documentary record.[55] When the hospital has been discussed, it has been identified as belonging to the cathedral chapter, despite a lack of

52 HStAD 115/36 (1329); HStAD C1 Nr. 89 f88r–89r, 99v–100r.

53 Willi Wagner, "Das Aufsichtsrecht Eberbachs über die ihm unterstellten Zisterzienserinnenklöster mit besonderen Berücksichtigung von Kumbd," *Landeskundliche Vierteljahrsblätter* 10 (1964), 160–172. HHStAW Abt. 22 Nr. 550.

54 HHStAW Abt. 22 Nr. 550, f. 4. A sixteenth-century account book holds abstracts of all transactions with St. Agnes judged to be significant, headed "Agnesen Kloster Scripta et Acta." The entry for 1310 simply reads: "Solvito debitum: 1310: Monasterio Eberbach debebat Archiepiscopo Moguntia 20 marcas quas Monasterio ad St. Agnes solvit."

55 See Weigl, *Städte und Spital*, 412–420; Bettina Toson, *Mittelalterliche Hospitäler in Hessen zwischen Schwalm, Eder, und Fulda* (Darmstadt: Hessiche Historische Kommission, 2012), 168; Dross, "Their Daily Bread," 65–67, as examples of works discussing hospitals as self-sustaining communities.

references to it in the chapter's surviving records.[56] Hitherto unexamined records of St. Agnes reveal that the women of this community were, in fact, responsible for managing Mainz's "new hospital." This has not previously been acknowledged although, in the eighteenth century, Georg Joannis claimed that, according to "a constant tradition," the central purpose of St. Agnes was that its sisters should care for the sick. He quotes the charter beginning "Nos Agnes abbatissa…" as "quite sufficient confirmation for this," although he dates it to 1367, rather than 1267.[57] The misdating could indicate that the charter to which Joannis refers was copied out and embedded in later, no longer extant documents produced by the sisters of St. Agnes, reaffirming their connection to hospital service. The chartulary of St. Agnes bears witness to the fact that they ensured their hospital had access to gardens and orchards, as well as rents from which the needs of the sick could be supplied. Largely, however, the sisters appear to have handled the hospital's administration internally.

The women of St. Agnes kept no (surviving) separate account books for the hospital; nor were external officials appointed for its quotidian management. This suggests that the "new hospital," located five minutes' walk from the cloister complex on the Dietmarkt, was viewed as an integral part of the community of St. Agnes. Ironically, this method of record-keeping obscures the role of St. Agnes in hospital administration. As the sisters' hospital and their administration of it developed from the late thirteenth century to the late fourteenth, the women of St. Agnes were active in managing the hospital and its surrounding properties, and in safeguarding its legal rights. The ways in which they did so demonstrate that they desired their hospital to thrive both as a space providing care, and as a community with the privileges of religious status.

There is evidence suggesting that the sisters administered an independent hospital complex from at least the 1270s onwards. A letter of 1290, issued by Archbishop Gerhard, uses vocabulary suggestive of the diversification, as well as the expansion of St. Agnes. In limiting new entries into the community, the archbishop uses interestingly flexible vocabulary for its members:

> [A]s it has come to our notice that the resources of your monastery are indeed tenuous and fragile (*tenues et exiles*,) insufficient for the comfortable sustenance of the many persons who serve God there. Having

56 Falck, *Mainz in seiner Blütezeit*, 52–54; Schaab, *Geschichte der Stadt Mainz*, 230–232; Falck, "Mainzer Hospitäler im Mittelalter," 414–415; StAWü MBVI 18, 19; Martinus-Bibliothek HS 3.

57 Georg Christian Joannis, *Rerum Moguntiacarum*, vol. 2, (Frankfurt am Main: J.M. Sande, 1722), 876–877. The misdating would be explained by Joannis' conviction that the monastery was not founded until 1290.

> deliberated over this, we wish to provide an opportune remedy for this, guaranteeing the tranquility of your monastery.[58]

Several particularities of this letter's phrasing merit closer examination. Firstly, there is the indication that, despite St. Agnes' ongoing financial difficulties, the community attracted many new members. Furthermore, the archbishop's language in describing these persons is notable for its flexibility. With no shortage of descriptive formulae for religious women at his disposal, Archbishop Gerhard chose instead to refer to "a multitude of persons seeking to become the servants of the Lord" in the community.[59] No mention is made of taking the habit, or becoming the handmaidens of God; not even the gender of the multitude of persons is specified. The language is characteristic of *donati*, which leads to the question of why those wishing to become "servants of the Lord" would have been drawn to the economically precarious community of St. Agnes.[60] Hospital service provides a plausible answer.

Despite the possessions with which the sisters of St. Agnes left the hospital on the Rhine, their early years were marked by financial difficulties. Their struggle to find a location for their community, and to accommodate a large number of persons, exacerbated these difficulties.[61] It is unlikely that the women would have had the resources to construct hospital buildings in their first years as an independent community; the desire to do so may be reflected in the frequent mentions of building projects in the episcopal indulgences which they obtained in the latter decades of the thirteenth century. These building projects, somewhat unusually, are not specified as limited to monastery or church.[62] The earliest record associating the women of St. Agnes with a hospital after their departure from the hospital on the Rhine is a rent agreement of 1267, preserved in the chartulary of Mainz's Augustinian house.[63] In this contract, the women identify themselves as "the nuns of St. Agnes at the hospital," suggesting that their new complex incorporated a space dedicated to the care of the sick-poor.[64] The "new hospital" of Mainz,

58 HStAD A2 115/24. "Tenues et exiles" was a standard legal formula, indicating the house's inability to adequately support itself from its revenues.

59 HStAD A2 115/24.

60 See Charles de Miramon, *Les "donnés" au Moyen Âge: une forme de vie religieuse laïque, v. 1180–v. 1500* (Paris: Cerf, 1999), 337–386, on *donati* in hospitals.

61 HStAD A2 115/24.

62 HStAD A2 115/14, HStAD A2 115/4, HStAD A2 115/13 (1285), HStAD A2 115/17 (1288).

63 No longer extant; transcribed in full in Baur, *Hessische Urkunden*, vol. 2, 204, Nr. 223.

64 Baur, *Hessische Urkunden*, 204. 18 May 1267.

though managed by the women of St. Agnes, was perceived by external authorities as in need of regulation as an independent religious house. The hospital's dedication to St. Alexius is a rare one, shared by several leper hospitals; Middle High German versions of the life of the saint confirm that his reputation in the region was as one dedicated to all the sick-poor among lepers and the blind, groups sometimes excluded from hospital statutes because of the intensive medical care they required.[65]

Several of Mainz's nineteenth-century historians testify to the existence of an archiepiscopal letter enjoining the sisters to manage their hospital according to the papally-devised rule of Santo Spirito. The letter appears to have been undated. Böhmer suggests that it may have dated to the archiepiscopate of Siegfried II, or corresponded with an unedited charter of 1254; Bodmann's confusion is even greater.[66] If we accept Böhmer's summary of the contents of the charter itself, we are given a *terminus post quem* for its dating. If the sisters were already located on the Dietmarkt, the charter must have been issued after 1279. The subsequent decade, which saw Archbishop Wernher von Eppstein busily engaged in the reform of religious houses, and the sisters of St. Agnes busily engaged with the building projects for which they canvassed support from prelates, seems the most likely period for the regulation of the hospital. The letter was probably issued as part of a wave of archiepiscopal reforms implemented in the 1270s–1280s.[67] The first mention of the rule in a surviving document comes in 1290, when Archbishop Gerhard alludes to the rule as being established, if only shakily, in the women's hospital. A letter from Archbishop Mathias, in 1326, suggests similar concerns.[68]

The rule of Santo Spirito was devised for a mixed religious community in a hospital serving diverse needs. Crucially, it had the stamp of papal

65 Maurizio Perugi, Saint Alexis: Genèse de sa légende et de la Vie française (Paris: Droz, 2014), 536–537

66 J.F. Böhmer and Cornelius Will, eds., *Regesta archiepiscoporum Maguntinensium. Register zur Geschichte der Mainzer Erzbischöfe von Bonifatius bis Heinrich II.*, vol. 2 (Innsbruck: Wagner, 1886), 203. Nr. 597. Böhmer summarizes the charter: "Siegfried II founds the cloister of St. Agnes on the Dietmarkt, in order to administer the hospital according to the model of the *hospitale de saxis* constructed by Pope Innocent [III] in Rome for brothers and sisters." Böhmer's use of the Latin suggests that he had the charter in front of him at some point; the fate of the document is unknown. Bodmann, *Rheingauische Alterthümer* I, 242, conflates the hospital with the hospital on the Rhine, and says that Siegfried II ordered the sisters to follow the rule of Santo Spirito, and equipped the hospital with various privileges.

67 Stephan Alexander Würdtwein, *Dioecesis Moguntina*, vol. I (Mannheim: Typis Academicis, 1768), 375–379.

68 HStAD A2 115/24; HStAD A2 115/35

approval, granting unambiguous religious status, and its attendant legal privileges.[69] The rule is unusually, explicitly inclusive in its provisions for daily life, and in specifying whom the house is to care for. All the poor who ask for admittance should be welcomed according to the ability of the house; orphans and pregnant women, both groups sometimes excluded from hospital statutes because of their special medical needs, are included, as are lepers.[70] The hospital managed by the sisters of St. Agnes may have been first located inside the cloister complex on the Dietmarkt; by the early fourteenth century, the women were connected to a "hospitale" on the Umbach.[71] The fact that a 1305 agreement over income from urban properties identifies two hospital buildings has hitherto been overlooked. Neither of the hospitals is identified by name, but their locations are demonstrably different.[72] Scholarship on similar charters and property descriptions in account books has convincingly shown that lists of possessions were made in the order in which they would be visited by those inspecting them or collecting rents.[73] The hospital which appears among private houses and fields in the semi-urban territory along the Umbach is not identical with

69 Drossbach, *Christliche caritas als Rechtsinstitut*, 34–35 et passim.

70 Drossbach, *Christliche caritas als Rechtsinstitut*, 122–125; Le Grand, *Statuts d'hôtels-dieu*, 25–26, Édouard Jeanselme, "Comment l'Europe, au Moyen Âge, se protégea contre la Lèpre," *Bulletin de la Société Française d'Histoire de la Médecine* 25 (1931), 106–107.

71 Several instances from the same period are known of the growth of hospitals out of spaces within monastery complexes; see Philippe Racinet, "Les infirmeries monastiques: perspectives de recherche," in *Hôpitaux et maladreries au moyen âge: espace et environnement: actes du colloque international d'Amiens-Beauvais, 22, 23 et 24 novembre 2002*, ed. Pascal Montaubin (Rouen: CAHMER, 2004), 21–34. On the location next to a source of running water as typical for hospitals of the region and period, see Andreas Saalwächter, "Ingelheimer Armen- und Krankenfürsorge im Mittelalter," in *Alt-Ingelheim: Kulturgeschichtliche Bilder aus der Vergangenheit Ingelheims und des Ingelheimer Grundes in gesammelten Schriften* (Ingelheim: Historischer Verein, 1958), 93–94; Wilhelm Frohn, *Der Aussatz im Rheinland: sein Vorkommen und seine Bekämpfung* (Jena: G. Fischer, 1933), 71–72, 151–152; Uhrmacher, *Lepra und Leprosorien*, 105––12.

72 HStAD 168/131. For the location of St. Alexius, see Heuser, *Namen der Mainzer Strassen*, 102. On hospitals dedicated to St. Alexius, see Otto Wimmer and Hartmann Melzer, *Lexikon der Namen und Heiligen*, 6th ed. (Innsbruck: Tyrolia-Verlag, 2002), TK; Nicholas Orme and Margaret Webster, *The English Hospital, 1070–1570* (New Haven: Yale University Press, 1995), 42, find a hospital dedicated to St. Alexius in Exeter; *Die Klapper* (1995), 2, discovers a St. Alexius leprosarium. Rotha Mary Clay, *The Medieval Hospitals of England* (London: Methuen, 1909), 245–246, observes that a dedication to the Holy Spirit, which might seem to be implied by the injunction of Archbishop Wernher in 1275, was often a secondary or joint dedication. Michel Pauly, "Für eine raumbezogene Hospitalgeschichte: Einführende Bemerkungen," in *Einrichtungen der sozialen Sicherung im mittelalterlichen Lotharingien*, Actes des 13es Journées Lotharingeinnes, 12–15 October 2004, ed. Michel Pauly (Linden: Section Historie de l'Institut Grand-Ducal, 2008), 12–13, identifies the question of hospital dedications as an issue calling for further study.

73 Lester, "Crafting a Charitable Landscape," 125–129.

Mainz's oldest hospital, which is reached by a narrow lane leading from the house Zum Spiegel, an identified burghers' residence near the cathedral.[74] The document recording the women's possession of property and rents surrounding—and potentially supporting—the site of the new hospital has been hitherto overlooked.

St. Agnes is on record as owning several houses in the district of the Umbach that could have been used as accommodation for the sick-poor. Two letters issued by Archbishop Mathias in 1326 suggest that year may have seen intensified efforts by the women of St. Agnes to expand the hospital community. First, on 23 March, the archbishop confirmed his purchase of multiple properties and revenues from the women of St. Agnes in a sealed charter. This was an atypical act of archiepiscopal support, undertaken "because of special favor" towards the chamberlain of Mainz, Rudolf zum Silberberg, possibly a patron of the community.[75] A letter of 24 May suggests that the need of the convent was specific, rather than ongoing. This charter, in a heavily abbreviated hand, asserts that Archbishop Mathias writes motivated by paternal affection. The archbishop has seen the "useful and comfortable works" of St. Agnes, but is concerned for the prosperity of the house. He forbids the women to add more persons to their community until their building projects—and the payment for those projects—have been completed.[76]

Mathias' language of "useful and comfortable works" resembles formulae concerning the works of mercy to which hospitals were obliged in both legal and theological thought.[77] The phrase is suggestive of the possibility that the building projects being undertaken—and possibly inspiring a new influx of sisters—were connected to the expansion of the hospital facilities of St. Agnes. Other documents from the 1320s and 1330s bear out this theory. A charter created in January of 1329 mentions the new hospital and St. Agnes getting rents in it, suggesting that it may have been constructed with their

74 HStAD 168/131. For a depiction of the relevant properties, see the Digitales Häuserbuch Mainz: http://www.mainz.de/WGAPublisher/online/html/default/hthn-8ubds9.de.o.

75 StAM U 1326 / 23 March.

76 HStAD A2 115/35.

77 On hospitals and works of mercy, see, for example, Adam J. Davis, "Hospitals, Charity, and the Culture of Compassion in the Twelfth and Thirteenth Centuries," in *Approaches to Poverty in Medieval Europe: Complexities, Contradictions, Transformations, c. 1100–1500*, ed. Sharon Farmer (Turnhout: Brepols, 2016), 35–37, 41; Carole Rawcliffe, *The Hospitals of Medieval Norwich* (Woodbridge: Boydell, 1995), 16–17; Joel Agrimi and Chiara Crisciani, "Charity and Aid in Medieval Christian Civilization," in *Western Medical Thought from Antiquity to the Middle Ages*, ed. Mirko D. Grmek (Cambridge, MA: Harvard University Press, 1998), 170–176.

involvement in mind from the outset.[78] A similar rent agreement, dated a year later, confirms that St. Agnes was entitled to draw the additional revenue of three marks "from the new hospital situated on the Umbach." The agreement covers multiple properties, including more houses near St. Agnes, a butcher's shop, and a fishpond, suggesting that the sisters' acquisition of property and income was anything but haphazard.[79] More telling even than this evidence of progressively growing rights in the hospital buildings is that the relevant entry in St. Agnes' chartulary is accompanied by a marginal note in a fifteenth-century hand, identifying the record as primarily relevant to "Sanct Allexien," the name by which the hospital became known.

Not until 1341 is there an unequivocal record of the convent's possession of buildings designed for use as a hospital. These new hospital buildings were located in the semi-rural belt of territory along the Umbach, only five minutes' walk from the cloister's location on the Dietmarkt.[80] The only copy of the relevant charter, dated 14 March, survives in a codex kept by St. Agnes as a chartulary-cum-account-book, compiled by multiple writers over the course of the fourteenth and fifteenth centuries. The hospital is described in the text as the "new hospital or hospice for strangers and pilgrims," suggesting that civic administration of the older hospital may have resulted in a privileging of the local sick-poor by that institution.[81] The women of St. Agnes appear anxious to affirm comprehensive rights in the hospital, including its possessions and the land on which it was built. In doing so, they reiterate their own claim to communal legitimacy, describing themselves as "the religious women, the abbess and community of the monastery of St. Agnes, known to belong to the Cistercian Order."[82]

The fact that the buildings were constructed under the auspices of a cathedral canon has led other historians of Mainz to identify this new hospital as belonging to the cathedral chapter.[83] None of the surviving records of the chapter mention the hospital except in property descriptions, nor incomes from it; they do not even record the possession of properties concentrated

78 StAM U / 18 January 1329/ I.

79 HStAD C1 A Nr. 89 20r–20v.

80 Heuser, *Namen der Mainzer Strassen*, 102.

81 HStAD C1 A Nr. 89 129v. Cf. Johnson, *Monastic Women*, 126–168, on patterns of patronage of religious houses by municipal elites.

82 HStAD C1 A Nr. 89 129v–130r.

83 Reinhold Rörig, *Die Mainzer Spitäler und Krankenhäuser: Ein Rückblick auf 2000 Jahre Krankenhausgeschichte* (Mainz: Schmidt, 1989), 36, claims without attribution that the hospital was founded by the chapter, and that it was a pilgrim hostel rather than a hospital for the sick-poor; Falck, "Mainzer Hospitäler im Mittelalter," in *Moguntia Medica*, 414–415, likewise claims that St. Alexius was founded by the cathedral chapter.

near the hospital.[84] By the time the women of St. Agnes purchased new buildings for the hospital in 1341, they had hired a provisor charged with its full-time supervision.[85] The presence of such an official is not an automatic indication that the women were not themselves engaged in hospital care. Their religious status need not have precluded their activities outside the cloister walls; indeed, porous claustration may have been the unspoken norm for many communities similar to St. Agnes. As Katherine Gill and Penelope Johnson have noted, the relative poverty of many houses made claustration an unattainable luxury.[86]

Following the acquisition of the hospital buildings in 1341, the women of St. Agnes appear to have undertaken further strategic acquisitions of property around both their monastery complex and the new hospital buildings. In 1348, in claiming the convent's rights on a house given to them by a married couple, Jakob von Rodenberg, who served the community as chaplain and legal representative, declared before the judges of Mainz that the gift had been designated for the public kitchen ("gemein kuchen") of St. Agnes.[87] Two things support the interpretation of this kitchen as a facility for the sick-poor, not merely for the convent and hospital staff. Firstly, gifts designated for the vowed members of St. Agnes—not uncommon in themselves—used the technical term "pitancie" to establish that the gift was a permissible supplement to the limited monastic diet.[88] Moreover, the husband and wife transferring the rents specified that the money was to be distributed by the portress of the community, and that if she did not do so, the responsibility was to pass to the priests of St. Agnes.[89] This dictation of terms to religious communities charged with providing for the sick-poor was far from uncommon in donations to hospitals.[90]

84 StAWü MBVI 18, 19, MRA Spitäler K 755/14; Martinus-Bibliothek HS 3.

85 HStAD C1 A Nr. 89 129v.

86 Penelope D. Johnson, *Equal in Monastic Profession: Religious Women in Medieval France* (Chicago: University of Chicago Press, 2009), 5–7, 106–111. Gill, "Scandala," 178. As Gill observes, "The fact that practice did not conform to precept is neither surprising nor, in itself, especially interesting. Why and how individual communities transgressed can be both."

87 HStAD C1 A Nr. 89, f. 41r–41v.

88 Baur, *Hessische Urkunden*, 748–750; StAM 13/310; cf. Paul Meyvaert, "The Medieval Monastic Garden," in *Medieval Gardens*, ed. Elisabeth Blair Macdougall (Cambridge, MA: Harvard University Press, 1986), 23–31.

89 HStAD C1 A Nr. 89, f. 41v.

90 For examples of conditional donations see StAM U / 18 September 1421; Alfred Hilgard, ed., *Urkunden zur Geschichte der Stadt Speyer* (Strassburg: Trübner, 1885), 216; HStAD C1 A Nr. 89, 50v–51r; Richard Dertsch, ed. *Die Urkunden des Stadtarchivs Mainz: Regesten*, Beiträge zur

Another mid-century transaction, initiated by St. Agnes, was the purchase of rights in a bakehouse located near the new hospital. Unusually, they acquired these rights despite the fact that another party made a claim to the same property, suggesting that St. Agnes set special value on the property, and on the opportunity to bake bread in large quantities for a growing community.[91] A charter written in June of 1345 identified its members as "the holy persons and women, the abbess and convent of the cloister of St. Agnes."[92] This is suggestive of the existence of a mixed community, since priests alone were habitually identified by their office. Records of new rights and possessions in 1352 and 1353 support the view of the mid-fourteenth century as a period of development.[93] A gift from a laywoman to the abbess and convent of Dalen, in 1356, contains further confirmation that the territory surrounding the hospital was still largely agricultural, and that its property was associated with St. Agnes.[94]

Even as the evidence for additional staff multiplies in the late fourteenth century, the women of St. Agnes still were active in managing the hospital, and defending its rights. A charter of 1385, confirming rents owed to the hospital of St. Alexius, and its rights in property by the Umbach, survives in the possession of St. Agnes.[95] Other records from the later fourteenth century are similarly oblique; and explanatory commentary is rare in the chartulary of St. Agnes. It is unknown, for instance, whether the rents owed to the hospital by a certain Sophia are recorded by St. Agnes by virtue of their rights over St. Alexius, or because Sophia entered the house as a vowed sister.[96] Few documents explicitly related to St. Alexius survive for the first half of the fifteenth century. Significantly, the next substantial record confirming the rights of the hospital, and the rights of St. Agnes over it, dates to 1466.

In 1463, long years of conflict over the position and rights of the archbishop within the city came to a conclusion with Diether von Isenburg's

Geschichte der Stadt Mainz 20 (Mainz: Stadtarchiv, 1963), Nr. 2272; HHStAW Abt 22 Nr. 438, f160v–161v; HStAD A2 168/792 (1441).

91 HStAD C1 A Nr. 89, f. 59v–60r. The legal rights were acquired in 1358. The bakehouse was identified as "zum Alten cappelen" on the *Graben* marking the city periphery. Dilo der Bareworthe had the first Bann over the Backhaus. Once again, the women's legal representative held a double function as a chaplain of the community.

92 HStAD C1 A Nr. 89, f. 128v, "den geistlichen luden und frawen der Eptissen und der Convent des Closters zu Sanct Agnesen."

93 HStAD A2 168/389 and HStAD A2 168/392.

94 HStAD A2 168/412.

95 StAM U 13 October 1385 .

96 HStAD C1 A Nr. 89, f. 11v. The original charter dates to 1370.

unsuccessful invasion of the city, and the establishment of Arnold von Nassau in the archiepiscopal dignity.[97] In the wake of this turbulent transition, the civic hospital returned to the direct administration of the archbishop. The women of St. Agnes, to whom hospital service had long been so significant, may have wished to preempt a similar fate for St. Alexius. The importance of the agreement to the community is indicated by the fact that it survives in triplicate: the original charter is both preserved, and copied into St. Agnes' chartulary, along with a confirmation obtained by the women a month after the initial legal process. The language of the document suggests that the community of St. Agnes, represented by their provost, may have created a legal fiction of lapsed rents to simplify their claim over the hospital and its attendant properties.[98] The confirmation of these rights, obtained a month later, is even more detailed in its provisions. St. Agnes asserts its rights over St. Alexius and adjacent properties, and of all the hospital's pledges and rents.[99] It is significant that these rights were affirmed when the legal status of Mainz's hospitals had been called into question by civic turmoil and archiepiscopal efforts to bring the city's religious houses more firmly under their control.[100] As late as the mid-fifteenth century, the sisters of St. Agnes saw their hospital as of symbolic and practical importance to their communal life.

Conclusion: Identifying St. Agnes

The bequest of a wealthy widow in 1304 is both the first lay donation to St. Agnes and, significantly, the first non-episcopal letter in which St. Agnes is identified as belonging to the Cistercian Order.[101] The charter of donation is unusual in referring to the women of St. Agnes as *sanctimoniales*, nuns.[102] The

97 Paul-Joachim Heinig, "Die Mainzer Kirche im Spätmittelalter (1305–1484)," in *Handbuch der Mainzer Kirchengeschichte: Christliche Antike und Mittelalter*, ed. Friedhelm Jürgensmeier, vol. 1 (Würzburg: Echter Verlag, 2000), 531–540; Wolfgang Dobras, "Münzerhausgenossen und andere Geschlechter. Bemerkungen zur Mainzer Oberschicht in den Bürgerkämpfen des 15. Jahrhunderts," *Mainzer Zeitschrift* 94/95 (1999/2000), 95–109.

98 StAM U / 15 October 1466. The charter is copied in HStAD C1 A Nr. 89 34v–35r.

99 This record survives only as copied into the women's chartulary; HStAD C1 A Nr. 89 47r–48r.

100 For more on the disputed archiepiscopal elections of the 1460s, and the resulting civil conflicts in Mainz, see Heinig, "Die Mainzer Kirche im Spätmittelalter," in *Handbuch der Mainzer Kirchengeschichte*, 536–549.

101 HStAD A2 115/31. The woman, Miltrudis, endows three altars "in Cenobio S(anc)te Agnetis in Magunt(ie) ord(in)is Cyst(erciensis.)"

102 HStAD C1 A Nr. 89, 19v; HStAD A2 168/148; HStAD A2 168/251.

term appears again in a confirmation of property rights sought by the sisters, who send their servant Wenzo to the judges of Mainz's secular court. In the 1310s and 1320s, a handful of similar procedures also identify the women as nuns, though sometimes with other terms used as if interchangeably: *puellae*, or *religiose domine*.[103] Many of their documents are in the vernacular, but although the term "Nonnen" was known, it was never used, authors preferring simply "Frauen," or occasionally "Schwestern."[104]

On the surface, these omissions and absences appear difficult to reconcile with the categorical identification contained in several of St. Agnes' episcopal letters: *ordinis Cisterciensis*. But as Heidi Febert, Letha Böhringer, and others have elegantly demonstrated, statements about the identity of female religious communities were more often polemical than declarative, especially in the thirteenth century.[105] In 1351, civic officials presided over a resolution of a property dispute between the women and one of their neighbors on the Dietmarkt, and in 1354, the abbess and convent issued a charter asserting their rights over a donation. The latter document is remarkable for its specificity in describing the gift of rents and grain, and the purposes for which it may be used within the convent—namely, to augment the ordinary portions of the nuns at meals. In return, the convent is to have their priests celebrate anniversary Masses for the donor and his parents.[106] In its fierce protection of the designated purpose of the gift—for food and for no other use—the charter is reminiscent of those issued to hospitals in the same period. Ecclesiastical officials in the fourteenth century limited the purposes for which religious institutions could legitimately accept donations while retaining their status. The intensifying efforts of fourteenth-century legislators to obtain gifts from the "dead hand" of the church did not exclude hospitals. Increasingly, canon law circumscribed the purposes for which hospitals could accept donations.

While the vocabulary used for the women of St. Agnes is notable for its lability, the women themselves consistently embraced, and even pursued,

103 StAM U 29 June 1317; StAM U 23 March 1326.
104 Barnhouse, "Disordered Women," 86–94.
105 Febert, "The Poor Sisters of Söflingen," 392–404; Felskau, "Von Brabant bis Böhmen und darüber hinaus," 75–76; Letha Böhringer, "Beginen und Schwestern in der Sorge für Kranke, Sterbende und Verstorbene: Eine Problemskizze," in *Organisierte Barmherzigkeit: Armenfürsorge und Hospitalwesen in Mittelalter und früher Neuzeit*, ed. Artur Dirmeier (Regensburg: Verlag Friedrich Pustet, 2010), 127–129; Kolpacoff Deane, "From Case Studies to Comparative Models," 55. See also Alison More, *Fictive Orders and Feminine Religious Identities, 1200–1600* (Oxford: Oxford University Press, 2018), particularly 109–133.
106 HStAD A2 168/401.

the identity of hospital sisters. Especially in the first years following their formation as an independent community, their association with hospital care was invoked by external authorities as well as in their own charters, a mark of identification in a time of transition. Even after being forced to leave Mainz's oldest hospital in 1259, the sisters continued the care of the sick in their new location on the Dietmarkt. Despite the declaration of the council and religious men of Mainz that the women should join the Cistercian Order, they did not formally do so before the late fifteenth century. The council's involvement in the split of the hospital's male and female staff indicates a desire on the part of civic authorities that the hospital should retain its religious status. The women's religious status continued to be a concern after they formed the independent community of St. Agnes. As part of a wave of reform measures imposed on religious houses by Archbishop Wernher in the 1270s–1280s, they were commanded to organize their hospital according to the papal rule of Santo Spirito. The selection of this rule is suggestive of the number and diversity of the sick-poor for whom the sisters cared.

Even after St. Agnes acquired rights over hospital buildings in the semi-agricultural neighborhood on the Umbach, the house maintained an infirmary large enough to have a chaplain dedicated to its altar. While the sisters maintained their identity as hospital sisters, their uncertain religious affiliation, coupled with their establishment in a prosperous and crowded mercantile neighborhood, resulted in a low level of contribution by lay donors. A campaign of acquiring indulgences—as Cistercian nuns—from European bishops, and the regulation of their hospital, set the women of St. Agnes on a more cordial footing with the laity of Mainz. Throughout the late thirteenth and fourteenth centuries, the women dedicated resources and energies to maintaining their identity as hospital sisters, even as they negotiated with ecclesiastical officials for affirmation of their religious status.

4 *Leprosaria* and the Leprous: Legal Status and Social Ties

Abstract

The place of lepers in medieval society has often been described as defined by segregation. Hospitals, in such narratives, appear as instruments of isolation, part of the desperate strategy of a society medically ignorant and indiscriminately terrified of the disease. The historiographical tendency to view medieval leprosy as a subject unto itself has prevented the recognition, let alone the analysis, of trends shared by all types of medieval hospitals. In canon law, *leprosaria* were one of four hospital types, and their institutional development shows that their legal status influenced their social relationships more than did medieval attitudes towards leprosy. I use the rich chartulary of Mainz's leper hospital alongside charters from leper hospitals throughout the central Rhineland.

Keywords: medieval hospitals, leper hospitals, medieval leprosy, history of leprosy

On a hot August Monday in 1358, a crowd gathered in front of the building where judgement was given in the village of Birgstadt. The village officials had come to witness an agreement between Gerlach and Else Hug, and the lepers who lived in the hospital of St. Georg just outside Mainz. The lepers and hospital staff, not present in Birgstadt, were represented by Emmerich Kuechener. The transaction was accompanied by some tension, as this was not a spontaneous act of charity on Gerlach and Else's part. Rather, they were affirming that a yearly rent of four measures of grain now belonged to the lepers by right, as a result of a sale that the couple had made when they were in financial straits. Gerlach and Else promised that they and their heirs would take full responsibility for the regular payment of the rent, and pledged property which would be made over to the lepers if the payment was defaulted on. The lepers and the hospital staff were reminded that

Barnhouse, Lucy C. *Hospitals in Communities of the Late Medieval Rhineland. Houses of God, Places for the Sick.* Taylor & Francis Group, 2023
DOI: 10.5117/9789463720243_CH04

they would be responsible for arranging to pick up the grain. The scribe recording this agreement affirmed that all these promises were made in the presence of the officials. Emmerich, the representative of the lepers, was largely responsible for the final form of the document: he formally requested that the Schultheiß testify that the pledges given were reasonable; and—perhaps with some asperity—told the scribe to write down all the particulars, reminding him of his oath to make a "public instrument" for the use of the lepers and the hospital staff, and to affix his customary sign thereto. As the scribe was sick, he got a student to do most of the writing for him, but added a postscript in his own hand, affirming that he himself had both seen and heard everything which was written down. Not only that, but he personally copied out the document, word for word, for the use of St. Georg at a later date.[1]

This legal proceeding, and the record of it, testify to the place of leper hospitals and the leprous in urban and extra-urban communities during the later Middle Ages. Of the total of forty-six items in St. Georg's chartulary, approximately a third contain evidence of the importance of oral culture and legal ritual in their creation. The court proceedings included the speaking of the terms of the agreement by the donors, in the presence of their heirs, of the hospital's representatives, and of municipal officials, before the results were recorded, often verbatim, by the scribe. As numerous scholars of legal history have argued, any legal process is also a social process.[2] Examining the records created by and for leper hospitals can offer a corrective to historiographical traditions that have too often considered *leprosaria* and the leprous in isolation.

Historiographical Debates

Despite the work of Carole Rawcliffe, François-Olivier Touati, and others, the historiography of medieval leper hospitals remains shaped by the durable notion that the desire to control leprosy and those who had been diagnosed with it was the primary engine of change for such houses, or the cause of

1 StAM 32/700, 1–3.

2 See, for example, Jiri Kejr, "Die Urkunde ale Beweismittel im Gerichtsverfahren in mittelalterlichen Böhmen," in: *The Development of Literate Mentalities in East Central Europe*, eds. Anna Adamska and Marco Mostert, Utrecht Studies in Medieval Literacy 4 (Turnhout: Brepols, 2004), 51–59; Shona Kelly Wray, Instruments of Concord: Making Peace and Settling Disputes through a Notary in the City and Contado of Late Medieval Bologna," *Journal of Social History* 42:3 (2009), 733–760.

their institutional stagnation.[3] While the scholarship on medieval leprosy continues to deepen and diversify, medievalists outside the discipline of history, non-medievalist historians of medicine, and some medieval historians continue to treat leprosy as a special case.[4] The documentary record, however, treats the condition of the leprous pragmatically; vocabulary of fear and horror recurs far more often in the historiography on medieval leprosy than in medieval sources themselves.[5] In literary texts, the leprous were uniquely suited to serve as an exemplary group because of the visibility of their disease, but the lepers of St. Georg, although prevented—either by illness or by attitudes towards it—from entering the courtroom, are visible in ways not primarily defined by their disease. Their suffering, moreover, is not glossed as punishment for sin or fetishized as particularly saintly, either by hospital donors or officials.

In contrast to more recent scholars, who glossed the alleged isolation of medieval lepers as sign and symptom of primitive medical and religious beliefs, historians in the late nineteenth and early twentieth centuries framed it positively. In the decades following the discovery of *Mycobacterium leprae* in 1877, scientists and historians looked to the past as they explored strategies of treatment, concluding that medieval Europe had instinctively followed policies similar to the quarantine believed necessary by nineteenth-century authorities. For Wilhelm Frohn, a medical historian who studied leprosy in the Rhineland, the eventual disappearance of leprosy from the archaeological record in early modern Europe testified to one of the greatest

3 For a historiographical overview, see Carole Rawcliffe, "Isolating the Medieval Leper: Ideas—and Misconceptions—about Segregation in the Middle Ages," in *Freedom of Movement in the Middle Ages: Proceedings of the 2003 Harlaxton Symposium*, ed. Peregrine Horden (Donington: Shaun Tyas, 2007) 229–248. Ludwig Falck, "Mainzer Hospitäler im Mittelalter," in *Moguntia Medica: Das medizinische Mainz von Mittelalter bis ins 20. Jahrhundert,* ed. Franz Dumont (Wiesbaden: B. Wylicil, 2002), 409–417, assumes that Mainz's leper hospitals were geared towards segregation.

4 See, for example, Christine Boeckl, *Images of Leprosy: Disease, Religion, and Politics in European Art* (Kirksville, MO: Truman State University Press, 2011), 45–49, and Mark Jackson, *The History of Medicine: A Beginner's Guide* (London: Oneworld Publications, 2014), 51, for claims that the leprous were generally feared. Kay Peter Jankrift, *Im Angesicht der "Pestilenz": Seuchen in westfälischen und rheinischen Städten (1349–1600)* (Stuttgart: Franz Steiner Verlag, 2020), 300–325, treats leprosy in an excursus.

5 Timothy S. Miller and John Nesbitt, *Walking Corpses: Leprosy in Byzantium and the Medieval West* (Ithaca: Cornell University Press, 2014), provides a salient example in its use of a fourth-century sermon title as representative; see also Irven M. Resnick, "The Jews and Leprosy," in *Marks of Distinction: Christian Perceptions of Jews in the High Middle Ages* (Washington, DC: Catholic University Press, 2012), 107.

achievements of the medieval world.[6] Segregation still appears in much scholarship as the sought-after norm, despite the copious evidence for the presence of lepers on the streets and in the squares of medieval cities.[7] Medieval leprosy has been described as not only a source of social stigma and subject of legislation, but a social issue of singular importance, even when nuanced and diverse reactions to the disease have been recognized.[8] As François-Olivier Touati has observed, views of the leper as Other within medieval societies have been closely bound up with the Other-ing of medieval society itself.[9]

The idea that leprosy held unique prominence in the medieval imagination of disease has proved resilient.[10] Michel Mollat has argued that the

6 Wilhelm Frohn, *Der Aussatz im Rheinland: sein Vorkommen und seine Bekämpfung* (Jena: G. Fischer, 1933), 3–6, 13–18. See also Jörn Henning Wolf, "Einführung," in *Aussatz-Lepra-Hansen-Krankheit: ein Menschheitsproblem im Wandel*, ed. Jörn Henning Wolf (Würzburg: Deutsches Aussätzigen-Hilfswerk), 1–16.

7 Nicholas Orme and Margaret Webster, *The English Hospital 1070–1570* (New Haven: Yale University Press, 1995), 23–31; Emmanuel Bodart, "L'étude des traces matérielles de l'activité hospitalière en Belgique: la rencontre de l'archéologie et l'histoire," in *Einrichtungen der sozialen Sicherung im mittelalterlichen Lotharingien*, 48. James Brodman, "Shelter and Segregation: Lepers in Medieval Catalonia," in *On the Social Origins of Medieval Institutions: Essays in Honor of Joseph F. O'Callaghan*, ed. Donald J. Kagay and Theresa M. Vann (Leiden: Brill, 1998), 35–45; Roberta Gilchrist, *Requiem: The Medieval Monastic Cemetery in Britain* (London: Museum of London Archaeology Service Monograph, 2005), 206–207; Laurinda Abreu and Sally Sheard, "Introduction," in *Hospital Life: Theory and Practice from the Medieval to the Modern*, eds. Laurinda Abreu and Sally Sheard (Oxford: Peter Lang, 2013), 3, 19; Clemens Lohmann, "Vom mittelalterlichen Spital zum modernen Klinikum: Die Entwicklungen bis 1945," in *Eine Stadt im Spiegel der Heilkunst: Streiflichter zu 850 Jahren Fritzlarer Hospitalwesen ; Festschrift des Hospitals zum Heiligen Geist, Fritzlar*, ed. Sabine Trosse (Kassel: LWV Hessen, 1998), 34–71.

8 Piers Mitchell, "The Myth of the Spread of Leprosy with the Crusades," in *The Past and Present of Leprosy: Archaeological, Historical, Palaeopathological and Clinical Approaches*, ed. Charlotte A. Roberts, Mary E. Lewis, and Keith Manchester (Oxford: Archaeopress, 2000), 171–172; Elma Brenner, "Outside the City Walls: Leprosy, Exclusion, and Social Identity in Twelfth- and Thirteenth-Century Rouen," in *Difference and Identity in Francia and Medieval France*, eds. Meredith Cohen and Judith Firnhaber-Baker (Farnham: Ashgate, 2010), 147–155.

9 François-Olivier Touati, *Maladie et Société au Moyen Âge: La lèpre, les lépreux et les léproseries dans la province ecclésiastique de Sens jusqu'au milieu du XIVe siècle* (Bruxelles: De Boeck & Larcier, 1998), 19; idem, "Histoire des maladies, histoire totale? L'exemple de la Lèpre et de la Société au Moyen Âge," *Sources et Travaux d'Histoire Haut-Pyrenéenne* 13 (1988), 3–5. See also Julie Orlemanski, "How to Kiss a Leper," *Postmedieval* 3 (2012), 146–148; Luke Demaitre, *Leprosy in Premodern Medicine: A Malady of the Whole Body* (Baltimore: Johns Hopkins University Press, 2007), 138–143; Rebecca Barnhouse, "Leeches and Leprosy: Medieval Medicine in Modern Novels for Young Readers," *Literature and Medicine* 21 (2002), 25–44.

10 See for example Demaitre, *Leprosy in Premodern Medicine*, 3–6, 74–83, 247–249; Miller and Nesbitt, *Walking Corpses*, 100–117; Damien Jeanne, "Leprosy, Lepers, and Leper-Houses: Between Human Law and God's Law, Sixth-Fifteenth Centuries," in *Social Dimensions of Medieval Disease*

medieval leper was conceptually prominent not as the ultimate Other, but as the paradigmatic *pauper*, the most easily recognizable of beggars on church porticoes and in saints' lives, poor Lazarus who was destined for the bosom of Abraham.[11] This framework points to a possible way of reconciling the apparent pragmatism with which medieval lepers are treated in charters and ordinances with the heightened emotional language of romances, saints' lives, and sermons. Concrete evidence for the incidence of medieval leprosy is scant, especially for the early medieval period, and attempts to calculate the average percentage of medieval populations affected have yielded widely varying results. Moreover, while the numbers of those suffering from the disease are notoriously difficult to determine, still more elusive is the percentage of those identified as lepers who resided within leper hospitals.[12] In focusing on leper hospitals, this chapter leaves aside the leprous who chose not to live in such institutions, and whose numbers and activities within urban and rural space are notoriously difficult to assess.[13]

The late medieval histories of the *leprosaria* of Mainz, Worms, Speyer, and Essen illustrate that *leprosaria* were neither practically nor symbolically isolated from the cities which supported them. It was not only leper hospitals that were situated in liminal locations; from 1236 onwards, Mainz's oldest hospital was built into the city walls; the city's leper hospital was located

and Disability, eds. Sally Crawford and Christina Lee (Oxford: Archaeopress, 2014), 69–79. For numerous examples of how leprosy has dominated post-medieval thought about the Middle Ages, see Carole Rawcliffe, *Leprosy in Medieval England* (Woodbridge: Boydell, 2006), 13–43.

11 Mollat, *Le Pauvre au Moyen Âge*, 44–60. For more on leprosy as metaphor, see Ortrun Riha, "Aussatz als Metapher. Aus der Geschichte einer sozialen Krankheit," in *Medizin in Geschichte, Philologie und Ethnologie: Festschrift für Gundolf Keil*, eds. Dominik Gross and Monika Reininger (Würzburg: Königshausen & Neumann, 2003), 89–104.

12 Carl Georg Bockenheimer, *Der Gutleuthof bei Mainz* (Mainz: Falk, 1882), 1–3; Charlotte A. Roberts, "The Antiquity of Leprosy in Britain: The Skeletal Evidence," in *The Past and Present of Leprosy: Archaeological, Historical, Palaeopathological, and Clinical Approaches*, eds. Charlotte A. Roberts, Mary E. Lewis, and Keith Manchester (Oxford: Archaeopress, 2000), 213; Mitchell, "The Myth of the Spread of Leprosy," 173–174. Schmidt, *Église Rouge*, 242, claims that the disease spread with alarming rapidity. For similar views, see Frohn, *Aussatz im Rheinland*, 1. Bruno Tabuteau, "Combien de lépreux au Moyen Âge? Essai d'étude quantitative appliquée à la lèpre: les exemples de Rouen et de Bellencombre au XIIIe siècle., *Sources, travaux historiques* 13 (1988), 19–23, offers an overview of literature on the subject.

13 Luke Demaitre, "O Brother Where Art Thou? Looking for the Real 'Pauper Lazarus,'" keynote address, *Leprosy and the "Leper" Reconsidered*, Montreal, Quebec, 20 September 2018; Lucy C. Barnhouse, "Good People, Poor Sick: The Social Identities of Lepers in the Late Medieval Rhineland," in *Leprosy and Identity in the Middle Ages: From England to the Mediterranean*, eds. Elma Brenner and François-Olivier Touati (Manchester: Manchester University Press, 2021), 189–191.

a mile outside the walls, but also managed a satellite house within them.[14] Recent scholarship has shown, moreover, that urban properties contributed to the social visibility of religious institutions; the evidence from the cities of the central Rhineland demonstrates that this was true for leper hospitals no less than for other houses.[15] The socio-spatial positioning of *leprosaria* was variable, rather than simultaneously determining and determined by fear of disease and of the sick.[16] The leprous were not treated as miserable outcasts; rather, their place in social, economic, and religious networks was defined by their status as religious persons. Looking at late medieval evidence, Carole Rawcliffe has noted a marked difference in attitudes towards those lepers who were obediently in hospitals—and thus regulated as religious persons—and those who were not.[17] In the later fifteenth and early sixteenth centuries, the leper hospital of Worms went so far as to elide the categories of the leprous and corrodians; a similar conflation is found in a seventeenth-century copy of the rule for Mainz's St. Georg.[18]

The place of the leprous in medieval society has often been described as defined by segregation. Segregation, it is argued, was designed to keep the wider population safe from contagion and the fear of contagion; and to keep the leprous safe from the endemic violence borne of such fear.[19]

14 On the implications of such locations, see Irina Metzler, "Liminality and Disability: Spatial and Conceptual Aspects of Physical Impairment in Medieval Europe," in *Medicine and Space: Body, Surroundings, and Borders in Antiquity and the Middle Ages*, eds. Patricia A. Baker, Han Nijdam, and Karine van 't Land (Leiden: Brill, 2012), 273–276.

15 See, for example, John Henderson, *Piety and Charity in Late Medieval Florence* (Oxford: Clarendon Press, 1994), 242–277; Miri Rubin, "Religious Culture in Town and Country: Reflections on a Great Divide," in *Church and City, 1000–1500: Essays in Honour of Christopher Brooke*, eds. David Abulafia, Michael Franklin, and Miri Rubin (Cambridge: Cambridge University Press, 1992), 3–10; Adam J. Davis, "Hospitals, Charity, and the Culture of Compassion in the Twelfth and Thirteenth Centuries," in *Approaches to Poverty in Medieval Europe: Complexities, Contradictions, Transformations, c. 1100–1500*, ed. Sharon Farmer (Turnhout: Brepols, 2016), 42; Carla Keyvanian, *Hospitals and Urbanism in Rome, 1200–1500* (Leiden: Brill, 2015), esp. 1–3, with notes.

16 Piera Borradori, "Etre lépreux autour de 1300," in *Le Pays de Vaud vers 1300*, eds. Piera Borradori and Nadia Pollini (Lausanne: Faculté des Lettres, Université de Lausanne, 1992), 105–109; Jean Grandin, "Recherches sur les maladreries dans l'Orne au Moyen Âge," *Cahiers Léopold Delisle* 23 (1974), 9–11; Anita Homolka, "Die Lebensgewohnheiten der Leprakranken im Spätmittelalter," in *Aussatz—Lepra—Hansen-Krankheit: ein Menschheitsproblem im Wandel*, ed. Jörn Henning Wolf (Würzburg: Deutsches Aussätzigen-Hilfswerk, 1986), 151-162.

17 Rawcliffe, *Leprosy*, 252–301.

18 StAW Abt 1B Nr 2011. StAM 0032/704, f175r–177v.

19 Frohn, *Aussatz im Rheinland*, 12, describes leprosy as a "constant and feared guest" in Europe from 1000–1500; in similar vein, see Édouard Jeanselme, "Comment l'Europe, au Moyen Âge, se protégea contre la Lèpre," *Bulletin de la Société Française d'Histoire de la Médecine* 25 (1931), 7–8, 33; Max Bär, "Das vormalige Siechenhaus bei Koblenz," *Mittelrheinische Geschichtsblätter* 4:2

Hospitals, in such narratives, appear as instruments of isolation, part of the desperate strategy of a medically ignorant society indiscriminately terrified of the disease.[20] Policies concerning lepers have been interpreted as part of a strategy of social exclusion employed by those in positions of power, despite a lack of direct evidence for such exclusion.[21] The infamous persecution of the leprous in 1321 has sometimes been taken as typifying medieval attitudes towards leprosy and the leprous.[22] Official responses to this persecution, however, focused on the rights of *leprosaria* and their residents. Much of what is known of this persecution, indeed, comes from a letter from a bishop in which he condemns public actions taken against leper houses and their property, saying that the innocent majority of lepers should not be held responsible for the actions of a few. The fact remains that these "few," like the Jews, were used as scapegoats. But that the consequences

(1924), 2–3; Siegfried Reicke, *Das deutsche Spital und sein Recht im Mittelalter*, vol. 2 (Stuttgart: Enke, 1932), 310–326; Marie-Louise Windemuth, *Das Hospital als Träger der Armenfürsorge im Mittelalter* (Stuttgart: Franz Steiner Verlag, 1995), 119–124; Françoise Bériac, *Histoire des lépreux au Moyen Âge. Une société d'exclus* (Paris: Imago, 1988). See also Sheila Zimmerman, "Leprosy in the Medieval Imaginary," *Journal of Medieval and Early Modern Studies* 38 (2008), passim; Roberta Gilchrist, "Christian Bodies and Souls: The Archaeology of Life and Death in Later Medieval Hospitals," in *Death in Towns: Urban Responses to the Dying and the Dead, 100–1600*, ed. Steven Bassett (Leicester: Leicester University Press, 1992), 101–103.

20 Michael W. Dols, "The Leper in Medieval Islamic Society," *Speculum* 58 (1983), 891–916. Gunther Risse, *Mending Bodies, Saving Souls: A History of Hospitals* (Oxford: Oxford University Press, 1999), 176–180; C. H. Talbot, *Medicine in Medieval England* (London: Oldbourne, 1955), 161; Nicole Brocard, *Soins, secours, et exclusion: Etablissements hospitaliers et assistance dans le diocèse de Besançon, XIVe et XVe siècles* (Paris: Presses Universitaires Franc-Comtoises, 1998), 233–258. Patricia H. Cullum, "Leperhouses and Borough Status in the Thirteenth Century," in *Thirteenth Century England, III: Proceedings of the Newcastle upon Tyne Conference 1989*, eds. P. R. Coss and S. D. Lloyd (Woodbridge: Boydell, 1991), 45–46. See Demaitre, *Leprosy in Premodern Medicine*, 134–138, for a debunking of the notion that the touch of a leper represented the ultimate horror.

21 Falck, "Mainzer Hospitäler im Mittelalter," 414; Danica Summerlin, *The Canons of the Third Lateran Council of 1179, Their Origins and Reception* (Cambridge: Cambridge University Press, 2019), 91, 100–112; Ephraim Shoham-Steiner, *On the Margins of a Minority: Leprosy, Madness, and Disability among the Jews of Medieval Europe*, translated by Haim Watzman (Detroit, MI: Wayne State University Press, 2014), 23–25. Touati, *Maladie et Société*, 332–334, reads Jacques de Vitry's sermons as an attempt to categorize and restrain. Andrew Louth, "The Body in Western Catholic Christianity," in *Religion and the Body*, ed. Sarah Coakley (Cambridge: Cambridge University Press, 1997), 27–30.

22 Miller and Nesbitt, *Walking Corpses*, 106–110, 151–154; Jürgen Belker-van den Heuvel, "Aussätzige: Tückischer Feind und Armer Lazarus," in *Randgruppen der Spätmittelalterlichen Gesellschaft*, ed. Bernd-Ulrich Hergemöller (Warendorf: Fahlbusch Verlag, 2001), 286–291; Frohn, *Aussatz im Rheinland*, 188–191. Cf. Uhrmacher, *Lepra und Leprosorien*, 47–56, for the argument that social and religious factors were more significant than leprosy itself in these persecutions.

should have taken this form of violent protest against the institutions is suggestive. Resentment of hospital policies or privileges—the collection of rents, or exemption from taxes—may have been cloaked in fear of the leprous themselves.[23]

In the central Rhineland, leper hospitals were connected to surrounding communities, and the religious status of such institutions affected the perception and treatment of the lepers resident there. Analyzing *leprosaria* alongside other hospitals affords the opportunity to reassess the often-alleged tension between fear of lepers and the frequency with which their service was extolled and embraced.[24] To this end I turn, firstly, to early medieval legal and hagiographical sources. Next, I analyze the relationship of lepers and leprosy to the institutional regularization of hospitals in the twelfth and thirteenth centuries. Leper hospitals enter the documentary record with increasing regularity from the first third of the thirteenth century onwards. The theory that this increase corresponded to an epidemic outbreak of the disease has been queried from at least the early twentieth century, but remains durable.[25] The multiplication of known hospitals has also been attributed variously to the growth of an urban underclass isolated from traditional support systems, and to late medieval growth in charitable donations on the part of laypersons anxious about the spiritual effects of their profit from the things of this world.[26]

23 Piera Borradori,"Etre lépreux autour de 1300," in *Le Pays de Vaud vers 1300*, eds. Piera Borradori and Nadia Pollini (Lausanne: Faculté des Lettres, Université de Lausanne, 1992), 110f.

24 Gilchrist, "Christian Bodies and Souls," 104–110; Idem, "Medieval Bodies in the Material World: Gender, Stigma, and the Body," in *Framing Medieval Bodies*, eds. Sarah Kay and Miri Rubin (Manchester: Manchester University Press, 1994), 43–46. On this question, cf. Jean-Luc Fray, "Hospitäler, Leprosenhäuser und mittelalterliches Straßennetz in Lothringen (ca. 1200–ca. 1500)" in *Auf den Römerstraßen ins Mittelalter: Beiträge zur Verkehrsgeschichte zwischen Maas und Rhein von der Spätantike bis ins 19. Jahrhundert*, eds. Friedhelm Burgard and Alfred Haverkamp (Mainz: Von Zabern, 1997), 407–426.

25 Jeanselme, "Comment l'Europe, au Moyen Âge, se protégea," 4; Grandin, "Recherches sur les maladreries," 5–7; Ana Rita Rocha, "Being a Leper in Medieval Portugal: The Lepers and the Leper House of Coimbra, Twelfth-Sixteenth Centuries," conference presentation, International Medieval Congress, Leeds, 5 July 2016; Jankrift, *Im Angesicht der 'Pestilenz,'* 143–144.

26 Françoise Bériac, "Les fraternités de lépreux et lépreuses," in *Doppelklöster und andere Formen der Symbiose männlicher und weiblicher Religiosen im Mittelalter*, ed. Kaspar Elm and Michel Parisse (Berlin: Duncker und Humblot, 1980), 203–211, makes a similar claim. See also Gilchrist, "Christian Bodies and Souls," 103; Grandin, "Recherches sur les maladreries dans l'Orne," 5–7. André Vauchez, "Lay People's Sanctity in Western Europe: Evolution of a Pattern (Twelfth and Thirteenth Centuries)," in *Images of Sainthood in Medieval Europe*, eds. Renate Blumenfeld Kosinski and Timea Szell (Ithaca: Cornell University Press, 1991), 23–25.

The increased visibility of leper hospitals was due in large part to external pressures for communities to record their rights as religious institutions, and to conform to the criteria for religious status created by ecclesiastical authorities.[27] A more coherent picture of the purpose of leper hospitals as imagined by their founders and administrators may be gained by comparing the statutes of *leprosaria* with monastic rules. Disease is never mentioned as grounds for the creation of such statutes.[28] When lepers are excluded by hospital statutes, it is as persons requiring specialized medical care, along with e.g. foundlings, those with burning sores, or pregnant women.[29] Moreover, legislation dedicated to limiting the contact of the leprous with the healthy is centered not on the issue of contagion, but on the principle of obedience to one's superior, central to religious life as vowed persons.[30]

Lepers, Leprosy, and the Rise of Hospitals

During the early Middle Ages, most leper hospitals were located in episcopal cities, with many of the sick remaining in informal groupings, or begging without a fixed place of abode.[31] The extent to which the leprous were cared for in other early medieval hospitals is elusive, although a letter of St. Jerome names the care of lepers alongside that of the other sick, and most hospitals were multipurpose institutions.[32] The famous ideal plan of the monastery of St. Gall designates spaces for the sick of the monastery, for other sick, and

27 See Mitchell, "The Myth of the Spread of Leprosy," 173; Michel Pauly, *Peregrinorum, pauperum ac aliorum transeuntium receptaculum: Hospitäler zwischen Maas und Rhein im Mittelalter* (Stuttgart: Franz Steiner Verlag, 2007), 74–80; Jankrift, Im Angesicht Der 'Pestilenz,' 301–307.

28 Angers, "La bourgeoisie de Falaise et ses lepreux à la fin du Moyen Âge," 217, makes much of the ways in which leper hospital statutes allegedly demarcated the leper from the rest of the population.

29 Léon Le Grand, *Statuts d'hôtels-Dieu et de léproseries: recueil de textes du XIIe au XIVe siècle* (Paris: Alphonse Picard et Fils, 1901), 25–26, 115. The theory of medical segregation is suggested by Cullum, "Leperhouses and Borough Status," 45–46. Touati, *Maladie et Société*, 604–605, speaks of "lepers in the shadow of leper hospitals."

30 StAM 32/704, printed in Bockenheimer, *Der Gutleuthof bei Mainz*, 20–21; StAW Abt 1 AI Nr I–0364. Cf. Le Grand, *Statuts d'hotels-Dieu*, 181–250 passim, especially 189, 192–193, 203, 225, 234.

31 Martin Uhrmacher, *Leprosorien in Mittelalter und früher Neuzeit* (Köln: Rheinland Verlag, 2000), 7–11; Bruno Tabuteau, "De l'expérience érémétique à la normalisation monastique: étude d'un processus de formation des léproseries aux XIIe-XIIIe siècles. Le cas d'Evreux," in *Fondations et œuvres charitables au Moyen Âge: Actes du 121e congrès national des sociétés historiques et scientifiques, section histoire médiévale et philologie, Nice, 1996* (Paris: CTHS, 1999), 89–96.

32 Franz Meffert, *Caritas und Krankenwesen bis zum Ausgang des Mittelalters* (Freiburg im Breisgau: Caritas Verlag, 1927), 60–64, 115–126.

for lepers.[33] Also situated in a monastery is the only non-biblical cautionary tale involving leprosy which I have found. The *vita* of a saintly abbot, in northern France, records that a certain monk, wishing not to live according to the strictures of the Benedictine Rule, paid a bribe to be found leprous. Naturally, the holy man was not deceived.[34] The appearances of lepers and leprosy in different genres of early medieval texts suggest a considerable range of ways to live as a leper, and ways lepers might be regarded.

The first evidence for a leper hospital in the archdiocese of Mainz comes from a transfer of rights over a community of lepers in the village of Klingelmunde.[35] In the mid-eleventh century, Gratian's synthesizing *Decretum* not only emphasized the legal obligation of all Christians to *hospitalitas*, but also drew a distinction between episcopally supported hospitals, which automatically had the privileges of *loca pia*, and those founded by laypersons.[36] This legal development may have provided the catalyst for Richolf and Danckmodis, count and countess of the Rheingau, to transfer a church and an associated leper house to the Benedictine house of Johannisberg in 1109. Although the charter of Richolf and Danckmudis is unusually early, it records, not the founding of the leper house, but the transfer of its administration, as was common in the region and beyond.[37]

33 Franz Irsigler, "Matriculae, xenodochia, hospitalia und Leprosenhäuser im Frühmittelalter," in *Einrichtungen der sozialen Sicherung im mittelalterlichen Lotharingien. Actes des 13es Journées Lotharingiennes (12–15 October 2004)*, ed. Michel Pauly (Linden: Section Historie de l'Institut Grand-Ducal, 2008), 337–338.

34 *MGH SS 15,2*, 670.

35 StAM U / 1109 (in StAM 14/310.) Printed in Valentin Ferdinand Gudenus, *Codex diplomaticus: exhibens anectoda ab anno DCCCLXXXI ad MCCC Moguntiaca, ius Germanicum, et S.R.I. historiam illustrantia* I, (Göttingen: Sumptu Regiae Officinae Librar. Academ., 1743), 40.

36 Peter Landau, "Die Leprakranken im mittelalterlichen kanonischen Recht," in *Staat, Kirche, Wissenschaft in einer pluralistischen Gesellschaft: Festschrift zum 65. Geburtstag von Paul Mikat*, eds. Dieter Schwab, Dieter Gießen, Joseph Listl, Hans-Wolfgang Strätz (Berlin: Duncker und Humblot, 1989), 568. For an overview of Gratian on this topic, with historiographical notes, see Thomas Frank, *Heilsame Wortgefechte: Reformen europäischer Hospitäler vom 14. bis 16. Jahrhundert* (Göttingen: V & R Unipress, 2014), 39–40.

37 On this vexed question see e.g. Margaret A. Seymour, "The Organization, Personnel, and Functions of the Hospital in the later Middle Ages," *The Bulletin of the Institute for Historical Research* 21 (1948), 249–250; Rudolf Virchow, "Der Hospititaliter-Orden des Heiligen Geist, zumal in Deutschland," in *Monatsberichte der Königlich Preussischen Akademie der Wissenschaften zu Berlin* 43 (1878), 340–341; and especially Reicke,1, vol. I, 73–92. Several leper houses in the region appear first in charters of donation, rather than foundation; see Uhrmacher, *Lepra und Leprosorien*, 210–211; Wernher, "Oppenheim," 309. For examples across Europe, see e.g. Bodart, "L'étude des traces matérielles de l'activité hospitalière," 26–27; Jasmin Kleemann, "Die Neuordnung des Heiliggeist-Hospitals im Jahre 1502," in *Himmel-Hölle-Fegefeuer: Jenseitsvorstellungen und Sozialgeschichte im spätmittelalterlichen Dortmund* (Dortmund: Stadtarchiv Dortmund, 1996),

The house in Klingelmunde already had properties dedicated to its upkeep, which it possessed on terms granted only to ecclesiastical institutions, and pastoral care routinely provided by an associated church. The account of the lepers of St. Bartholomäus bears out the theory that the legal status of hospitals as religious institutions was to some extent taken for granted in the twelfth century, becoming a subject of dispute only incrementally.[38] It is worth noting that the charter only survives because of the need of a religious foundation to confirm its property rights in the later Middle Ages.[39] Ambiguity surrounding the circumstances of hospital foundation could lead to legal difficulties, as it was episcopal foundation that conferred unambiguous status as a religious institution.

Direct archiepiscopal involvement is not visible in the case of St. Bartholomäus, although the mention of Archbishop Ruthard as having dedicated the church may have been intended as a claim to legitimacy via archiepiscopal patronage. Such attempts at control and regulation could be resented by hospital communities as an imposition, or welcomed for the legal privileges they conferred.[40] The twelfth century saw an increase in

137; Daniel Le Blévec, *La Part du Pauvre: l'assistance dans les pays du BasRhône du XIIe siècle au milieu du XVE siècle*, vol. 1 (Rome: École française de Rome, 2000), 822–830; Albert Bourgeois, *Lépreux et Maladreries du Pas-de-Calais* (Arras: Commission Départementale des Monuments Historiques du PasdeCalais, 1972), 34–37; Meinert, *Die Hospitäler Holsteins*, 79; Monika Eschner-Apsner, "Geistliche Institutionen und Hospitäler," in *Caritas im Bistum Trier: Eine Geschichte des Helfens und Heilens*, ed. Roland Ries and Werner Marzi (Trier: Kliomedia Verlag, 2006), 78–79; Damien Jeanne, "Le groupe de lépreux de Saint Lazare de Falaise," in *Lépreux et sociabilité du Moyen Âge aux temps modernes*, ed. Bruno Tabuteau (Rouen: Publications de l'Université de Rouen, 2000), 39–41; Kälble, "Sozialfürsorge und kommunale Bewegung," 242–246; Watson, *Fundatio, Ordinatio, et Statuta*, 13, equates the date of hospital foundation with its emergence into the written record. On difficulties in establishing the circumstances and date of foundation for monastic houses, see e.g. Maria Magdalena Rückert, "Zur Inkorporation südwestdeutscher Frauenklöster in den Zisterzienserorden. Untersuchungen zu Zisterzen der Maulbronner Filiation im 12. und 13. Jahrhundert," in *Studien und Mitteilungen zur Geschichte des Benediktinerordens und seiner Zweige* 111 (2000), 387–393; Franz Josef Felten, "Abwehr, Zuneigung, Pflichtgefühl. Reaktionen früher Zisterzienser auf den Wunsch religiöser Frauen, zisterziensisch zu leben," in *Female vita religiosa between Late Antiquity and the High Middle Ages: Structures, Developments, and Spatial Contexts*, eds. Gert Melville and Anne Müller (Berlin: LIT, 2011), 398–401; Phillips, *Beguines in Medieval Strasbourg*, 254–255.

38 Touati, *Maladie et Société*, 405. Cf. Christian Probst, "Das Hospitalwesen im hohen und späten Mittelalter und die geistliche und gesellschaftliche Stellung des Kranken," in *Medizin im mittelalterlichen Abendland*, ed. Baader and Keil (Darmstadt: Wissenschaftliche Buchgesellschaft, 1982), 260–262.

39 StAM 14/310.

40 Beriac, "Les fraternités de lépreux et lépreuses," 203–211; Rotha Mary Clay, *The Medieval Hospitals of England* (London: Methuen, 1909), 15–16; Pauly, *Peregrinorum, pauperum ac aliorum transeuntem*, 113.

episcopal pressure for regular observance by religious houses of all kinds, including hospitals. Within the charter, the leper house of St. Bartholomäus itself appears both as a *curte leprosorum,* suggesting a community perhaps with its own arable land, and as a *leprodochium.* The term *leprodochium* does not appear to have been at any time standard vocabulary, appearing only in a handful of early medieval saints' lives and chronicles.[41] Its use seems intended to identify the house as a place offering therapeutic care, borrowing its Greek ending from the term *xenodochium*, used for hospitals and hospices in much conciliar legislation.[42] The gift of the properties in Klingelmunde included vineyards and fields intended for the support of the church and leper house, and although the charter had few legal terms, it specified that the vineyards of the leper house were exempt from tithes.[43]

Legal and literary texts alike suggest that hospital life became the desired norm for the majority of lepers from the late twelfth century onwards. Why this was so has been much debated. Among other factors, the growth of new religious movements in the high Middle Ages certainly affected the conceptualization of charitable work as holy labor.[44] Care for the leprous, too, became increasingly prominent in saints' lives. Edmund Kealey has suggested that this prominence is indicative of the high visibility of the leprous, and the extent to which public opinion focused on them as potential objects of revulsion or compassion.[45] As Luke Demaitre has pointed out, moreover, thirteenth-century "leprosy saints" do not overcome fear of contagion, or heal lepers, but overcome fear or revulsion of the leprous, presenting a moral lesson to the healthy.[46] Robert Jütte describes the lives

41 *Acta Sanctorum Aug.* III, col. 0093A0095C, the life of Radegund, describes the Frankish queen as exhibiting charity to the sick-poor, and especially lepers (*charitate in pauperes, præcipue leprosos.*) The word does not occur in the MGH.

42 The word was seen by Manfred Stimming, *Mainzer Urkundenbuch*, vol. 1 (Darmstadt: Verlag des Historischen Vereins für Hessen, 1932), 353–354, Nr. 446, as evidence against the charter's authenticity. Stimming echoes Zedler, and asserts that the charter was a seventeenth-century forgery of the Jesuits, who had recently made a gift of St. Bartholomäus and vineyards. This is disproved by its presence in StAM 14/310.

43 StAM U / 1109.

44 Adam J. Davis, *The Medieval Economy of Salvation: Charity, Commerce, and the Rise of the Hospital* (Ithaca: Cornell University Press, 2019), 115–118.

45 Edward J. Kealey, *Medieval Medicus: Physicians and Health Care in England, 1100–1154* (Baltimore: Johns Hopkins University Press, 1981), 41–43, 89–95. See also Vauchez, "Lay People's Sanctity in Western Europe," 27–31; Boeckl, *Images of Leprosy*, 83–89.

46 Demaitre, *Leprosy in Premodern Medicine*, 247–249. Cf. Courtney Krolikoski, "Saints and Sinners: The Role of the Saint in the Life of the Leper Before the Thirteenth Century," *Annual of Medieval Studies at CEU* 18 (2012), 66–67, who claims that the medieval leper "was stripped of his or her previous life and set outside the boundaries of his or her previous society."

of the leprous during this period as marginalized and stigmatized, but not necessarily undesirable because of the Christian "caritas" model which prioritized the serving of the lowliest.[47] The links between the care of lepers and religious life need not, however, be explained solely in terms of devotion.[48]

Many scholars have attributed the apparent multiplication of leper hospitals to an increased incidence of the disease, sometimes using the heightened language of crisis and catastrophe.[49] The historiographical pattern of studying leper houses separately from other hospitals has obscured the fact that hospitals of all types, not merely *leprosaria*, enter the historical record in greater number and frequency in the late twelfth and early thirteenth centuries.[50] Attempts to bring hospitals into conformity with canon law would account for both why and how hospitals enter the written

47 Robert Jütte, "The Social Construction of Illness in the Early Modern Clinic," in *The Social Construction of Illness*, eds. Jens Lachmund and Gunnar Stollberg (Stuttgart: Franz Steiner Verlag, 1992), 33.

48 Anne E. Lester, "Cares Beyond the Walls: Cistercian Nuns and the Care of Lepers in Twelfth and Thirteenth Century Northern France," in *Religious and Laity in Western Europe 1000–1400: Interaction, Negotiation, and Power*, eds. Emilia Jamroziak and Janet Burton (Turnhout: Brepols, 2006), 204–206. Cf. Risse, *Mending Bodies*, 173–178. Probst, "Das Hospitalwesen im hohen und späten Mittelalter, 260–274, passim; Frohn, "Aussatz im Rheinland," 205–213; Uhrmacher, *Leprosorien im Mittelalter*, 26–30; James Brodman, *Charity and Welfare*, 8–27.

49 Carl Johann Heinrich Villinger, "Wormser Hospitäler. Ein Beitrag zur Geschichte der Wormser Caritas im Mittelalter," *Jahrbuch für das Bistum Mainz* 2 (1947), 180–185; Nicolas Norbert Huyghebaert, "L'origine ecclésiastique des léproseries en Flandre et dans le Nord de la France," *Revue d'histoire ecclésiastique* 58 (1962), 850–852; Frohn, *Aussatz im Rheinland*, 217; Resnick, "The Jews and Leprosy," 105–107; Miller and Nesbitt, *Walking Corpses*, 119–121; Irwin W. Sherman, "Leprosy, the Striking Hand of God," in *The Power of Plagues* (Washington, DC: American Society of Medicine Press, 2006), 306. For an assessment of the figure of 19,000 leper hospitals, see Bruno Tabuteau, "Vingt mille léproseries au Moyen Âge? Tradition française d'un poncif historiographique," *Memini: Travaux et documents* 15 (2011), 119–128; Michel Pauly und Martin Uhrmacher, "Die Koblenzer Hospitäler in zentralörtlicher Perspektive," in *Zwischen Maas und Rhein: Beziehungen, Begegnungen und Konflikte in einem europäischen Kernraum von der Spätantike bis zum 19. Jahrhundert*, ed. Franz Irsigler (Trier: Universität Trier, 2006), 334–340.

50 See for example Wolfgang W. Schürle, *Das Hospital zum Heiligen Geist in Konstanz; ein Beitrag zur Rechtsgeschichte des Hospitals im Mittelalter* (Sigmaringen: Jan Thorbecke Verlag, 1970), 70–75; Paul Bonenfant, "Les premiers 'hospitia' de Bruxelles au XIIe siècle," *Annales de la Société belge d'histoire des hôpitaux* 11 (1973), 3–7; Kay Peter Jankrift, "Hospitäler und Leprosorien im Nordwesten des mittelalterlichen Regnum Teutonicum unter besonderer Berücksichtigung rheinischwestfälischer Städte," in *Europäisches Spitalwesen. Institutionelle Fürsorge in Mittelalter und Früher Neuzeit*, eds. Martin Scheutz, Andrea Sommerlechner, Herwig Weigl, and Alfred Stefan Weiß (Munich: R. Oldenbourg Verlag, 2008), 298; Farmer, "The Beggar's Body," 159–161; Touati, *Maladie et Société*, 247–307.

record. The proliferation of records for hospitals shows not a new kind of institution springing fully formed from a cultural preoccupation with charity, but rather, preexisting communities working to achieve recognition under a new set of legal parameters.

Leper Hospitals and Their Communities

The extant records of the leper hospital of Mainz—and those in comparable cities of the Middle Rhineland—show both *leprosaria* and their resident lepers as active in relationships with their neighbors. Evidence from the province of Mainz shows that hospitals functioned as guarantors of lepers collective rights, providing legal and social stability. Moreover, the leprous could receive such legal protection and therapeutic care within multipurpose institutions, as well as *leprosaria*. The social interpretations of leprosy were both contingent and diverse. Not the least of the variables contributing to these interpretations was the relationship of individual lepers to the hospitals where they received or resisted the rights and responsibilities of religious status.[51] Thus the growth of leper hospitals can be taken as an index of changing social realities for individual lepers.

The earliest evidence for an independent hospital devoted exclusively to the leprous in Mainz does not predate the mid-fourteenth century. There are several indications, however, that such a hospital existed earlier. Nineteenth-century historians of Mainz unanimously place the earliest reference to a leper hospital for the city in 1261.[52] The fullest description of this document identifies it as a record of the gift of a grain rent from the Cistercian convent of Altmünster to "the priest of the leper house [*Siechenhaus*]."[53] Regrettably, printed editions made in the eighteenth and nineteenth centuries do not contain even a register for this charter.[54] Dieter Staerk has suggested that

51 See Barnhouse, "Good People, Poor Sick," 323–324, 334–335.

52 Karl Schaab, *Die Geschichte der Stadt Mainz* (Mainz: F. Kupferberg, 1841), vol. 2, 415; Bockenheimer, *Der Gutleuthof bei Mainz*, follows Schaab, and identifies the house as St. Georg. According to Bockenheimer, records for the origins of the house were no longer extant at the time of his writing. Rörig, *Mainzer Spitäler*, 32, identifies the record of 1261 as a charter belonging to Altmünster; on what evidence he does so is unclear, as Schaab is not so specific.

53 Schaab, *Geschichte der Stadt Mainz*, vol. 2, 415. Quotation marks his. Frohn, *Aussatz im Rheinland*, 68–69, follows Schaab in identifying this record as the first for lepers in Mainz.

54 Ludwig Baur, *Hessische Urkunden: Die Provinz Rheinhessen von 963–1325*, vol. 2 (Darmstadt: Der historische Verein für das Grossherzogthum Hessen, 1862); Franz Joseph Bodmann, *Rheingauische*

Mainz had two *leprosaria*, asserting that the reference from 1261 refers to a house by a different gate than the Gautor, where the hospital of St. Georg stood.[55] Other records concerning the early history of medieval leprosy in Mainz appear to have been lost since the nineteenth century; Bockenheimer, whose work remains widely relied upon, says that "the sources showed that [lepers] were permitted to visit churches."[56]

Through the first third of the thirteenth century, and at least intermittently afterwards, Mainz's oldest hospital cared for lepers alongside its other sick. The hospital's 1236 statutes make explicit the fact that the hospital excluded no class of persons for medical or other cause, and comparison with other hospital statutes demonstrates that this was not merely formulaic.[57] Moreover, as late as 1369, a testament specifies that the hospital cared for lepers.[58] The "little house" by the hospital, referred to in several charters as part of the hospital complex, appears to have been actively used by the hospital community itself. The house is traditionally known by the moniker "zum Roten Kopf," "the ruddy head." This, and the lepromatous deformations visible on identifying signs for the house from the early modern period, are consistent with the high medieval iconography of leprosy.[59] A charter from another hospital in the region, moreover, records the existence of a "Krankenhaus" and a "Siechenhaus" as adjoining facilities in the same hospital complex.[60] As the formula "Kranken und Siechen" was used in the Rhineland to denote the sick and lepers as separate but linked groups, the buildings in Mainz would seem to have been designed to house the leprous separately from other sick persons, while allowing them to be served by the

Alterthümer oder Landes und Regimentsverfassung des westlichen oder Niederrheingaues im Mittlern Zeitalter, (Mainz: Florian Kupferberg, 1819).

55 Dieter Staerk, "Gutleuthäuser und Kotten im südwestdeutschen Raum. Ein Beitrag zur Erforschung der städtischen Wohlfahrtspflege in Mittelalter und Frühneuzeit," in *Die Stadt in der europäischen Geschichte. Festschrift Edith Ennen*, eds. W. Besch, F. Irsigler, et al. (Bonn: L. Röhrscheid, 1972), 529–533.

56 Bockenheimer, *Der Gutleuthof bei Mainz*, 4.

57 StAM 6 (30) 4. Le Grand, *Statuts d'hotels-Dieu*, 25–26, 115; Charlotte A. Stanford, *Commemorating the Dead in Late Medieval Strasbourg: The Cathedral's Book of Donors and its Use (1320–1521)* (Farnham: Ashgate, 2011), 268–269. See discussion above in Chapter 2.

58 StAM U 14 May 1379 includes a gift "to the leprous sick [maleden siechen] in the Heilig Geist Spital located by the Rhine in Mainz."

59 Boeckl, *Images of Leprosy*, 24–44; Orlemanski, "How to Kiss a Leper," 142–146; Touati, "Histoire des maladies, histoire totale?" 12–13; William B. Ober, "Can the Leper Change His Spots? The Iconography of Leprosy," *American Journal of Dermatopathology*, Part I, 5/1 (1983), 43–58; Part II, 5/2 (1983), 173–186; Frohn, *Aussatz im Rheinland*, 140–147.

60 Fordham University, Walsh Library Special Collections: Gemunde Document 16.

same staff.[61] The Templar house in Mainz also offered care for lepers until its rights were disputed, and eventually bought out, by another hospital.[62]

In Worms, Speyer, and Strasbourg, episcopal cities of comparable size to Mainz within the ecclesiastical province, independent leper hospitals enter the records in the first half of the thirteenth century, at the same time that many hospitals were responding to the codification of religious status in the *Liber Extra* of 1234. The rule of Santo Spirito, which was followed by the new hospital under the aegis of the sisters of St. Agnes, also allowed for the accommodation of lepers.[63] Further suggestive evidence for the accommodation of lepers in the city and archdiocese of Mainz is provided by a significant silence: no regional councils, archiepiscopal communications, or hospital records contain rites or regulations indicating that lepers were outcast or isolated.[64] Under the jurisdiction of archbishops unusually active in the standardization of liturgical practice and religious observance, this is a notable omission.

Speyer's St. Georg was endowed with the bequest of a private citizen, Ulrich Klüpfel, in 1259. The hospital received not only properties and revenues in two villages, but the right of patronage over a parish, enabling it to be a selfsustaining community in conformity with the directives of Lateran III for the liturgical and sacramental functions available to every such hospital.[65] In subsequent years, the council would take over the administration of the hospital, and free it explicitly from taxes, in accordance with the house's religious status. In 1262, the hospital procurators successfully petitioned the bishop for the right to have Masses celebrated within the hospital.[66] The foundation of Strasbourg's Église Rouge is of uncertain date; the extant episcopal privileges of 1234 indicate its previous existence. It became much more clearly regulated from 1309 onwards, with its passage into civic control. More restrictive regulations were introduced in the fifteenth century, but there were still so many exceptions as to make isolation useless, had it ever been a goal.[67] In Worms, the first reference to an independent leper

61 On the linked terms "Kranken und Siechen" see Benjamin Laqua, *Bruderschaften und Hospitäler während des hohen Mittelalters: Kölner Befunde im westeuropäischvergleichende Perspektive* (Stuttgart: Hiersemann, 2011), 109–113, 168–169, 207–209.

62 Bodmann, *Rheingauische Alterthümer*, vol. I, 200.

63 For a more detailed discussion of the rule of Santo Spirito and its adoption by the women, see above, Chapter 3.

64 Bockenheimer, *Der Gutleuthof bei Mainz*, 4–5, was the first to observe this absence.

65 Alfred Hilgard, ed., *Urkunden zur Geschichte der Stadt Speyer* (Strassburg: Trübner, 1885), 67 (charter of 5 January 1259).

66 Hilgard, ed., *Urkunden zur Geschichte der Stadt Speyer*, 71, 9, 72, 18, 25.

67 Archives de Strasbourg 1AH 215–217, 1 AH 7432.

hospital does not appear until the year 1321, when the "good people [guten leuten]" appear as the recipients of an annual gift of grain; the same gift is made to the "sick in the hospital," suggesting the possibility of a recent separation of, and still active connection between, the two communities.[68] Moreover, the leprosarium and the hospital appear as beneficiaries in a list of religious houses, moving from the cathedral and ancient foundations of the city, through mendicants and canons, to beguine houses and hospitals.

The account book of Worms' leper hospital contains methodically organized records of income owed and revenues received, but no indications of when properties were acquired. The entries are organized geographically, revealing that the hospital's holdings were concentrated in vineyards, fields, and gardens, with urban property as a secondary concern. Extensive grain revenues, and the management of a granary and bakehouse, are also suggestive of the hospital's active involvement in local markets.[69] The one dated entry is from the late fifteenth century, a period roughly contemporary with the hand in which the bulk of the entries are written.[70] The scope of the work suggests that it served as a compilation; but of how many decades' acquisitions and donations it is impossible to say.[71] The account book of Speyer's leper hospital, similarly, was created from extant records in 1584, making the organizational principle useless for analysis of the hospital's medieval organization and administration. Few of the records originated in the medieval period. The earliest dates are for the 1380s, though the hospital is known to have flourished before then, and there are many undated entries.[72]

The internal records of the central Rhineland's *leprosaria* testify not only to their prosperity, but also to their integration in local markets, and visibility in urban environments. These institutions had socio-spatial locations that were far from isolated, and in variable positions relative to the symbolic and geographic centers of their respective cities.[73] This contradicts the

68 Heinrich Boos, ed., *Urkundenbuch der Stadt Worms*, vol. 2 (Berlin: Duncker und Humblodt, 1890), 112.

69 StAW Abt. 1B Nr. 2011, fol. 6v, 33v.

70 StAW Abt. 1B Nr. 2011

71 StAW Abt. 159 Nr. 431/1 contains excerpts from the hospital's inventories of possessions from 1486 through 1787, compiled in the late eighteenth century. The entries take the form of neatly numbered brief abstracts of document contents, and contain no clues to the dating of the documents referred to.

72 StASp III 122–3 B.

73 On shifts in location like that of the civic hospital, reflecting shifts in administrative control, see e.g. Stanford, *Commemorating the Dead in Late Medieval Strasbourg*, 269–270. As observed in Pauly und Uhrmacher, "Die Koblenzer Hospitäler in zentralörtlicher Perspektive," 340–342, determining the precise location of early medieval hospitals is often an impossibility. Brocard,

frequent claim that the liminal location of leper hospitals marked them as intrinsically different from other institutions dedicated to the sick-poor.[74] The discussion here concentrates on hospitals rather than the less formal leper communities that did not enjoy religious status, though it is worth noting that the chartulary of Essen's leper hospital unusually refers to the hospital residents as "the lepers in the huts," perhaps referring to an earlier mode of institutional organization.[75]

The leper hospital of Worms was a focal point of a neighborhood despite being on the outskirts of the city.[76] The hospital's location outside the city walls was shared with the "new hospital" founded in the thirteenth century. Both this, and the fact that the location *extra muros* is not used as a characteristic descriptor in donation charters or contracts, indicate that this peripheral location was not seen as central to the lepers' collective identity. Moreover, the lepers of Worms appear enmeshed in the city's property markets.[77] In Speyer, the leper hospital was located in the street of the salt merchants, at the heart of the city's mercantile and liturgical activity. In Mainz, the leper hospital managed both a location on the main road leading west out of the city, and a chapel within Mainz where the sick were also cared for, in addition to numerous leased properties. Such social and economic interactions were not unique to this region. Rouen's

Soins, secours, et exclusion, 247–258. See also Simon Roffey, "Treating Leprosy: St. Mary Magdalen, Winchester," *Current Archaeology* 267 (2012), 12–18.

74 Walter Schneider, "Die Hospitäler im Raum Alt-Tirol: Probleme einer Pass- und Übergangsregion," in *Funktions-und Strukturwandel spätmittelalterlicher Hospitäler im europäischen Vergleich*, ed. Michael Matheus (Stuttgart: Franz Steiner Verlag, 2005), 90–3. Cf. Brenner, "Outside the City Walls," 141–3; Neeb, "Zur Baugeschichte des Hospitals zum Heiligen Geist," 57; Uhrmacher, *Leprosorien im Mittelalter*, 37–9; Joseph P. Huffman, "Potens et pauper: charity and authority in jurisdictional disputes over the poor in medieval Cologne," in *Plenitude of Power: The Doctrines and Exercise of Authority in the Middle Ages. Essays in Honor of Robert Louis Benson* (Aldershot: Ashgate, 2006), 118.

75 Stadtarchiv Essen Rep. 100, Nr. 2147.

76 For use of the leper hospital as a geographical marker, see Boos, ed., *Urkundenbuch der Stadt Worms* 235, 238, 240, 271. For comparative secondary references, see Schaab, *Geschichte der Stadt Mainz*, 413; Karl Baas, *Mittelalterliche Gesundheitsfürsorge im Gebiet des heutigen Rheinhessens*, Veröffentlichungen aus dem Gebiete der Medizinalverwaltung (Berlin: Richard Schoetz, 1931), 34–36; Erich Hinkel, *Das Gau-Algesheimer Hospital. Beiträge zur Geschichte des Gau-Algesheimer Raumes*, (Carl-Brilmayer-Gesellschaft: Gau-Algesheim, 1987), 1, for a regional pattern of hospital foundations along the Rhine in the late thirteenth century. See *Spätmittelalter am Oberrhein*, 85, for discussion of the extramural economic activities in Worms. Michael Matheus, "Vom Bistummstreit zur Stiftsfehde: Mainz 1328–1459," in *Mainz: die Geschichte der Stadt*, 178–181, emphasizes the close social and economic ties among the great episcopal cities of Mainz, Worms, and Speyer.

77 *Boos, ed., Urkundenbuch der Stadt Worms* vol. II, 15, 22, 112, 156, 195, 401, 442.

Mont-aux-Malades, like Mainz's St. Georg, remained integrated in the city's economic life, owning numerous houses and properties in the city. They also hosted an annual fair, the popularity of which indicates that contagion must not have been a pressing fear. The leper hospital of Holstein, like that of Mainz, had a dual location inside and outside the city walls.[78]

Located approximately ten minutes' walk beyond a city gate, Mainz's leper hospital, dedicated to St. Georg, was strategically situated on the great road to Paris. Within the city, St. Georg held several properties, concentrated in a few neighborhoods. In addition to possessions in the Stephansberg, St. Georg held interests in several properties along the Kirschborn, a canal running through a busy neighborhood that might be described in modern zoning parlance as mixed-use. St. Georg held rents on houses at the heart of the Kirschgarten, near bakehouses, bathhouses, and private residences, ensuring that, symbolically at least, the interests of the lepers were central in the business of Mainz. That this location was significant is suggested by the fact that rents on the house "Zum Wilden Gans" were retained by the hospital through several generations and even a change of name of the property itself.[79] The chartulary entries pertaining to the property suggest a longer and better documented history for St. Georg's possession of it than that which now survives. A charter of 1427, for example, contains both a brief history of the house's tenants and a marginal note that "now it has been leased to a haberdasher."[80]

Associated still more intimately with the hospital was the chapel of St. Georg, identified according to its location either as "in die Marktstrasse" or "auf dem Schweinmist." Though the only historian to identify the chapel as belonging to the leprosarium does not cite evidentiary support for the claim, extant documents bear out the interpretation of the chapel and the hospital as linked communities.[81] A bequest preserved in St. Georg's

78 Brenner, "Outside the City Walls," 139–140; Meinert, *Die Hospitäler Holsteins*, 69–72. For the debate on the socio-spatial location of hospitals, see Andreas Puth," 'Our and the Empire's Free City on the Rhine': Visualizing the Empire in the Mainz Kaufhaus Reliefs," in *Mainz and the Middle Rhine Valley*, eds. Ute Engel and Alexandra Gajewski (Leeds: British Archaeological Association, 2007), 89–90.

79 StAM 32/700, f54v–55r. Rents on the property were shared with the hospital sisters of St. Agnes, at least from the early fifteenth century; HStAD C1 A Nr. 89, f. 54v–55r.

80 StAM 32/700, f. 18. [1427]

81 Baas, *Mittelalterliche Gesundheitsfürsorge*, 35, identifies the St. Georgskapelle by the Schweinmist, first named 1297 (charter of 14 May in StAM 13/282, f. 50v) as belonging to the leper hospital. Rita Heuser, *Namen der Mainzer Strassen*, 240, mistakenly identifies the chapel of St. Georg as being within the hospital complex outside the Gautor; Fritz Viktor Arens, *Die Kunstdenkmäler der Stadt Mainz* (Berlin: Deutsche Kunstverlag, 1962), 68, says that the chapel

chartulary, for instance, is made to “the priest who is chaplain and says Mass for the leprous of Mainz in the city.”[82] A similar bequest, including the chapel alongside other hospitals, survived in St. Georg’s possession.[83] The chapel also appears in connection with a community of “clusenern,” resident or active there.[84] The presence of such women suggests that the chapel could have provided a place of care, as well as worship.[85] The record linking the women with the chapel specifies that they may make full use of a garden and its produce, particularly useful for communities providing food and medicine for the sick-poor.[86]

The association of the leprosarium with the chapel and those who served it is corroborated by the discussion of a “cloister” and “chapel” of St. Georg, in a separate location from the St. Georg which is reached “by the public road,” in the *liber vitae* of the Liebfrauen canonry.[87] The location of the St. Georg chapel near the pigs also indicates a possible connection of the hospital with hygienic hazards. The chapel’s location near the property of the Antonine friars (whose the pigs almost certainly were), and not far from the hospital of St. Alexius, suggests that there was a belt of charitable institutions along the Ambach.[88] In the case of St. Georg, this concentration of property also

became associated with beguines; there is no evidence for the latter assertion, which Arens probably took from the statement of Schaab, *Geschichte der Stadt Mainz*, 361.

82 StAM 32/700, f14–15.

83 StAM U / 19 September 1431.

84 StAM U / 19 September 1431. The title of “clusenern” need not have denoted a community of strictly cloistered women; see Christian-Frederik Felskau, “Von Brabant bis Böhmen und darüber hinaus. Zu Einheit und Vielfalt der ‘religiösen Frauenbewegung’ des 12. und des 13. Jahrhunderts,” in *Fromme Frauen—unbequeme Frauen? Weibliches Religiosentum im Mittelalter*, ed. Edeltraud Klueting (Hildesheim: Georg Olms Verlag, 2006), 75–76; Walter Simons, “Beginnings: Naming Beguines in the Southern Low Countries, 1200–1250,” in *Labels and Libels*, 44. Cf. Elizabeth Makowski, “When is a beguine not a beguine? Names, Norms, and Nuance in Canonical Literature,” in the same volume, 83–98.

85 Letha Böhringer, “Beginen und Schwestern in der Sorge für Kranke, Sterbende und Verstorbene: Eine Problemskizze,” in *Organisierte Barmherzigkeit: Armenfürsorge und Hospitalwesen in Mittelalter und früher Neuzeit*, ed. Artur Dirmeier (Regensburg: Verlag Friedrich Pustet, 2010), 127–131; Walter Simons, “Beginnings: Naming Beguines,” 43; Felskau, “Von Brabant bis Böhmen,” 98–99.

86 HStAD A2 168/546 (1390). The presence of a vowed community connected to the chapel is claimed by Schaab, *Geschichte der Stadt Mainz*, 361. Jennifer Kolpacoff Deane, “Geistliche Schwestern: the pastoral care of lay religious women in medieval Würzburg,” in *Partners in Spirit: Women, Men, and Religious Life in Germany, 1100–1500*, ed. Fiona J. Griffiths and Julie Hutchin (Turnhout: Brepols, 2014), 243, notes that chapels could provide centers for informal groupings of lay religious women.

87 StAM 013/287, f16r-v.

88 Lester, “Crafting a Charitable Landscape,” 141, has described similar patterns for the towns of northeastern France.

enabled the hospital to cultivate multigenerational relationships with its donors.

Surviving evidence for leper hospitals not associated with cities indicates that, although such institutions may have been more economically precarious than those in larger urban centers, they cultivated similar relationships with their neighbors. The 1344 testament of a parish priest in Oppenheim includes both the multipurpose hospital and the leprosarium of the village among numerous charitable bequests. Thirty poor persons and beggars are to be given alms on his anniversary, indicating a concern with the sick-poor.The sick lying in the hospital of Oppenheim, and the "lepers in the chapel of St. Nicholas at the gate of the same," each receive the same sum.[89] The will of Conrad, a priest in Spangenberg, is still more specific, arranging for gifts of eggs and herrings to the leprous in the village's hospital. He charges the hospital administrators with fulfilling the terms of his bequest, using vocabulary that conforms to the requirements of canon law.[90] Whether or not Conrad regularly provided spiritual services to the hospital is not specified, although the hospital was clearly served by a priest as required by Lateran III. In any case, he had a thorough knowledge of the needs of the hospital and its residents. The oral testimonies recorded in his will indicate that the lepers and the leper hospital were embedded in a network of religious persons and institutions. Heimerich Fischbach, the hospital representative, and several civic officials of Spangenberg, among others, testify to the validity of the charter created at Conrad's insistence. The shifting use of the first person indicates that pledges to witness the fulfillment of Conrad's wishes were taken orally, as well as written down, attested with the seals of the city, the hospital representative, and a priest.[91]

Living by the Rules: Regulating the Rhineland's Leper Hospitals

The clearest contrast between multipurpose hospitals and *leprosaria* is found in the emergence of their rules. Although leper hospital rules do not have distinctly different priorities from those of multipurpose institutions, leper hospital rules in the Rhineland first appear much later than those of their multipurpose counterparts, which accompanied waves of

89 HHStAW Abt 22 Nr. 438, 34v–39r.
90 HStAM Urk 86 Nr 887.
91 HStAM Urk 86 Nr 887.

thirteenth-century religious legislation. This may reflect a relatively lax approach to twelfth-century developments in canon law; northern French statutes show a wave of leper hospital statutes devised in the late twelfth and early thirteenth centuries, and a later one, following the Council of Vienne.[92] In the archdiocese of Mainz, service to the leprous appears to have endured longer as an independent signifier of religious identity, and guarantor of religious privileges.

The first rule for the leper hospital of Worms was issued in 1440 by the Bürgermeister and council of the city. No mention of a previous rule is made, nor are existing customs explicitly referred to except as regarding internal practices, though the wording suggests that the rule supplemented customs internal to the hospital.[93] The hospital's population appears to have been diverse: the language of the rule provides evidence that men, women, and adolescents of both genders resided in the leper house, and that they came from the surrounding region as well as the city itself. Although they are referred to as the "poor sick set apart [*armen siechen ausgesetzt*,]" there are no indications that they were shunned by the healthy population of Worms. The central concern of the rule is obedience; the hospital's lepers are accused of frequently wandering about without leave. The directions for the lepers' conduct in the city are shaped by hygienic concerns: they are not allowed access to the kitchen or the running water of the house, and should also avoid the street, "as is the custom."[94] The statutes appear chiefly concerned, however, with internal organization, predicated on the religious status of the house and its residents.

The rule of Worms emphasizes that the lepers owe to the house their obedience in life, and their property after death; they are admonished to be content with the amount of their maintenance, even if this has to be temporarily decreased because of the house's poverty.[95] There are the expected prohibitions on sexual relationships between patients, but also indications that accusations of such relationships should not be lightly believed.[96] Infraction of the rules is to be punished with losing the privileges of the house, indicating that segregation cannot have been the ultimate goal of

92 Le Grand, *Statuts d'hôtelsDieu*, 181–223 for the earlier phase, 224–252 for the latter.

93 StAW Abt 1 AI Nr I–0364.

94 StAW Abt 1 AI Nr I–0364.

95 StAW Abt 1 AI Nr I–0364.

96 For similar prohibitions, cf. Le Grand, *Statuts d'hôtels-Dieu et de léproseries*, passim; it is worth noting that they are not limited to leper hospitals. See Rawcliffe, *Leprosy*, 86.

such houses.[97] If the lepers sit on the street or go into the city, to the churches or elsewhere, they must wear their grey felt hats and old clappers. They are directed, for the sake of hygiene, to avoid bakehouses, bathhouses, "and all other places that a leper should avoid."[98] The lepers' distinctive clothing is portrayed as a form of identification—fulfilling the requirement for religious persons to wear a habit—rather than an inalienable marker of disease.[99] While it is clearly concerned with particulars of local circumstances and public hygiene, the rule echoes religious language, and priorities, common to numerous hospital statutes from the preceding centuries.

In Essen as in Worms, the leprosarium was overseen by burghers of the city, while being bound by canon law. The case of Essen further demonstrates that civic authorities might use canon law to reinforce the institutional identity and institutional power of hospitals they managed. Rather than seeing religious status as an impediment to their authority, they used it as a tool. The founding narrative of Essen's leper hospital, crafted in the 1470s, invokes both ecclesiastical privileges and the agency of council members as authoritative. While unusual in its amplitude, this document is far from atypical in its concerns, defining the revenues and types of donation to which the hospital is entitled, and defining the hospital's social purpose as consisting in the care and comfort of the leprous. One of the notable things about Essen's narrative is that it scrupulously records preexisting legal privileges. Originals do not survive; but independent charters attest to the existence of the leper hospital as an established institution from the second half of the thirteenth century. Moreover, the records copied into the foundation narrative track an evolution of privileges and priorities consistent with late medieval social and legal developments, rather than seeming to respond with suspicious aptitude to contemporary concerns.[100] Marginalia marking passages related to particular properties and privileges suggest that the unusual document was used in legal contexts; this interpretation is strengthened by the fact that the chartulary of Mainz's leper hospital was used in a similar way, according to internal evidence.

Although the communal autonomy of lepers is often spoken of as a prerogative eroded under external pressures from the later thirteenth century

97 StAW Abt 1 AI Nr I–0364. Infractions may be punished by the provisor by removing wine or meat for two or three days.

98 StAW Abt 1 AI Nr I–0364.

99 StAW Abt 1 AI Nr I–0364.

100 Stadtarchiv Essen Rep 100, Nr 2148.

on, Mainz's St. Georg retained its legal privileges without intervention from either ecclesiastical or secular authorities until the end of the fifteenth century. The city council of Mainz was involved in appointing hospital staff, but on the evidence of St. Georg's chartulary, these men do not seem to have aggressively intervened in the policies of the hospital or the decisions of its residents.[101] Such intervention on the part of Mainz's ecclesiastical authorities comes only after the archbishops had reasserted their rights to exercise political authority over the city, in 1462. The first known rule, issued in 1488, was long preserved by the hospital; the original no longer survives, although Bockenheimer claims to have seen it in the nineteenth century.[102] That the hospital's relationship to Mainz's authorities became a concern only after the reassertion of the archbishops' political power is suggested by the fact that the rule contains, alongside injunctions of obedience to the sick, a strongly worded command to the staff. "All the staff and representatives of the hospital's lepers, are commanded on their oath to diligently observe and enforce all articles, and to fulfill the following, as every leper of the house has promised to do, and has sworn by the saints."[103] The importance of hospital staff as guarantors of order was also long a theme of conciliar legislation.[104]

When St. Georg finally had rules imposed on it, statutes were handed down by the archbishops in 1488, 1493, and 1512. This flurry of regulation cannot be attributed to alleged late medieval decline; there was scarcely time between edicts for lapses in observance. Questions of who had the right to examine for leprosy (and collect the fee for so doing!) were prioritized over those of separation, or even internal regulation. A number of points suggest that the assertion concerning the hospital's traditional independence in 1488 was accurate.[105] Firstly, St. Georg's property was unusually concentrated in geographic scope, lying within a radius of roughly twelve kilometers of the hospital. Such concentration of property may have been embraced as a deliberate strategy to increase ease of administration, a particularly pressing desirability for institutions where those who supervised the fields and vineyards may not all have been able-bodied.[106] Furthermore, once

101 StAM 32/700, f4–5, 8.

102 The rule is printed in Gudenus vol. 1, 942. Bockenheimer, *Gutleuthof*, 11, says that the original survives, but does not say where.

103 StAM 0032/704.

104 Ziegler, *Medieval Healthcare and the Rise of Charitable Institutions*, 101–117.

105 StAM 32/704; StAM U / 6 June 1493; StAM 3 October 1512.

106 Bettina Toson, *Mittelalterliche Hospitäler in Hessen zwischen Schwalm, Eder, und Fulda* (Darmstadt: Hessiche Historische Kommission, 2012), 98–100, adduces the parallel case of the

the lepers of St. Georg joined the hospital, they appear to have exercised considerable agency in that community.

Although the ordinances of 1488 limit the rights of the lepers of St. Georg to inspect those seeking admittance to their community, their own infraction of the house's rules is to be punished with loss of their privileges there.[107] This indicates that, even after the plague, contagion and segregation were not the primary concerns of authorities; and that residence in the leper hospital conferred recognized legal privileges. The archbishop evinced concern that such privileges were granted (for a fee!) all too readily by the hospital. The ordinances forbid the admittance of anyone, "whether male or female citizen of Mainz, inhabitant of Mainz or outsider, noble or nonnoble, religious or secular, man or woman, who is burdened with the sickness of leprosy and wishes to purchase a half or whole pension there," without the consent of Mainz's preeminent ecclesiastical and civic authorities.[108]

The walls of St. Georg were porous enough to allow ongoing relationships not only with those with whom they negotiated for supplies of wine and grain, but with those whom the hospital asked to appear as witnesses to their business transactions in court. Whether or not these men and women were connected to staff and patients by blood must remain speculative, though there are indications that the lepers of St. Georg may have continued in proximity to their friends and kin after death. A 1493 decree issued by Archbishop Berthold, and surviving in the possession of Mainz's university, contains an emphatic double prohibition concerning the use of the hospital cemetery. The lepers of St. Georg were to be buried there "and not elsewhere," and the cemetery was to be reserved for members of the hospital community.[109] This suggests that hospital donors sought burial within the enclosure—a practice well known for hospitals, as well as for other religious houses—and that lepers or their families might seek to restore the sick to their parishes, if only through burial in their parish churchyards. Archbishop Berthold's letter acknowledged that the lepers of St. Georg might wish to be buried next to their parents, or elsewhere. In such cases, they were to make arrangements with the hospital staff [*Pfleger und Vormünder*], confirming that this burial took place with their knowledge and permission. This remarkable exception to the rule of the community's

St. Georg leper hospital in Melsungen. See also Pauly and Uhrmacher, "Die Koblenzer Hospitäler in zentralörtlicher Perspektive," 346–347.

107 StAM 0032/704.

108 StAM 0032/704.

109 StAM U / 6 June 1493. This privilege is also contained in the statutes of 1488, StAM 0032/704.

stability shows both the importance of the principle of religious obedience, and acknowledgment of the complex social identities of the leprous.[110]

Conclusion

Medieval leper hospitals were affected primarily by the law that defined them, like other hospitals, as religious institutions, rather than by fear or loathing for a poorly understood disease. Prescriptive sources governing *leprosaria* spoke of the leprous as unable to live together with the healthy; but it should not be forgotten that similar sources spoke of monastic institutions and persons as being isolated from the world.[111] The rhetoric concerning hospitals should be treated with a similar skepticism. Documents of practice from the Rhineland show leper hospitals as active participants in religious, economic, and social networks. Few such records survive from the early Middle Ages; but the symbolic use of leprosy as a figure of sin, it has been argued, does not reflect a social view of lepers as sinners. Rather, legal texts suggest familiarity with leprosy, rather than fear; and hagiographical texts show lepers as cared for by family and friends, before their miraculous cures.

Evidence from the twelfth and thirteenth centuries indicates that lepers were often cared for alongside the other sick in multipurpose hospitals, a practice that began to wane in the mid-thirteenth century. Throughout the late Middle Ages, some lepers appear to have chosen to live independently, peripatetic or congregated in loosely organized communities at crossroads. These lepers we glimpse only obliquely, known by their gathering places, or as the recipients of food and clothing distributed by religious houses. The majority of those identified as lepers, however, apparently entered into leper hospitals. They took vows in so doing, surrendering their individual rights to property and inheritance in exchange for collective rights, and the privileges of the hospital. Their collective rights were acknowledged not only as significant in local contexts, but as tied to the privileges of leper hospitals as religious institutions. Leper hospitals emerge from the records as distinctive but not isolating places of care, where residents were given a common identity more through routines of liturgy and regimens of care than by their medical condition.

110 StAM 0032/704.

111 On the myth of monastic isolation, see Constance Hoffman Berman, *The Cistercian Evolution: The Invention of a Religious Order in Twelfth-Century Europe* (Philadelphia: University of Pennsylvania Press, 2000), 23–33.

The diverse socio-spatial locations of *leprosaria* in the archdiocese of Mainz—both outside and inside the walls, and possessing significant urban properties—show these institutions as continuously embedded in the socioeconomic networks around them. The ways in which lepers engaged with their healthy neighbors outside the hospital, and with the economic hubs of their urban environments, were affected by considerations of hygiene and good order. Isolation, however, never appears as the ultimate goal of administrators, nor revulsion as the default reaction of citizens. Leper hospitals appear connected in diverse ways to urban communities. They were included alongside their multipurpose counterparts in bequests; like other hospitals and monastic houses, they cultivated multigenerational relationships with their neighbors and donors. These patterns demonstrate that the legal parameters of hospital life, rather than social attitudes towards leprosy as disease, were formative in the development of institutions for the leprous.

5 "For all miserable persons": Small and Extra-Urban Hospitals

Abstract
This chapter examines small hospitals in the central Rhineland, concluding that, no less than more prominent institutions, such hospitals were integrated in their communities as religious houses. This chapter takes on both small and ephemeral hospitals in urban environments, and hospitals which flourished outside cities. The infrastructure of urban bureaucracy appears to have been a crucial factor in assuring the survival of medieval hospital records. The scattered and fragmentary evidence from extra-urban hospitals in the central Rhine region, however, offers glimpses of active and prosperous houses integrated with their communities, understood and functioning in similar ways to their urban counterparts.

Keywords: medieval hospitals, canon law, leper hospitals, medieval poverty

The leper hospital of Spangenberg is known to us only through a single record, of the mid-fourteenth century. In this document Conrad, a priest of the hospital, makes a will in favor of the hospital and its sick, in terms revealing much about the hospital's functions. Conrad sets, for "the comfort and health of his soul," a sum designated for alms, to be distributed by the hospital master. Some of these alms are to be generally distributed, while twelve sick, permanently resident in the hospital, are to be given eggs and herrings. Notably, Conrad specifies that no one except these twelve sick—not even the hospital master or a hospital priest—is to receive these alms, echoing the prescriptions of the Council of Vienne.[1] These prescriptions are

1 HStAM Urk 86 Nr 887. Joseph Alberigo, Joseph A. Dossetti, Pericles Joannou, Claude Leonardi, and Paul Prodi, eds., *Conciliorum Oecumenicorum Decreta,* 3rd ed. (Bologna: Istituto per le

Barnhouse, Lucy C. *Hospitals in Communities of the Late Medieval Rhineland. Houses of God, Places for the Sick.* Taylor & Francis Group, 2023
DOI: 10.5117/9789463720243_CH05

witnessed both by the hospital master and by members of the council of Spangenberg.[2] The case of Spangenberg provides an extreme example of the paradox of the small hospital: characterized by a fleeting and fragmentary presence in the documentary record, such institutions nevertheless appear as thriving institutions, useful to their communities and acknowledged within them as providing both therapeutic and spiritual services.

Hospitals Beyond Cities

Hospitals have often been spoken of as institutions that helped to define medieval cities, and contributed to their centrality.[3] But what of hospitals that boasted no such institutional influence? Small medieval hospitals and those located outside urban centers have received comparatively little scholarly attention. Their omission distorts the picture of how medieval hospitals were part of communities and networks. Where nonurban hospitals have been studied, it has usually been in connection to pilgrimage routes.[4]

scienze religiose, 1973), 351; on the diet of lepers, see Elma Brenner, *Leprosy and Charity in Medieval Rouen* (Woodbridge: Boydell, 2015), 93–99; Nicole Brocard, *Soins, secours, et exclusion: Etablissements hospitaliers et assistance dans le diocèse de Besançon, XIVe et XVe siècles* (Paris: Presses Universitaires Franc-Comtoises, 1998), 277–281; Rawcliffe, *Leprosy in Medieval England* (Woodbridge: Boydell, 2009), 213–232; on hospital diet and its therapeutic use more generally, Daniel Le Blévec, *La Part du Pauvre: l'assistance dans les pays du Bas-Rhône du XIIe siècle au milieu du XVE siècle,* vol. 1 (Rome: École française de Rome, 2000), 786–805; Kerr, *Monastic Hospitality*, 121–153; Joel Agrimi and Chiara Crisciani, "Charity and Aid in Medieval Christian Civilization," in *Western Medical Thought from Antiquity to the Middle Ages*, ed. Mirko D. Grmek (Cambridge, MA: Harvard University Press, 1998), 182–192; Paul Meyvaert, "The Medieval Monastic Garden," in *Medieval Gardens*, ed. Elisabeth Blair Macdougall (Cambridge, MA: Harvard University Press, 1986), 32–33; Timothy S. Miller, *The Birth of the Hospital in the Byzantine Empire* (Baltimore: Johns Hopkins University Press, 1985), 15–24; Christine Jéhanno, "L'Alimentation hospitalière à la fin du Moyen Âge: l'Exemple de l'Hotel-Dieu de Paris," in *Hospitäler in Mittelalter*, 107–130.

2 HStAM Urk 86 Nr. 887.

3 Michel Pauly, "Hospitäler im Mittelalter-wann und wo gehörte das Hospital zur Stadt?" in *Was machte im Mittelalter zur Stadt? Selbstverständnis, Außensicht und Erscheinungsbilder mittelalterlicher Städte,* eds. Kurt-Ulrich Jeschke and Christhard Schrenk (Heilbronn: Stadtarchiv Heilbronn, 2007), 245–269, esp. 261–262; Pauly and Uhrmacher, "Versorgungsgebiet," 211–254; Pauly and Uhrmacher, "Die Koblenzer Hospitäler," 346–347; Fray, "Institutions hospitalières médiévales et problématique historienne de la centralité," 352–354. Jesko von Steynitz, *Mittelalterliche Hospitäler der Orden und Städte als Einrichtungen der Sozialen Sicherung* (Berlin: Duncker und Humblot, 1970), 103–106.

4 Bodart, "L'étude des traces matérielles de l'activité hospitalière en Belgique," 48–51; Fray, "Hospices et hôpitaux médiévaux," 195–196, distinguishes between urban hospitals and those "isolated" on pilgrimage and travel routes.

Gerardo Doti's study of hospitals in the Piceno region of Italy is exceptional in its consideration of both urban and rural hospitals. He notes enormous variation in the size and structure of hospitals, not always connected to their location.[5] Small and extra-urban hospitals provided useful services for pilgrims and others, particularly for the increasingly diverse and mobile populations of the later Middle Ages. The limited surviving documents from such institutions makes it difficult to reconstruct evidence for their quotidian practice.[6] While hospitals in small towns or villages often lack robust documentation, surviving records indicate that they, like their prosperous civic counterparts, cultivated connections between cities and their hinterland.[7] Despite the paucity of surviving sources, it is possible to construct a picture of how hospitals functioned in extra-urban environments.

Many medieval hospitals are known only through single references; it is entirely probable that many more have, as Doti claims, left no trace in the surviving sources. Sethina Watson has recently referred to known hospitals as "the tip of a lost iceberg."[8] Only a fraction of medieval hospitals were the prosperous urban institutions on which much historiography has focused, which makes the study of their smaller counterparts desirable despite its challenges. Large cities were often distinguished by the presence of multiple hospitals; often, however, only the most prosperous institutions have left substantial extant sources. This chapter includes institutions which, despite little presence in the documentary record, were integral and vital to networks of charity and healthcare in urban environments. Cities were not essential to the creation and the survival of active hospitals. They have, however, proved vital to the preservation of hospital history. Hospitals located in and near small towns, rather than thriving cities, were less likely to be associated with economic and bureaucratic infrastructures with a vested interest in preserving hospital records. Their properties and resources, too, were less likely to be significant to successive generations. But extant records indicate that they were vital to

5 Gerardo Doti, "La rete degli hospitalia nel Piceno," in *L'accoglienza religiosa tra tardo antico ed età moderna*, 50–53.

6 See Carole Rawcliffe, *The Hospitals of Medieval Norwich* (Woodbridge: Boydell, 1995), 135–149.

7 Le Blévec, *La Part du Pauvre*, 587–588; Rubin, "Religious Culture in Town and Country," 3–10; Pauly, "Für eine raumbezogene Hospitalgeschichte," calls for more interpretative work to be done on how hospitals connected medieval cities to their hinterland, and where hospital networks thrived.

8 Watson, *On Hospitals: Welfare, Law, and Christianity in Western Europe, 400-1320* (Oxford: Oxford University Press, 2020), 6–7, n. 9; on the challenges of studying small hospitals, see Brocard, *Soins, secours, et exclusion*, 39–41.

their communities, providing pastoral services and receiving donations as religious institutions.

The sources on small hospitals of the archdiocese of Mainz consist largely of passing references to such hospitals as geographical markers, as well as charters surviving in the records of more durable institutions. The only records for Bingen's leper hospital, for instance, are devoted to confirming its privilege to levy a bridge toll. This is indicative of the hospital's importance to the town and its trade in the later Middle Ages, but allows no further analysis of its social ties. No medieval documents for the hospitals of Ingelheim and Bacharach survive; their histories are reconstructed using records of the early modern period.[9] Such documents survive chiefly in the possession of prosperous monastic houses or of civic governments. Some few records pertaining to the medieval hospitals of the region also survive in full or partial transcription in the notebooks of Bodmann, Mainz's archivist at the turn of the nineteenth century.[10]

Several "hospitia" in the region are attested for the fourteenth century, in contexts indicating that they formed part of support networks for the sick-poor. A 1343 letter from Archbishop Heinrich von Virneburg to his tax collector, Conrad, records the intake of wine by his guesthouses (*hospitia*) in Frankfurt; Eberhard, chamberlain of Mainz, together with his wife Irmentrudis and son Phillip, sold goods including guesthouses in the villa of Treisen to the canonry of St. Peter.[11] The will of a widow, Luchardis, specifies that such "hospitia et herbergas" are to be free of "precarias, angarias...exactiones, consuetudines, vel jura generis cuiuscumque," confirming that such houses could receive the legal status of hospitals.[12] That a wealthy woman felt no need to specify the names or locations of the hospitals involved in her bequest is itself suggestive. Clearly, Luchardis expected her heirs and executors to know such institutions well. Both the local officials who took oaths affirming the privileges attendant on

9 Andreas Saalwächter, "Ingelheimer Armen- und Krankenfürsorge im Mittelalter," in *AltIngelheim: Kulturgeschichtliche Bilder aus der Vergangenheit Ingelheims und des Ingelheimer Grundes in gesammelten Schriften* (Ingelheim: Historischer Verein, 1958), 93–97; Susanne Schlösser, "Das Bacharacher Hospital. Ein Beitrag zu seiner mittelalterlichen und frühneuzeitlichen Geschichte," in *Bacharach und die Geschichte der Viertälerorte Bacharach, Steeg, Siebach und Manubach*, ed. Friedrich Ludwig Wagner (Bacharach: Verein für die Geschichte der Stadt Bacharach, 1996), 327–332.

10 HStAD C1 A Nr. 68; C1 A Nr. 78.

11 HStAD C1 A Nr. 78, 95, 109–110.

12 HStAD C1 A Nr. 68, 14–5. Luchardis, widow of Phillip, lord of Bolandia, makes over all her/their goods in Isenheim to the dean and chapter of Liebfrauen. Luchardis herself was present at the making of the contract.

the properties, and the canons who inherited Luchardis' wealth, must have known what and where these houses were. At least some of them may have been informal communities of lepers, known to have been present among the villages surrounding Mainz, but this must remain speculative.[13]

A tantalizing glimpse at the management of small hospitals is provided by a single account book folio, preserved only because it was used as a protective cover for a luxuriously illuminated *Glossa Ordinaria*. There are several indications—besides the record's survival in the possession of the Cistercian house of Eberbach—that this unidentified hospital, known as "Mappin," was located near Mainz. The hand is characteristic of the region; Mainz measurements are used in referring to quantities of grain; Mainz's emblem, the wheel, is drawn in the margin; and the installation of a new *magister* for the hospital takes place on the feast day of St. Martin.[14] The 1308 appointment of a Brother Wolfram as *magister* of the hospital in Mappin involves an exchange of livestock, arable land, and sacks of grain. The hospital buys oxen from Wolfram, while he buys measures of grain with which to sow his new land, rendering proceeds to the hospital.[15] These complicated transactions are suggestive of an arrangement by which the incumbent *magister* was provided, de facto, with a modest income by the hospital. The hospital would have needed a legal loophole to accomplish this; Brother Wolfram may simultaneously have held an external post, rather than having taken vows as a member of the hospital. One example of such a situation, although with unwaged staff, is found in the case of the canons of Liebfrauen acting as hospital staff for St. Barbara in Mainz. The hospital of Mappin had close relationships with its administrative staff. In 1318, Ludwig, a brother of the house, bequeathed in his will enough wool (and thread!) to provide a year's new clothing for the entire community, as well as some old clothes, cushions, and other wool, which was sold for a hefty sum.[16]

13 On such communities, see Lucy C. Barnhouse, "Good People, Poor Sick: The Social Identities of Lepers in the Late Medieval Rhineland, in: *Leprosy and Identity in the Middle Ages: from England to the Mediterranean,* eds. Elma Brenner and François-Olivier Touati (Manchester: Manchester University Press, 2021), passim.

14 Bodleian MS Laud Misc. 102, f1. The codex itself was produced in the twelfth century, but the relevant folio, recording events from the early fourteenth century, was obviously put in much later. Archbishop Laud's acquisition of the volume in the first third of the seventeenth century provides only a distant *terminus ad quem*.

15 Bodleian MS Laud Misc. 102, f1r.

16 Bodleian MS Laud Misc. 102, f1r.

The name of Mappin is not found in reference works, but the hospital must have been located not far from the city of Mainz.[17] An itemization of grain revenues from 1318 contains revenues in Bingen and Lorsch, and also in the villages of Bretzenheim and Algesheim, located in Mainz's environs. A reference to "the lord abbot and the visitators" suggests that the hospital was affiliated with the Cistercians, perhaps under the protection of Eberbach, where the record survives.[18] The community of Mappin was responsible for the management of a guesthouse and of a hospital dedicated to the poor. The guesthouse must have been of considerable size, as it held 24 beds "as much good as bad," and six great beds for the use of visiting nobility, in addition to blankets, hand towels, sheets, and pillows.[19] The hospital, too, was generously proportioned, with two floors and twenty-eight beds (with twenty-eight cushions) for the use of the poor. It may be inferred that the vowed staff resided on the upper floor of the hospital, since eight further beds were "in the cloisters in the upper house."[20] This remarkable survival both echoes conciliar language in recording what it possessed *ad usus pauperum*, and demonstrates the vitality of an early fourteenth-century hospital. Other records from the middle Rhineland indicate that Mappin's priorities and hospital management were representative: the hospital's revenues and outlay are reckoned in wine and grain; its possessions testify to the provision of shelter, food, and clothing for the sick-poor.

Mappin's documentation of an administrative transfer between staff, and of the material furnishings of the hospital, is unusual; but it seems reasonable to suppose that the realities it records were not atypical. A similar financial relationship between Mainz's hospital and its hospital master is illustrated by a dispute arising between the heirs of Conrad zum Römer and the hospital after Conrad's death. In 1322, Conrad's daughter and the hospital provisors went before the judges of Mainz, and many prestigious witnesses, to resolve the division of the former hospital master's property, including household goods. In the end, it was determined that only Conrad's utensils were to go

17 Böttcher, ed., *Germania Sacra*, 522; Friedhelm Jürgensmeier, ed., *Germania Benedictina: Die Männer- und Frauenklöster der Benediktiner in Rheinland-Pfalz und Saarland* (St. Ottilien: EOS Verlag, 1999); Jürgensmeier, *Die Mönchs- und Nonnenklöster der Zisterzienser in Hessen und Thüringen* (St. Ottilien: EOS Verlag, 2011).

18 On Cistercians and care for the sick-poor, see e.g. Watson, *Fundatio, Ordinatio, Statuta*, 178–179 (a leper hospital); Léon Le Grand, *Statuts d'hôtels-Dieu et de léproseries: recueil de textes du XIIe au XIVe siècle* (Paris: Alphonse Picard et Fils, 1901), 73, on the hospital of Lille; Lester, "Cares Outside the Walls," passim.

19 Bodleian MS Laud Misc. 102, f1v.

20 Bodleian MS Laud Misc. 102, f1v.

to his daughter, who was liable to pay a third of the debts her father had left owing to the hospital. The document resolving the dispute was witnessed by members of other families connected to the hospital; the dispute itself reveals that the rights of hospitals and hospital staff could be ambiguous even in the years following the Council of Vienne.[21]

Hospitals' religious status, rather than their size or prosperity, appears to have been the decisive factor in determining outside intervention. The Order of St. John provided one of the most stable models for hospital rules in the later Middle Ages, but this did not guarantee the prosperity of individual houses. The Hospitallers' house in Sachsenhausen appears as the subject of several letters from the center of the order, suggesting that the community may have been engaged in defending its rights around the year 1280.[22] The late thirteenth century also saw the provisors of the mixed gender hospital in Bingen taking initiative in a legal case. The Rupertsberg convent, on the other side of the dispute, may have originally had responsibility over the hospital, giving rise to the argument over whether the hospital or the convent was entitled to certain properties. Bodmann calls this Bingen hospital "the hospital of the Holy Spirit," but there is no internal evidence for such a dedication or affiliation. The presence of an Augustinian friar may indicate that the hospital had a relationship with Bingen's Augustinian house, as St. Agnes did with the friary in Mainz.[23] These records suggest that small hospitals, no less than more prosperous institutions, were affected by the efforts of Mainz's archbishops to reform the observance of religious houses in the 1270s–1290s.

Small Urban Hospitals

The establishment of the privately-founded hospital of St. Barbara reveals a keen awareness of the criteria for religious status in the mid-fourteenth century. The founder, Voltzo, a canon of Liebfrauen, is described as endowing the hospital in the knowledge that it is "a good and pious work to gather the sick and poor, pilgrims and exiles, and to succor their poverty, provide for their wants, and have pity on their afflictions."[24] This language defines the activities of the hospital broadly, while presenting all these activities as

21 HStAD C1 78, 40r-v.
22 HStAD C1 A Nr. 78, 94, 96.
23 HStAD C1 A Nr. 78, 60.
24 HStAD A2 120/1 (15 November 1353).

included under the canonical mandate that hospitals should be exclusively devoted to the care of the sick-poor. Voltzo's legal circumspection becomes even clearer in the description of the process by which he acquired the buildings to be used by the hospital. Each of the properties is listed with the assurance that he purchased them outright with his own money, and even these straightforward property transactions are described as being inspired by love of God and God's poor. One of the houses was owned by an apothecary and his wife, and thus likely to have been equipped with facilities suitable for the compounding of medicines. This suggests that Voltzo purchased the properties with a view to converting them into a hospital.[25] These properties, once legally united, were donated for the exclusive use of the hospital, described as a "public residence and shelter or *xenodochium* for all sick, poor, pilgrims, and vulnerable persons coming to this house from any place whatsoever."[26] The care these persons are to receive is explicitly defined as consisting in the provision of food and other necessities, echoing the language of fourteenth-century councils.[27]

The surviving records of Liebfrauen contain little direct information on the management of the hospital. Their record of endowments does, however, contain several references to the hospital as a point of orientation in the inspection of the canonry's properties. The codex, originally compiled by Henricus Medenbach in 1472, contains copies of charters dating back to the midfourteenth century. Three mentions of a hospital suggest that hospital territory is being referred to metonymically; the lack of specific geographical locations makes it likely that the hospital is St. Barbara, rather than an unidentified other hospital. The hospital held several acres of property along well traveled roadways in Mainz's agricultural belt, indicating that it supported itself at least partially by the consumption and sale of grain, whether this property was designated for St. Barbara's use by donors, in no longer extant charters, or by the canons of Liebfrauen, whose task it was to manage the hospital. That the latter might be the case in times of need is indicated by the marginal gloss "Et Barbare" in a late hand on a list of revenues. The hospital did have lay staff, in addition to the supervising canons; a Fridericus Melbecher von Geylhusen, identified as a servant of St.

25 HStAD A2 120/1. Charters concerning the apothecaries of Mainz indicate that special permission was required to build specialized equipment for the distillation of medicines (*electuariis.*) Cf. Hans Dadder, "Die frühe Entwicklung des stadtmainzischen Apothekenwesens bis zur Apothekerordnung Erzbischof Albrechts II. von Brandenburg," in *Das Apothekenwesen von Stadt und Erzstift Mainz* (Frankfurt am Main, Govi-Verlag, 1961), 18–24.

26 HStAD A2 120/1.

27 HStAD A2 120/1.

Barbara, appears in 1369 in the witness list of a contract between a canon of Liebfrauen and a tenant of the house.

The prosperous canonry of Liebfrauen appears to have been well known in Mainz for its regular provision of alms. Numerous donations from laypersons and clergy of diverse social standing are designated for the provision of food and clothing for lepers, poor scholars, and the indigent and infirm who gathered at the community's gate.[28] Voltzo may well have been engaged in the provision of such services even before endowing a separate establishment for the support of the sick-poor. In its extant records, St. Barbara appears both as an *eleemosynarium*, the word used for almshouse in the Council of Vienne, and under the much older word of *xenodochium* (literally: a house for strangers,) the Greek word used for the first European hospitals in the early Middle Ages.[29] Extant evidence makes clear that St. Barbara was governed by a set of statutes devised by the founding canon himself. These, unfortunately, do not survive; but multiple confirmations of them by the archiepiscopally appointed judges of Mainz do. Also surviving is the lengthy document issued by the judges of Mainz at the canon's request, approving the foundation of the hospital, and detailing its designation for the uses of the sick.

The agreement drawn up by Mainz's judges under Voltzo's direction is notably detailed in its specifications about the administration of the hospital, and in its emotional rhetoric of charity. Health is invoked in both its physical and its spiritual senses; Voltzo frequently speaks of his decisions about the hospital as being made *salubriter*. This vocabulary appears both in the hospital's foundation documents of 1353, and in the confirmation of its statutes and properties issued in 1361, suggesting its importance.[30] The

28 StAM 013/284, 69f, contains the fullest entries for the 1480s and onwards.

29 Jean Imbert, *Histoire des hôpitaux français: contribution à l'étude des rapports de l'église et de l'état dans le domaine de l'Assistance Publique: les hôpitaux en droit canonique du décret de Gratien à la sécularisation de l'administration de l'Hôtel-Dieu de Paris en 1505* (Paris: J. Vrin, 1947), 46–50; Reicke, *Das deutsche Spital und sein Recht*, 3–13; Franz Irsigler, "Matriculae, xenodochia, hospitalia und Leprosenhäuser im Frühmittelalter," in *Einrichtungen der sozialen Sicherung im mittelalterlichen Lotharingien. Actes des 13es Journées Lotharingiennes (12–15 October 2004)*, ed. Michel Pauly (Linden: Section Historie de l'Institut Grand-Ducal, 2008), 323–326; Franz Meffert, *Caritas und Krankenwesen bis zum Ausgang des Mittelalters* (Freiburg im Breisgau: Caritas Verlag, 1927), 60–64.

30 HStAD A2 120/1, StAM 6/30, f19–f24. The latter folia comprise three copies of St. Barbara's foundation charter, with an indulgence for its support. These documents, no longer extant, appear to have survived in the possession of the city's oldest hospital after St. Barbara's destruction in the Thirty Years' War. On the depredations of hospitals located outside the walls during the Thirty Years' War, see Barbara Günther, "100 Jahre Totenregister St. Barbara Hospital in Mainz (1700–1798)," *Archiv für mittelrheinische Kirchengeschichte* 40 (1988), 333.

instructions for the hospital's organization are given in the public forum of the court "so that no doubt may arise concerning its governance" after Voltzo's death. This formulation suggests that he was personally involved in the leadership of the hospital, a hypothesis supported by the model provided for the transmission of leadership between successive generations of administrators. The management of St. Barbara is to be taken on by two canons of Liebfrauen in perpetuity, with one in a position of seniority. Upon the death or retirement of the elder, the other is to be promoted, and another canon appointed to the secondary position.[31] This strategy prioritizes St. Barbara's institutional continuity over the convenience or aspirations of appointees from the mother house. Future administrators are advised that they should accomplish the *pia opera* of serving the hospital and the sick in such a manner that they might merit heavenly joy.[32] Such pious rhetoric clearly leans on that of conciliar legislation; in so doing, it claims for St. Barbara an institutional security that could often be precarious for such small houses.

A number of small hospitals within and around the city of Mainz were evanescent. St. Alban certainly cared for the sick, and managed an active hospital in the 1320s.[33] A 1288 charter records the donation of a spousal couple, designated for bread, wine, flesh, and fish to be distributed by the "master of the sick," with leftover funds to be given to the poor.[34] No independent records for a hospital attached to the house survive, but a charter of 1331 references "the field of the sick of the monastery of St. Alban"; in the same year, "the master of the sick of St. Alban" appears as the recipient of a rent of chickens.[35] Since the monastery had been destroyed in 1329 in the wars over the archiepiscopal election, this supports the idea that a separate hospital survived.[36] A 1384 letter belonging to the St. Katherine hospital mentions the hospital master of St. Alban as a holder of properties adjacent to their own.[37] If the hospital of St. Alban had dedicated buildings, records of these have not survived; but it did have a large and well-paid enough staff that "the maid (*ancilla*) of the hospital master of St. Alban" was able to donate a

31 HStAD 120/1.

32 HStAD 120/1.

33 The hospital master appears in 1327 as a witness in the closing of a dispute involving the prosperous and influential Cistercian monastery of Eberbach, printed in Rossel, *Urkundenbuch Eberbach*, vol. 2, 829 (nr. 832.)

34 StaWü Mainzer Urkunden Nr. 5072.

35 StAM U / 1331 Juni 26; StAM 13/231.

36 See Schmid, *Die Abtei St. Alban vor Mainz*, 146–160.

37 HStAD 168/527.

pound to the Liebfrauen foundation in 1373.[38] Another small hospital appears to have been managed by the canonry of St. Johannes.[39] In the chartulary of St. Johannes, an entry from 1285 records a gift from a chaplain in Kastel, on the anniversary of his ordination; among the diverse parcels of land he made over to St. Johannes were four acres designated as a gift to the hospital; this is the first record of such a hospital's existence.[40] The only other explicit reference to their hospital is a note that property in the village of Vilzbach, just outside Mainz, was made over to the provisors of "our hospital, called *ad coronam* or *hospitium Krone*."[41] The fact that the hospital had a sign to identify it—in Latin and the vernacular—indicates its usefulness to the surrounding community. Elsewhere in the chartulary, the hospital appears as a geographic marker; a burgher's testament makes clear that St. Johannes was known for the daily distribution of alms, which could well have taken place at the site of their hospital.[42] Another donation to St. Johannes, by a married couple, identifies their residence as "opposite the hospital and next to Peter the baker."[43] Since, elsewhere, other hospitals in Mainz are identified by name, and since no baker is known to have been located next to either the Heilig Geist Spital or the hospital of St. Agnes, it may be presumed that the hospital in question is the one managed by St. Johannes.

The apparent paradox of internal evidence for St. Johannes' administration of a hospital, and the hospital's invisibility in external documents, can be resolved if we accept the premise that the hospital did not have legal status as an independent institution. By the mid-thirteenth century, according to conciliar decrees issued by the archbishops of Mainz, monastic institutions were required to have facilities of care for the sick-poor.[44] Such facilities could vary considerably in size; this is suggested not only by instances of independent communities originating within monastery complexes, but also by the legal stipulation that monastic hospitals did not themselves

38 StAM 013/284, 6. For more on poor and anonymous donors to this foundation, see Lucy C. Barnhouse, "'A Certain Poor Woman': Vulnerability and Visibility among Hospital Donors and Tenants," *Medieval People: Social Bonds, Kinship and Networks* 36 (2022): 133–154.

39 Ludwig Falck, *Mainz in seiner Blütezeit als Freie Stadt (1244–1328)*, Geschichte der Stadt Mainz III (Düsseldorf: Verlag Rau, 1973), 51, counts a hospital of St. Johannes as an independent institution in his brief survey of Mainz's medieval hospitals, claiming that St. Johannes had a separate hospital master and master of the sick in 1356. I was unable to find evidence of this.

40 StAM 13/231, 49–50 (pages numbered by archive.)

41 StAM 13/231, 31.

42 StAM 13/231, 3–7.

43 StAM 13/321, 114–115.

44 Giovan Domenico Mansi, *Sacrorum conciliorum nova et amplissima collectio*, vol. 23 (Florence: Antonio Zatta, 1759), col. 1080–1106.

possess the legal privileges of religious institutions.[45] Had the hospital of St. Johannes, located outside the walls of Mainz, functioned as an independent institution, it would have had to compete with the hospital of St. Katherine, a late medieval addition to Mainz's hospital landscape.

Until 1655, the hospital of St. Katherine was located in Vilzbach, by the Rhine, just outside the walls of Mainz.[46] Its date of foundation, as is the case for so many medieval hospitals, is unknown, but may be tentatively placed in the mid-fourteenth century. A reference to a certain "Elsa of St. Katherine" in the 1379 will of a male relative may refer to a sister of the mixed gender community.[47] St. Katherine's first certain appearance in the written record, in 1384, shows an established and reasonably prosperous institution. Its staff members (*Pfleger*) Orte zur Eiche and Heinz Schüler, who appear as its legal representatives, are both burghers of Mainz, and the hospital has its own seal. The transaction they conclude with the cathedral chapter is a lease of almost seventy-five acres of land, distributed in the outskirts of Mainz, on both sides of the Rhine. In exchange, Orte and Heinz agree that they and their successors shall make an annual payment to the cathedral chapter of thirty-six measures of good, dry grain.[48] The property's substantial size suggests that it may have been intended to serve as St. Katherine's main property base. Such an interpretation is supported by the silence of the written record concerning the hospital before this date, even as a geographical marker or as a neighboring property-holder.

The first known rule for St. Katherine dates to 1471, and was apparently created in response to archiepiscopal efforts to reinforce and extend their power over the city's religious institutions.[49] The rule prioritizes the

45 Gregory IX, *Decretals*, Liber III, Title XXXV, Cap VI, UCLA Digital Library Program. *Corpus Juris Canonici (1582)* http://digital.library.ucla.edu/canonlaw, last accessed April 23, 2020; Hostiensis, *Summa Aurea*, 1151–1152, http://works.bepress.com/david_freidenreich/35/, last accessed April 23, 2020. Johannes de Imola, *In Clementinas* (Venice: Johann von Köln and Johann Manthen, 1480), col. 322.

46 The mapping of St. Katherine's properties suggests that the hospital was in the neighborhood of the Winterhafen, which was flattened by bombs during the Second World War. See Heuser, *Namen der Mainz Strassen*, 578.

47 StAM U 14 May 1379.

48 HStAD A2 168/527 (18 January 1384.) The seal is now missing.

49 StAWü Mz. Urk. Geist. SchR. 22/5 (1471). Another copy of the hospital's regulations survives in StAWü MRA Spitäler K 755/14. For the political upheavals of Mainz in the 1460s, and their consequences for the city's religious institutions, see Kai-Michael Sprenger, "Die Mainzer Stiftsfehde 1459–1463," in *Mainz: Die Geschichte der Stadt*, 205–225; Michael Kläger, "Das Stadtbild im Wandel," in *Beiträge zur Mainzer Geschichte* 28 (1988), 18; Saalwächter, "Ingelheimer Armen und

obligations of poverty and obedience for all men and women entering the hospital community as vowed staff. All those who entered the hospital swore to abide by the terms of the rule, and to obey the hospital master, presumably elected from among their number. Moreover, they promised to surrender all their property, which would then be held and used in common by the hospital staff. The rule also enjoins the service of the sick, using the language of the works of mercy. Not only are the hospital master and the brothers and sisters of St. Katherine to "generously receive all the poor and miserable persons who seek the hospital in their need," but they are also explicitly commanded to give goods not necessary to the hospital—such as extra bedclothes—to those who could make good use of them.[50] Though this specificity is unusual, there is evidence for hospitals' regular provision of alms both in Mainz and in the nearby small town of Ingelheim.[51] The religious obligations of the staff are framed using the terms of the works of mercy. All of these characteristics of the rule support the claim of St. Katherine to the legal privileges of an independent religious institution.

The legal status of the hospital is also reflected in the administrative guidelines of the rule. The hospital master is commanded not to sell, alienate, or lease any of the hospital's revenue, echoing the language of *Quia contingit*.[52] Violation of these terms is punishable with the loss of office. The presence of multiple burghers and artisans named in the rule of St. Katherine as having authority to consult in the appointment of the hospital master suggests that St. Katherine may have been a private foundation. Hospital property and administration are clearly both concerns of the named laymen. The two bakers among their number may have been involved in the supply of the hospital as well as its oversight. The bake oven of Vilzbach, moreover, had its own path directly opposite St. Katherine's chapel.[53]

Krankenfürsorge," 94, makes clear that the destructive effects of the feud over the archbishopric were not limited to the seat of Mainz itself.

50 StAWü Mz. Urk. Geist. SchR. 22/5 (1471).

51 Jean Imbert, *Histoire des hôpitaux français: contribution à l'étude des rapports de l'église et de l'état dans le domaine de l'Assistance Publique: les hôpitaux en droit canonique du décret de Gratien à la sécularisation de l'administration de l'Hôtel-Dieu de Paris en 1505* (Paris: J. Vrin, 1947), 15–17; StAM U / 18 August 1386; StAM 13/231, 3–7; Karl-Heinz Henn, "Mittelalterliche Spitäler in Ingelheim: Krankheiten und Nöte lassen Standesschranken fallen," *Heimat am Mittelrhein* 47 (2002), 2.

52 StAWü Mz. Urk. Geist. SchR. 22/5 (1471).

53 Richard Dertsch, ed. *Die Urkunden des Stadtarchivs Mainz: Regesten,* vol. 2, (Mainz: Stadtarchiv, 1963), 197, Nr. 1404. The oven is also mentioned in connection with St. Katherine in Dertsch, *Die Urkunden des Stadtarchivs Mainz*, vol. 3, 99, Nr. 2010.

The creation of the scrupulously thorough rule at this comparatively late date may be explained by the turbulence of the 1460s, when Diether von Isenburg and Adolf II von Nassau were rival claimants to the archiepiscopal dignity. Diether, the candidate representing Mainz's civic elite, was elected over the papal candidate, Adolf, and reelected due to anxieties that his territory might be lost to the province. Although many of Diether's policies proved unpopular, his efforts to bring the city's religious institutions under a tighter rein may well have been welcomed by municipal elites.[54] The likelihood of an external rather than an internal stimulus for the rule's creation is suggested by the fact that St. Katherine appears as a recipient of donations from the midfourteenth through the midfifteenth century.[55] St. Katherine is also mentioned in the chartulary of St. Georg, demonstrating ties among the city's hospitals.[56] In 1400, the priest of St. Katherine is recorded as owing rents on his house to the Heilig Geist Spital.[57] St. Katherine's position in the hierarchy of the city's hospitals was a matter of more importance to some donors than to others. A burgher's 1369 will gave three beds to the Heilig Geist Spital, and "seiner klynster bette," his smallest bed, to St. Katherine.[58] Those living nearer to St. Katherine, or in the village of Vilzbach itself, were more generous; Rudolf zum More, another burgher, gave the same modest sum to the sick-poor of St. Katherine, of the Heilig Geist Spital, and of the hospital on the Ambach, managed by the women of St. Agnes.[59] St. Katherine was a significant property- holder in the village, and the few internal records that do survive show that it was knowledgeable about its neighbors and tenants, and connected to other religious institutions. Its ties were concentrated in a narrower geographic and social compass than those of Mainz's larger hospitals, but its comparative obscurity in the extant records may not imply a lack

54 Friedhelm Jürgensmeier, "Erzbistum Mainz," in *Die Bistümer des Heiligen Römischen Reiches von ihren Anfängen bis zur Säkularisation*, ed. Erwin Gatz (Freiburg im Breisgau: Herder, 2003), 416. StAWü MBVI 19 f5r; MartinusBibliothek HS 3, f72v and f87r. StAWü MBVI 71r–76r, a series of privileges obtained by the civic council from Archbishop Diether, bears testimony to his fraught relationship with civic elites.

55 Earlier references are vague and unsubstantiated. Dertsch, *Die Urkunden des Stadtarchivs Mainz,* vol. 1, Nrs. 417, 436, 446, 488; Dertsch, *Die Urkunden des Stadtarchivs Mainz,* vol. 2, 223, Nr. 1488.

56 StAM 700/2, 14. Dertsch, *Die Urkunden des Stadtarchivs Mainz,* vol. 3, 12–13, Nr. 1784.

57 Dertsch, *Die Urkunden des Stadtarchivs Mainz,* vol. 3, 323, Nr. 2688.

58 StAM 13/121, 153–157; Dertsch, *Die Urkunden des Stadtarchivs Mainz,* vol. 3, 44–45, Nr. 1864–1865.

59 StAM U / 24 April 1404.

of contemporary success.[60] In this, St. Katherine was typical of small hospitals in the region.

Hospitals in Religious and Ecclesiastical Networks

A bequest from a patrician couple of Mainz in the thirteenth century sheds light on the performance of liturgy in hospitals, and provision both spiritual and physical for the sick-poor. In 1266, Humbert zum Widder, a burgher of Mainz, and his wife Elizabeth, gave a farm in Oppenheim to the hospital of the same town. It is specified that the hospital staff may dispose of the property as they wish; a further ration of grain, wine, and cash is designated "for the maintenance of the priests who celebrate Mass for the sick-poor in that hospital and provide spiritual care for them in other ways."[61] Humbert and Elizabeth also give twenty measures of grain in exchange for the promise that their anniversaries will be observed with the burning of lamps day and night in the room where the sickpoor receive care. The choice of grain, presumably for direct use by the sick-poor, may reflect an awareness of the legal limitations on gifts made to hospitals as religious institutions, even as the designations for the support of priests and provision of anniversary services shows that the hospital was valued for its religious privileges. This gift may have been intended to help Oppenheim's hospital provide care commensurate with recently acquired civic dignities. After decades of somewhat turbulent history, Oppenheim had joined the Rheinischer Städtebund formed by Mainz and Worms in 1254.[62] But the lack of surviving documentation for the hospital suggests that, while the city emulated its larger and more prosperous neighbors, its hospital failed to do likewise.

Surviving records of landowning and exchange by Mainz's small hospitals indicate that such institutions had ties to their neighbors and to other religious institutions in the city, as well as to each other. The same dynamism is seen in hospitals elsewhere in the archdiocese. The few records surviving for the hospital of Fritzlar, a cathedral town north of Frankfurt, make

60 StAM U / 27 August 1423 (confirming an agreement made in Lent of the previous year) and StAM U / 25 April 1437 record agreements between St. Katherine and the Carthusian convent of Mainz, which was located nearby; see the Digitales Häuserbuch Mainz, http://www.mainz.de/microsite/digitaleshaeuserbuch/kartenteil/index.php, last accessed July 27, 2023.

61 HStAD A2 197/25.

62 Karl Schaab, *Geschichte des großen rheinischen Städtebundes, gestiftet zu Mainz im Jahre 1254 durch Arnold Walpod* (Mainz: Kupferberg, 1854), 8–13.

its history appear to be an untold success story. From the thirteenth to the fifteenth centuries, the hospital appears in archiepiscopal charters at moments of transition or tension in its institutional history, as well as in a handful of donation records. In 1229, Siegfried II took the hospital "under his protection and that of the blessed Martin," confirming the hospital's status as a religious institution.[63] The next appearances of a hospital in Fritzlar occur in 1308. The letter issued by Archbishop Peter von Aspelt speaks of the hospital as a new construction, but the record created by the hospital community itself makes clear that this was not a new foundation. The hospital sisters, having made an agreement with the burghers of Fritzlar, assert their rights to a priest, a chapel, and a cemetery in a new location.[64]

The new location is identified as near a bridge, which would have been a favorable location for alms collection. The move to a location outside the city walls may well have been prompted by lay dissatisfaction with the hospital's occupation of increasingly scarce and valuable urban property, as in the case of St. Agnes in Mainz. The archbishop's letter, in speaking of the growth and expansion of the hospital, supports such a hypothesis. Archbishop Peter's charter also indicates tensions concerning the hospital's privileges as a religious institution; the archbishop writes that, by his "special grace," the hospital may maintain its own priest, and a cemetery within the city.[65] Both charters draw on the legitimizing language of canonists and councils in speaking of the hospital's dedication to the care of the sick and the performance of the works of mercy.[66] Fourteenth-century donation charters for the hospital similarly emphasize the hospital's functions both of long-term care and of alms distribution.[67]

Like Mainz's oldest hospital, that of Fritzlar was dedicated to the Holy Spirit, but had altars dedicated to regional saints, including Martin ("confessor and our patron") and to Katherine, Dorothy, and Barbara, two of whom were notably also associated with the hospitals of Mainz.[68] An archiepiscopal

63 J.F. Böhmer and Cornelius Will, eds., *Regesta archiepiscoporum Maguntinensium. Register zur Geschichte der Mainzer Erzbischöfe von Bonifatius bis Heinrich II.*, vol. 2 (Innsbruck: Wagner, 1886), 255, nr. 328 identifies the hospital as dedicated to the Virgin Mary, but the transcription in Gudenus I, 556, makes it clear that it is the hospital altar that is dedicated to Mary.

64 Stephan Alexander Würdtwein, *Dioecesis Moguntina*, vol. I (Mannheim: Typis Academicis, 1768), 483–484. Würdtwein identifies the hospital sisters as "die klosterjungfrauen des hospitalis." The extent to which this unusual macaronic formulation may echo the charter directly is difficult to say.

65 Würdtwein, *Dioecesis Moguntina*, 483.

66 Würdtwein, *Dioecesis Moguntina*, 483–484.

67 Würdtwein, *Dioecesis Moguntina*, 492–504.

68 Würdtwein, *Dioecesis Moguntina*, 480.

charter of 1476 makes clear that these altars were meaningful foci of devotion for those in the hospital's wider community, as well as for its residents. Shortly after his second election to the see of Mainz in 1475, Archbishop Diether von Isenburg (r. 1459–1461, 1475–1482) specified, presumably at the request of the hospital staff, that the altars were sufficiently endowed for the support of a priest, and that his duties could be performed without prejudice against the priest of the parish in which the hospital was situated.[69] The agency of Fritzlar's hospital community is more directly visible in another charter obtained from Archbishop Diether, this one in 1481. This charter confirms an extensive list of properties and privileges, from the *jus patronatus* of the hospital, to their privileges of celebrating Masses, to their rights to properties and revenues given by a burgher family of Fritzlar. The archbishop confirms all these rights, and affirms that the hospital is entitled to all manner of "constructions, foundations, and endowments" undertaken for the sake of divine worship, the salvation of souls, and just and pious vows.[70] The late medieval documentary history of Fritzlar's hospital, while slight in proportion to its apparent prosperity, is more abundant than that of many others. It is characteristic in that documents concerning the hospital's legal privileges comprise the majority of its records.

The period of institutional formalization in the 1220s–1230s brought a hospital in Gotha into the documentary record; but following a period of several legal transfers, it fades once more into obscurity. A papal request to Archbishop Siegfried II resulted in the grant to the hospital of its own crypt and chapel in 1229.[71] According to this record, the hospital was founded by Ludwig (husband of St. Elisabeth) and his mother; the dates concerned, however, suggest that their patronage may have been to an already existing community, perhaps through donations made in connection with Ludwig's departure on crusade. Archbishop Gerhard I gave an indulgence of twenty days to supporters of the hospital, identifying it as a hospital for the poor.[72] Although the hospital survived throughout the later Middle Ages, its records have not.

69 Würdtwein, *Dioecesis Moguntina*, 480. On Diether von Isenburg and medical care, see Hermann Reifenberg, "Die 'Ansprache' be der Krankensalbung nach Mainz Diözesanbrauch seit dem Mittelalter," *Mainzer Zeitschrift* 60/61 (1965/66), 62.

70 Würdtwein, *Dioecesis Moguntina*, 480–481.

71 J.F. Böhmer and Cornelius Will, eds., *Regesta archiepiscoporum Maguntinensium. Register zur Geschichte der Mainzer Erzbischöfe von Bonifatius bis Heinrich II.*, vol. 1 (Innsbruck: Wagner, 1886), 201, Nr. 576.

72 Böhmer and Will, *Regesta archiepiscoporum Maguntinensium*, vol. 2, 343, Nr. 212. The editors mention no original charter.

The hospital of Oppenheim was a thriving institution in the thirteenth and fourteenth centuries, although none of its internal records survive. A multipurpose institution, it was led by a prior, with a staff of clerical and lay brothers; these men kept the hours, as well as caring for the sickpoor. The fact that the hospital had only one altar suggests that it was comparatively small, but several priests customarily administered the sacraments there. A 1325 property dispute offers an unusual glimpse at a case where a prosperous burgher appears to have had recourse to the hospital in serious illness. A certain Fritzo of Ostersheim having died in the hospital, his moveable and immoveable properties, including a house opposite the hospital, became the subject of dispute between his brother and the house of Eberbach. Fritzo's testament is referred to, but not extant. The charter records the "dissent and rancor" between opposing parties, and the intervention of Fritzo's executors as "friendly mediators." At stake are properties in part neighboring the hospital "where the said Fritzo died."[73]

It has been speculated that the hospital emerged from the direct oversight of a monastery in the mid-twelfth century, and was the object of archiepiscopal reforms in the mid-thirteenth. Surviving evidence is inconclusive, but such an institutional trajectory would fit regional patterns.[74] Like the house of St. Agnes in Mainz, the hospital of Oppenheim was included in the wave of reform imposed on religious houses by Archbishop Wernher von Eppstein in the 1280s. The rights granted to the hospital at that time were confirmed by Archbishop Peter von Aspelt in the early fourteenth century, indicating that the hospital was vigilant in maintaining its privileges.[75] The fifteenth-century records of the papal penitentiary make clear, moreover, that the hospital property was recognized as having religious immunity.[76]

The hospital of Oppenheim was also integrated in networks of religious houses, with ties both to the prosperous convent of Marienkrone in Oppenheim itself, and to the canonry of St. Stephan, in Mainz. When, on 28 October

73 HStAD A2 186/6. None of the witnesses "specially called to hear these things" are named as hospital staff, nor is any further information about Fritzo's illness given.

74 Carl Wernher, "Das Hospital zum Heiligen Geiste," in *Oppenheim: Geschichte einer alten Reichsstadt* (Oppenheim am Rhein: Oppenheimer Druckhaus, 1975), offers partially speculative background on the civic and leper hospitals in Oppenheim. The reconstruction is incomplete, and imperfectly clear. Cf. Karl W. Heyden, "Die Hospitäler in Oppenheim," *Oppenheimer Hefte* 1 (1990), 14–36; Susanne Schlösser, "Armen und Krankenfürsorge im Gebiet des heutigen Rheinhessen," *Archiv für hessische Geschichte und Altertumskunde* 49 (1991), 61–84.

75 Stephan Alexander Würdtwein, *Dioecesis Moguntina*, vol. I (Mannheim: Typis Academicis, 1768), 375–381; Böhmer and Will, *Regesta archiepiscoporum Maguntinensium*, vol. 1, 410, nr. 503.

76 Romana Repertoria Online, *Repertorium Germanicum* IV 12467, http://www.romanarepertoria.net/993.html

1280, Archbishop Wernher intervened to reform the hospital in Oppenheim and to give it new statutes, he did it together with the provost of St. Victor and the cantor of St. Stephan, who appear as joint issuers of the charter.[77] Moreover, the archbishop specifies that his guidelines for reform, focusing on the appointment of the hospital priest, have been created in accordance with suggestions made by the abbess of Marienkrone, a prosperous foundation that Wernher had brought into line with Cistercian observance some years earlier, in 1265.[78] The incumbent priest is not censured for his conduct; he was presented by the archbishop himself. It is specified, however, that in future the hospital priests are to be jointly presented by the abbess of Marienkrone and the provost of St. Victor, with the archbishop's consent, almost certainly granted as a formality.[79] The involvement of the abbess and the provost provides a glimpse of how hospitals could be integrated in regional religious networks. This integration was, of course, sometimes fraught; the last medieval record I have found concerning the hospital of Oppenheim concerns a dispute between a hospital priest and the community of Marienkrone.[80]

Small Leper Hospitals

The Middle Rhineland was dotted with small *leprosaria* along the river that led from the house of Melaten in Köln, through Bacharach and Bingen, to the great cities of Mainz, Worms, and Speyer. Few of their records survive, however; the existence of many houses is known only through singular charters.[81] Oppenheim boasted a leprosarium in addition to its multipurpose hospital; allegedly, the first records for it record episcopal indulgences for visiting and donating to it, clearly affirming its privileges as a religious

77 Würdtwein, *Dioecesis Moguntina I*, 375.

78 Böhmer and Will, *Regesta archiepiscoporum Maguntinensium*, vol. 1, 410, nr. 503; Wolfgang Seibrich, "Monastisches Leben von ca. 1200 bis zur Reformation," in *Handbuch der Mainzer Kirchengeschichte: Christliche Antike und Mittelalter*, ed. Friedhelm Jürgensmeier, vol. 2 (Würzburg: Echter Verlag, 2000), 692–697.

79 Würdtwein, *Dioecesis Moguntina I*, 378–379.

80 Romana Repertoria Online, *Repertorium Germanicum* V 01274, http://www.romanarepertoria.net/993.html

81 Martin Uhrmacher, *Lepra und Leprosorien im rheinischen Raum vom 12. bis zum 18. Jahrhundert* (Trier: Porta Alba Verlag, 2011), 97–99. Uhrmacher, who described these hospitals as a "string of pearls," comprising their own network, omitted the leper hospital of Mainz from his valuable catalog of them.

institution.[82] The only extant records I have found relating to the hospital date to the fifteenth century: a single donation, which treats it as well known to the surrounding community, and a reference to the hospital priest in the registers of the papal penitentiary. The donation charter, issued by a married couple, makes donations to multiple religious institutions in Oppenheim, and gifts to be distributed in alms, in addition to the money designated "for the feeding of the poor sick in the leper hospital of Oppenheim."[83] St. Goar is widely reputed to have had a thriving leper hospital. The saint's association with the cure of lepers makes this probable; but the earliest extant record unambiguously referring to the presence of lepers in the town dates to the sixteenth century.[84] A visitation of St. Agnes, in 1496, refers to a "Brother Johannes, chaplain from St. Goar," who may have been a brother in the hospital there.[85]

A surviving record of income reveals that there was a moderately prosperous leper hospital in Friedberg in the later fourteenth century. The prosperity of this hospital appears to have been on the upswing around the year 1400, as several entries in the fragmentary *Salbuch* of Mainz's oldest hospital contain records of revenue originally paid by individuals, and later taken over by the lepers. The fact that the same family was originally responsible for the revenues suggests that the same community of the leprous replaced them as tenants.[86] This community of lepers was separate from the multipurpose hospital in Friedberg, which paid in slightly larger cash revenues at the Michaelmas ingathering. It is, furthermore, worth noting that the lepers of Friedberg are invariably referred to as themselves the holders and managers of property, apparently sharing the late medieval autonomy of Mainz's community of St. Georg. The economic power—and initiative—of leper hospitals is also illustrated by a 1322 contract between Count Ulrich von Regenstein and the leprosarium of Derneburg. The somewhat unusual involvement of a nobleman in the hospital's affairs is explained by the fact that the property which the lepers and their provisor have decided to sell

82 Wernher, "Das Hospital zum Heiligen Geiste," 309, reports that Gerhard II offered a forty-day indulgence in 1297, which was later confirmed by the Bishop of Worms.

83 StAM U / 18 September 1421. See also Romana Repertorium Online, *Repertorium Germanicum* VIII 02576, http://www.romanarepertoria.net/993.html

84 Sankt Goar MU 53 is a record of 1527 that refers to lepers being taken into hospital. See Frohn, *Aussatz im Rheinland*, 130, and Staerk, *Gutleuthäuser und Kotten*, 534.

85 HHStAW Abt. 22, 523 is a codex from the Cistercian monastery of Eberbach, dating to the early sixteenth century (some time after 1519) and containing copies of earlier records. Fols. 101r–102v contain the relevant visitation record.

86 HStAD C2 504/1.

was a donation made by the previous Count von Regenstein.[87] The language of canon law permeates the document, with the property and its legal rights being described as "given over to and taken over by the aforesaid lepers." The property is sold for a lump sum to be converted for the use of the lepers, for whom the money is currently more desirable than a farm. The farm itself is sold to another hospital, located closer to the property in question, and therefore perhaps better able to manage it.[88] The detailed terms in which Count Ulrich affirms his consent to the transaction suggests the possibility that the original gift was made in consideration of the particular needs of the leper hospital at the time. The repeated emphasis on the rights of the lepers themselves echoes the terms of the Council of Vienne, which declared that donations to hospitals could only be put to the services of the sick.[89]

Conclusion: Size and Significance

It can be difficult to discern whether the rates of survival reflect the contemporary significance of late medieval hospitals with anything like accuracy. The geographical and chronological spread of such records can yield a picture that is at least suggestive, if fragmentary. Wills, statutes, charters of donation, and ecclesiastical privileges suggest that the hospitals of small towns, like the more prominent ones of prosperous cities, were integrated in their communities as religious institutions. Their legal status could lead to conflict with parochial or civic officials, but also enabled their participation in religious networks, and their receipt of donations from a wide cross-section of the laity. No less than multipurpose hospitals, small *leprosaria* appear as successful institutions, contradicting the historiographical narrative claiming that such houses were likely to be obscure, ill-kept, and poverty-stricken.[90] Small hospitals of all types, like

87 HStAD A14 949.

88 HStAD A14 949.

89 Imbert, *Histoire des hôpitaux français*, 140–147; Brundage, *Medieval Canon Law*, 139–140.

90 Belkervan den Heuvel, "Aussätzige: Tückischer Feind und Armer Lazarus," 276; Courtney Krolikoski, "Saints and Sinners: The Role of the Saint in the Life of the Leper Before the Thirteenth Century," *Annual of Medieval Studies at CEU* 18 (2012), 67, 73–74; Beck, *Untersuchungen über die frühere Verbreitung des Aussatzes*, 12–32; Nicole Bériou, *Voluntate Dei Leprosus: les lépreux entre conversion et exclusion aux XIIème et XIIIème siècles* (Spoleto: Centro Italiano di studi Sull'altro Medioevo, 1991), 68–70; Boeckl, *Images of Leprosy*, 50–66 et passim; Borradori, "Etre lépreux autour de 1300," 105–113; Dols, "The Leper in Medieval Islamic Society," 891–893; Rafael Hyacinthe, *L'Ordre de Saint-Lazare de Jerusalem au Moyen Âge: Milites Christi* (Millau: Conservatoire Larzac Templier et Hospitalier, 2003), 30–42.

their larger counterparts, survive in the documentary record in ways affected by their religious status. When the criteria for this status were consolidated in the first third of the thirteenth century, many hospitals emerged into the record for the first time. Episcopal interventions account for many of these records, as well, as do charters created to confirm rights acquired by hospitals from ecclesiastical authorities, from their neighbors, or from donors. Reconstructing a full history of such hospitals may be impossible; but the composite history offered here aims to show the importance of acknowledging such hospitals as part of regional landscapes and networks.

6 Hospitals and their Networks: Recreating Relationships

Abstract
This chapter, devoted to analysis of hospitals' social networks, reveals that location and wealth both affected how hospitals cultivated relationships with donors and neighbors. The thirteenth-century popularity of hospitals with the laity—as founders, benefactors, and staff—has often been described as a manifestation of lay piety paralleling the rise of new religious movements. That the phenomena are connected is indubitable, but lay hospital foundations, or lay entrance into hospital service, have been too often treated as the result of mere devotion. Consequently, judgments on the success or failure of hospitals' so-called true purpose have too often been made according to anachronistic views on the relative worthiness of different groups—the poor versus the aged, for example—to receive care.

Keywords: medieval hospitals, religious institutions, donations, almsgiving

The Documents in the Case

In 1396, Wernher de Indagine, who served as the rector of the "new hospital" of Mainz managed by the sisters of St. Agnes, made his will; it provides insight into the social functions of late medieval hospitals. Though Wernher's possessions were modest, he bequeathed them with a specificity characteristic of much wealthier testators. Wernher did not wish his involvement with hospitals to end at his death; he left a furlong of arable land to the hospital in the village of Butzbach, near his birthplace, "to be converted to serve the pious uses of the sick."[1] He specified that a measure of the grain yielded by

1 StAM 13/231, f98r. Although the particle implies that Wernher was of an influential family, I can find no record of the surname "Indagine," "Imidagine," "Jundagine," or plausible vernacular equivalents in the records of Mainz.

Barnhouse, Lucy C. *Hospitals in Communities of the Late Medieval Rhineland. Houses of God, Places for the Sick.* Taylor & Francis Group, 2023
DOI: 10.5117/9789463720243_CH06

the land should be awarded to the priest or lay minister of the hospital, in exchange for annual commemoration of Wernher and his parents in the Mass.[2] Wernher left the same quantity of land, with the same direction that its produce should be used by the sick, to the hospital in his native Münzenberg. The final stipulation was that Wernher could repurchase either furlong of land, for a set price that would then be used as a pension for his support in whichever of the mentioned hospitals he chose. Presumably, this eventuality was foreseen in case Wernher felt that age and infirmity prevented him from discharging his office in the hospital of Mainz.[3] It can be surmised that Wernher chose the hospitals of Butzbach and Münzenberg, rather than the one where he served, as his places of commemoration—and eventual retirement and death—in order to be close to his place of birth, where he may have had more remaining kin.

In specifying that his gifts should be employed "for the pious uses of the sick," Wernher echoed the language of ecclesiastical councils and papal letters, as discussed in Chapter 1. The use of this vocabulary acknowledged—or claimed!—the hospitals' legal identity as religious institutions, and made their rights to the land and its produce unambiguous. The other specifications of Wernher's testament, however, demonstrate that the functions of late medieval hospitals were often broader than serving the physical needs of the sick-poor in the ways outlined by canon law. This points to ongoing late medieval tensions concerning the categories of those whom hospitals could legitimately serve. Hospitals' taking in of corrodians has sometimes been deplored as a sign of degeneracy, but Wernher appears to have perceived this as one of their services to the sick-poor and infirm.[4] Moreover, the liturgical commemoration provided by hospitals, and the prayers of hospital

2 StAM 13/231, f98r.

3 StAM 13/231, f98r-v.

4 Angers, "La bourgeoisie de Falaise," 222–223; Falck, *Die Geschichte der Stadt Mainz*, vol. II, 166–167; Ute Mayer and Rudolf Steffens, *Die spätmittelalterliche Urbare des Heiliggeist-Spitals in Mainz* (Stuttgart: Franz Steiner Verlag, 1992), 25; Ulrich Knefelkamp, *Das Heilig-Geist-Spital in Nürnberg vom 14–17. Jahrhundert: Geschichte, Struktur, Alltag* (Nürnberg: Verein für Geschichte der Stadt Nürnberg, 1989), 218–235, 359–362; Wolfgang W. Schürle, *Das Hospital zum Heiligen Geist in Konstanz; ein Beitrag zur Rechtsgeschichte des Hospitals im Mittelalter* (Sigmaringen: Jan Thorbecke Verlag, 1970), 70–80; Siegfried Reicke, *Das deutsche Spital und sein Recht im Mittelalter*, vol. 1 (Stuttgart: Enke, 1932), 66–67; Ulrich Knefelkamp, *Das Gesundheits und Fürsorgewesen der Stadt Freiburg im Breisgau im Mittelalter* (Freiburg im Breisgau: Herder, 1981), 41. Benjamin Laqua, *Bruderschaften und Hospitäler während des hohen Mittelalters: Kölner Befunde im westeuropäisch-vergleichende Perspektive* (Stuttgart: Hiersemann, 2011), 43–44, sounds a welcome note of caution. See Hans Liermann, *Handbuch des Stiftungsrechts. Vol. 1: Geschichte des Stiftungsrechts* (Tübingen: J. C. B. Mohr, 1963), 71–77, on the formation of legal expectations of corrodians.

communities (including and especially their sick members) were also valued by those in their social networks.

This chapter examines the connections between hospitals and their staff, neighbors, and donors; as the case of Wernher demonstrates, these groups could and did overlap. In the central Rhineland and beyond, hospitals cultivated relationships with donors and tenants that were multilayered, and sometimes intimate.[5] Account books and charters—and the annotations made on them by generations of hospital staff—reveal that hospitals' use of resources took account of their long-term viability as institutions; of the needs of the sick; and of the needs of their tenants and donors. Hospitals participated in regional economies in diverse ways, purchasing exotic ingredients for medicines, and selling as well as consuming the grain and wine they cultivated.[6] Moreover, like monastic houses, they provided diverse spiritual services for the laity, including the performance of memorial Masses. Looking at the individuals—from prosperous burghers to poor widows—who entered into relationships with Mainz's hospitals, can elucidate the hospitals' respective positions in local economic, social, and religious networks.

Comparison of the surviving records of Mainz's hospitals sheds light on how these institutions managed and perceived their privileges and possessions. This chapter uses records relevant to the hospitals of Worms, Speyer, and the Mainz institutions of the Heilig Geist Spital, St. Alexius, St. Barbara, and St. Georg. Few original charters survive in the possession of the institutions themselves, with the exception of St. Agnes. This is due to nineteenth-century classification: since St. Agnes was classified as a religious institution, while the documents of Mainz's hospitals were stored separately, different fates befell them at the time of the Napoleonic invasions, catastrophic to Mainz's archives.[7] Some charters documenting hospital possessions survive in the municipal records of Mainz, or in the holdings of monastic institutions, whether preserved in Mainz or Darmstadt. Internal evidence indicates that charters were often commissioned—and jealously guarded—by medieval hospitals. The initiative in ecclesiastical courts, where hospitals applied for affirmation of their privileges as religious

5 Stefan Sonderegger, "The Financing Strategy of a Major Urban Hospital in the Late Middle Ages (St. Gallen, 15th Century)," in *Assistenza e solidarità in Europa Secc. XIII-XVIII = Social Assistance and Solidarity in Europe from the 13th to the 18th centuries: atti della "Quarantaquattresima Settimana di Studi," 22–26 aprile 2012*, ed. Francesco Ammannati (Florence: Firenze University Press), 225–226.

6 StAM 33/1.

7 Wolfgang Wann, "Die alten Mainzer Archive," *Archivalische Zeitschrift* 60 (1964), 111–112.

institutions, always lay with the plaintiff.[8] Most of the extant medieval records belonging to the hospitals of the central Rhineland are chartularies and account books, the latter often based on oral testimony, as well as other documents. The differing forms of such records can be used productively in the analysis of how these institutions cultivated and managed their possessions. Hospital foundations were motivated by awareness of the needs of transportation networks and civic communities, as well as by charitable impulses. The needs of hospital networks were more often determined locally than by papal fiat.[9]

Charters and chartularies, individual testaments, *vidimus* records issued by municipal courts, and hospital account books all testify to the fact that hospitals' status as religious institutions affected their interactions with donors and tenants. Despite the statutes regulating hospitals as self-contained communities, their residents maintained unbroken social relationships with contacts outside the hospital, whether these were predicated on preexisting social or familial bonds, on practical exchanges, or the collecting of alms.[10] Useful work on the connections between the performance of charity and the performance of civic identity has focused on the activities of late medieval almshouses and confraternities.[11] In analyzing such connections

8 James A. Brundage, *Medieval Canon Law* (New York: Longman, 1995), 129–134. On hospitals' initiative in legal processes see e.g. Thomas Frank, *Heilsame Wortgefechte: Reformen europäischer Hospitäler vom 14. bis 16. Jahrhundert* (Göttingen: V & R Unipress, 2014), 15; Letha Böhringer, "Beginen und Schwestern in der Sorge für Kranke, Sterbende und Verstorbene: Eine Problemskizze," in *Organisierte Barmherzigkeit: Armenfürsorge und Hospitalwesen in Mittelalter und früher Neuzeit*, ed. Artur Dirmeier (Regensburg: Verlag Friedrich Pustet, 2010), 147–150; S. Jennifer Stemmle, "From Cure to Care: Indignation, Assistance, and Leprosy in the High Middle Ages," in *Experiences of Charity, 1250–1650*, ed. Anne M. Scott (Farnham: Ashgate, 2015), 59–61. Cf. Gabriel Cros-Mayrevieille, *Les frères donnés à la léproserie du bourg de Narbonne* (Toulouse: Privat, 1930), 28–30.

9 Maria Pia Alberzoni, "Norditalienische Pilgerhospize im 12. und 13. Jahrhundert," in *Wege zum Heil: Pilger und Heilige Orte an Mosel und Rhein*, eds. Thomas Frank, Michael Matheus, Sabine Reichert (Stuttgart: Franz Steiner Verlag, 2009), 290–292; Gisela Drossbach, "Hospitäler in Patrimonium Petri," in *Europäisches Spitalwesen*, 91–104; Sheila Sweetinburgh, *The Role of the Hospital in Medieval England: Gift-Giving and the Spiritual Economy* (Portland, OR: Four Courts Press, 2004), 106–112; Lester, *Creating Cistercian Nuns*, 39–42, 211–216; Sara Ritchey, *Acts of Care: Recovering Women in Late Medieval Health* (Ithaca: Cornell University Press, 2021), 1–34.

10 Weigl, "Städte und Spital," 420–425.

11 Frank Rexroth, "Zweierlei Bedürftigkeit. Armenhäuser und selektive caritas im England des 14. bis 16. Jh.," in *Sozialgeschichte Mittelalterlicher Hospitäler*, eds. Neithard Bulst and Karl-Heinz Spiess (Ostfildern: Jan Thorbecke Verlag, 2007), 11–37; Knefelkamp, *Das Gesundheits und Fürsorgewesen der Stadt Freiburg*, 41; Palmer, "The Church, Leprosy and Plague," 86; Cochelin, "Bourgeoisie et léproseries de la principauté de Liège," 15–18; Miri Rubin, *Charity and Community in Medieval Cambridge* (Cambridge: Cambridge University Press, 1988), 238–288; Monika

for hospitals, and the rhetoric and uses of hospital donations, this chapter makes use of network studies and charter analysis. These methods have proven fruitful in expanding and refocusing histories of monastic houses, and of manuscript circulation, but remain comparatively under-used by historians of medieval hospitals.[12]

This chapter considers the agency of medieval hospitals through their administrative policies, which illustrate their use and understanding of their privileges as religious institutions. There follows a discussion of the identity of Mainz's hospital staff, illuminating the social connections on which the institutions could draw. Surnames are known for so few of Mainz's hospital staff that the majority can be presumed to have been local. Lastly, I turn to the known donors of Mainz's hospitals, making a comparative analysis of those connected to the hospitals over time. Due to the notoriously labile vocabulary of such transactions, I have not limited myself to documents where the language of donation is explicitly used.

Property Administration and Communal Agency: Mainz's Civic Hospital in Perspective

Hospitals, although they could be dominant players in regional economies, functioned themselves as contained economic units where, e.g. grain acquisition would have a more or less direct effect on the food, clothing, and services available to the sick.[13] Hospitals in the Lower Rhine kept rent records organized both by location and by date due, from the beginning of the calendar year onwards, at intervals of approximately six weeks. The

Eschner-Apsner, ed., *Mittelalterliche Bruderschaften in europäischen Städten. Funktionen, Formen, Akteure* (Frankfurt: Peter Lang, 2009).

12 See the influential Barbara Rosenwein, *To Be the Neighbor of St. Peter: The Social Meaning of Cluny's Property, 909–1049* (Ithaca: Cornell University Press, 1989), 60–62; more recently, Julie Hotchin, "Reformatrices and Their Books: Religious Women and Reading Networks in Fifteenth-Century Germany," in *Communities of Learning: Networks and the Shaping of Intellectual Identity in Europe, 1100–1500*, ed. Constant J. Mews and John N. Crossley (Turnhout: Brepols, 2011), 251–291; Emilia Jamroziak, "Spaces of Lay-Religious Interaction in Cistercian Houses of Northern Europe," *Parergon* 27 (2010), 37–58; Montserrat Cabré, "Women or Healers? Household Practices and the Categories of Healthcare in Late Medieval Iberia," *Bulletin of the History of Medicine* 82 (2008), 18–51.

13 See Dross, "Their Daily Bread," 51, 54–55. Dross notes that scandals in hospital finance were often talked about in terms of the sick. Cf. Benjamin Thompson, "From 'Alms' to 'Spiritual Services:' The Function and Status of Monastic Property in Medieval England," in *Monastic Studies, II. The Continuity of Tradition*, ed. Judith Loades (Bangor, Gwynedd: Headstart History, 1991), 227–261.

method of recording, as well as the frequent intervals, suggests that the hospital chose this date distribution to ensure a ready flow of resources. The hospitals of Mainz had staff who were dedicated to pursuing collective policies and protecting their collective rights; nor were they exceptional in this.

Over the course of the thirteenth and fourteenth centuries, many hospitals worked to consolidate their properties, allowing able-bodied hospital residents to easily tend fields and gardens.[14] This strategic policy also affected hospitals' networks of neighbors, donors, and tenants. Mainz's hospitals held properties of varying types, in varying patterns of distribution. Geographical concentration or a preponderance of a certain type of property—flexible rents or profitable vineyards, for instance—can shed light on the needs and priorities of hospital communities. Notably, a 1331 charter concerning the religious privileges of St. Agnes lists the *colonos* and *cultivores* of the convent and hospital alongside the women themselves as members of the community.[15] A hospital's resources affected both the institution's capabilities and the social networks it cultivated. The evidence suggests that hospitals sought to cultivate relationships with particular donors, as well as to acquire particular types of donations.[16]

Records of property administration offer a window on the communal agency and communal influence of Mainz's hospitals. Such documentation becomes regular for Mainz's oldest hospital in the early fourteenth century; this is a pattern consistent with trends across Europe, as urban economies and the written record both expanded.[17] The hospital's account books bear

14 Bayrische Akademie der Wissenschaften, *Monumenta Boica* (Munich: Bayrische Akademie der Wissenchaften, 1763), VI 78 (12 December 1322); Vogt, *Regesten der Erzbischöfe von Mainz*, nr. 2024. Joseph P. Huffman, working with evidence from Köln, suggests that concentrations of hospital property and influence might align with parish boundaries. Pers. comm, 2015.

15 HStAD C1 A 78, f71v (1331).

16 See, for example, Sonderegger, "The Financing Strategy of a Major Urban Hospital," 215–216, and Brigitte Pohl-Resl, *Rechnen mit der Ewigkeit: Das Wiener Bürgerspital im Mittelalter* (Munich: Oldenbourg Verlag, 1996), 22–33.

17 Pohl-Resl, *Rechnen mit der Ewigkeit*, 142–143, argues that property administration was one of the chief ways in which hospitals exercised influence within the walls of the urban centers with which they were associated. On hospitals and urban economies, see for example Sethina Watson, *Fundatio, Ordinatio, and Statuta: The Statutes and Constitutional Documents of English Hospitals to 1300* (Oxford: D.Phil., 2003), 222; Sonderegger, "The Financing Strategy of a Major Urban Hospital," 213; Lester, "Crafting a Charitable Landscape," 130–135. On the emergence and expansion of hospitals' traces in the written record, see Ernst-Adolf Meinert, *Die Hospitäler Holsteins im Mittelalter: Ein Beitrag zur mittelalterlichen Stadtgeschichte* (Neumünster, Wachholtz Verlag, 1997), 14–15; on documentary culture generally, Rouse and Rouse, *Authentic Witnesses*, 1, 7–9. On the interrelation of urban networks and texts, see Franz-Josef Arlinghaus, "Point of

witness to ongoing and conscientious management. In volumes from 1315 and 1366, and one from 1395 surviving only in fragmentary form, the hospital organizes the records of its property and income both by location and by date. These volumes provide more than snapshots; interlinear and marginal glosses, as well as full entries added in other and later hands, demonstrate that these account books were heavily used by multiple members of the hospital community, and illustrate that hospital staff were attentive to the condition of their property and the needs of their tenants. The administrative staff of the hospital clearly had a good working knowledge of the hospital's properties, not only in Mainz, but in nearby villages as well. This knowledge may have been gained through personal investigation, or through conference with other members of the hospital staff who inspected the villages where the hospital held property, and thus knew the terrain and its legal boundaries.

All three of the hospital's account books use similar formatting, designed to facilitate reference in both property assessment and rent collecting, to judge by the marginalia. Possessions inside the city of Mainz are consistently listed first, with subheadings for the dates on which rents were due. Determining the dates on which revenues were received may itself have been a component of resource management, assuring a regular flow of cash and foodstuffs for the hospital.[18] Within Mainz, the routes of inspection taken by successive generations of hospital staff can be identified with some accuracy, due to the presence of named houses. The properties outside Mainz are described in a sequence moving geographically outwards from the city. Insofar as can be determined, the properties were also described in the order in which an inspecting official would tour them, moving along roads where landmarks were often given relative to other propertyholders. Such descriptions, laying out relations of properties and those who lived and worked in them, were a way in which lay persons "created" the space around them.[19] Similar descriptions are found in the charters of other hospitals in Mainz and beyond.[20] Addenda to the account books provide summary records of what revenues were expected on which dates, preserving the division between properties inside Mainz and in outlying villages. That this division was reflected in the deputization of different staff members

Reference: Trust and the Function of Written Agreements in a Late Medieval Town," in *Strategies of Writing*, eds. Petra Schultert, Marco Mostert, and Irene van Renswoude (Turnhout: Brepols, 2008), 286–288, 297.

18 See Dross, "Their Daily Bread," 52–55; Pohl-Resl, *Rechnen mit der Ewigkeit*, 137–143.

19 Lester, "Crafting a Charitable Landscape," 125–129.

20 StAM 33/2, f29. See also HStAD A2 168/392 (1353); HStAM Urk 86 Nr. 1233.

to inspect and collect from these properties must remain a speculation, but it is not an improbable one.

Of Mainz's hospitals, the Heilig Geist Spital held the most rents and properties in the urban center. The acquisition of such valuable holdings may well have been facilitated by the fact that the hospital was an established institution before the city's late medieval expansion, and by the hospital's connection to the influential and prosperous council. Such connections remain largely speculative, however; charters recording dates of sale or donation to the hospital are scarce. When recording their rights and possessions, hospital staff appear to have been less concerned with the origin of their claims than with identifying their property, their neighbors, and, in the case of rents, those who shared claims to revenue on a given house or courtyard.

Similar strategic patterns of acquisition and maintenance are visible in hospitals of comparable size and function; the surviving charters belonging to Essen's civic hospital also bear witness to a concentration both of properties and donors. The hospital appears to have cultivated two centers of property: one in the city, centered on the hospital itself, and one just outside the city walls. The hospital's donors are frequently recorded as giving the hospital arable land in the latter neighborhood, suggesting that the hospital may have solicited such donations, or that such lands were acquired with the intent of giving them to the hospital. In the latter half of the fourteenth century, 91 men and women made gifts of lands, cash rents, and grain to Essen's hospital and its staff. With few exceptions, these donors did not belong to the urban patriciate, but approximately a third of them enjoyed burgher status. Their donations, sometimes amounting to as much as several acres of land, or an annual revenue of grain sizable enough to sell in the marketplace, reflected both their status and their commitment to the institution. The donors to Essen's hospital were, moreover, a remarkably cohesive group. Approximately a third of them (33 of 91) specified that their heirs were party to their transactions; 38 of the 91 named persons donated alongside their spouses; and 35 gave as part of familial groupings, defined as transactions with three or more named persons as donors, rather than in cases where individuals are identified solely as the heirs of the principal donors. Essen was, of course, a much smaller city than Mainz. Even so, such a high concentration of family loyalty appears unusual, both when compared to donations to Mainz's hospital, and to donations to other religious houses in Essen.[21]

21 For the donors to Mainz's hospital, see the discussion elsewhere in this chapter; for donors to other institutions in Essen, see Thomas Schilp, "Totengedenken des Mittelalters und kulturelles

The Heilig Geist Spital's move to the walls of the city was followed by a concerted and rapid program of property acquisition to form a base of useful properties surrounding the hospital.[22] The hospital's fourteenth-century account books contain numerous records of land and revenues held "among the lower butchers" and "by the herring stalls."[23] The concentration of hospital properties among the butchers and the fish stalls of the city suggests that administrators prioritized pragmatism over prestige. The hospital fed its residents fish and flesh according to season; it appears also to have cultivated multifaceted relationships with its suppliers. Elsewhere in Mainz, the types of properties the hospital held, and the neighborhoods where they were located, were diverse. This suggests that the hospital's acquisition of urban property and revenues was influenced more by those who chose to donate to the hospital than by a policy pursued by staff.[24]

The records of the Heilig Geist Spital are extensive enough to permit the discernment of patterns in tenant naming. Inspection records for the villages along the Rhine where they had properties frequently include full names for tenants and neighbors, as well as comparatively detailed property descriptions.[25] The hospital's location on the Rhine appears to have been used to its economic as well as its hygienic advantage. Several tenants were commercially involved in river traffic, including a sailor named Cruger, of Bacharach, and a number of sailmakers. One of the latter, a woman named Nese, was both a tenant and, later in life, a hospital resident; she may be identical with the woman who bequeathed her property to the hospital and its staff in 1400.[26] Within Mainz itself, identifications rely heavily on local knowledge. The presence of "Kettchens," "Hennekins," and "Gretes" in the records reveals frustratingly little about the social composition of the hospital's networks. The fact that nicknames were adequate to identify so many, though, testifies to the intimacy of social contacts between these

Gedächtnis: Überlegungen zur Perspektive der Memoriaforschung für das Frauenstift Essen," in *Pro Remedio et Salute Anime Peragemus: Totengedenken am Frauenstift Essen im Mittelalter*, ed. Thomas Schilp (Essen: Klartext Verlag, 2008), 19–36.

22 For more detail, see Chapter 2.5, "Space, Identity, and Liturgy: The Hospital's New Location."

23 See StAM 33/2, f36; StAM 33/1, 68, 69; StAM 33/2, 5, 21, 31; StAM U / 29 June 1401 II. See also Heuser, *Mainzer Strassen*, 338–339, for the extent of this neighborhood.

24 Pace Meyer and Steffens, *Die spätmittelalterliche Urbare des Heiliggeist-Spitals*, 56–57.

25 See, for example, StAM 33/2, 79–85.

26 StAM 33/2 and StAM 33/4; Meyer and Steffens, *Die spätmittelalterliche Urbare des Heiliggeist-Spitals*, 230; U /16 October 1400. For hospitals' use of rivers as avenues of trade, see Peter Linehan, "A Tale of Two Cities: Capitular Burgos and Mendicant Burgos in the Thirteenth Century," in *Church and City, 1000–1500: Essays in Honour of Christopher Brooke*, eds. David Abulafia, Michael Franklin, and Miri Rubin (Cambridge: Cambridge University Press, 1992), 81–110.

tenants and the hospital.[27] Such dependence on close social ties is even more visible in the city's other hospitals.

The Women of St. Agnes and the New Hospital

When the women of St. Agnes established themselves on the Dietmarkt, a hub for trade in grain and livestock, they gradually acquired houses and rents in the vicinity of their convent. By the early fourteenth century, they began to develop a second pole of geographical focus: the hospital they managed on the Umbach, known simply as "the new hospital." Located in a periurban district, the hospital was approximately five minutes' walk from the convent. A legal agreement from 1348, drawn up at the behest of the abbess and the sisters of St. Agnes, illustrates the importance which the community laid on the creation and preservation of legal records. The document is created "forasmuch as we have learned of a praiseworthy custom, introduced for the certainty of the present, and the memory of those in the future, that people's deeds are rendered in writing, so that by this means, if necessary, both parties may return to it to avoid difficulties, to say nothing of trouble and expense."[28] This pragmatic prologue was anything but formulaic. The women further state that they have drawn up the record for the benefit not only of all those who might see and hear its contents, but for all who have an interest in the transaction... or believe themselves to have an interest in it. It is hard not to read the tone of this explanation as acidulous.

The transaction itself—the receipt of a perpetual income of two pounds in exchange for the offering of anniversary Masses, as called for in the will of a parish priest—is fairly straightforward. The number of altars involved has been reduced by the consent of the priest's executors, after consultation with the chaplain of St. Agnes; this charter establishes that, if the relatives of the deceased are dissatisfied and wish to reclaim the incomes, they must pay St. Agnes a lump sum. The importance of the transaction is attested by the presence of two seals, both of which are identified as belonging to St. Agnes. Another point of interest is that the *custodissa* of the community is mentioned numerous times as the individual responsible for contact with donors and oversight of proper use of incomes. It is tempting to see, in the unusual degree of activity foreseen for the holder of this office, the influence of hospital administration as a community responsibility. Other suggestive

27 StAM 33/1, StAM 33/2

28 HStAD A2 115/42.

evidence is found in the number of priests identified as connected with St. Agnes, even as the women complained of finding adequate income with which to support them.[29]

The women of St. Agnes were zealous not only in recording their rights, but also defending them in court. Urban properties, paths of access, wells, and latrines were frequent subjects of dispute. In 1379, for instance, Friederich Bender and Henchin Rodenscheiben came before a judge to confess that a latrine was theirs to use only by special favor of St. Agnes and not by law. A representative of St. Agnes' staff was sent to confirm that this was the nuns' good will and pleasure.[30] The language of several letters resolving such disagreements indicates that ongoing, informal, and possibly bitter negotiations often preceded the intervention of external authorities. When, in 1420, the civic building inspectors (*Baumeister*) Götze zum Jungen and Johann Luchtwiß mediated a controversy concerning St. Agnes' convent and their neighbor Hermann von Heidelberg, they spent time listening to both parties (presumably separately,) and visited the site. Having resolved the argument in the women's favor, Götze and Johann concluded that the letter should close all dispute between the parties, "and all malice should flow out into this letter."[31] The same metaphor of discord flowing into a letter, like water into a good channel, is used in a similar boundary dispute concerning a property owned by St. Agnes near the Fischporte by the Rhine. St. Agnes' neighbor is commanded to lower his wall, "as the above-mentioned women will not suffer it any longer," an atypical specification indicating that the women themselves were involved in discussions with the inspectors, and perhaps in observation of the property.[32]

The most persistent disputes over St. Agnes' property concerned possessions surrounding their hospital. A four-way dispute over an orchard, in 1468, resulted in the *Baumeister* holding sessions to listen to the testimony and counter-testimony of all parties involved, as well as seeing all their letters, registers, and charters, and assessing their respective plans for the property.[33]

29 HStAD A2 115/42. See also HStAD A2 168/339, a charter of 1343.
30 HStAD C1 A Nr. 89, 126v–127r (late November 1379). See Lucy C. Barnhouse, "From Helpful Gardens to Hateful Words: Moral and Physical Health-scaping in the Late Medieval Rhineland," in *Disease and the Environment in the Medieval and Early Modern Worlds*, ed. Lori Jones (London: Routledge, 2022), 52–64.
31 HStAD C1 A Nr. 89 folio 58r; folio 108v–109r (September 1432) makes clear that the effort was not permanently successful, but the women were again legally confirmed as having rights to the disputed properties.
32 HStAD C1 A Nr. 89 folio 104r. The original, dating to 1411, reads: "...das die obergenannte frauwen nit lenger liden wollent."
33 HStAD C1 A Nr. 89 folio 88r–89r.

In the event, St. Agnes retained the orchard near the hospital. The first extant charter recording convent possessions in and around the hospital survives in a copy in St. Agnes' account book. The date of 1330 indicates that the women held interests in the hospital before outright ownership of the land and buildings was transferred to them in 1341. They gathered rents on multiple houses, as well as on a fishpond, a butcher's, and an artisans' workshop. All these properties surround "the new hospital on the Umbach," which is identified by a later hand in the chartulary margin as "Sanct Allexien."[34] The women's acquisition of diverse properties concentrated around the hospital suggests the cultivation of resources dedicated to maintaining the hospital buildings, and to providing for its community.[35]

In addition to the fishpond and the butcher's, other adjacent properties may have supplied ingredients for medicinal recipes. Rights in the property "with courtyard, houses, garden, and fruit trees," and a gate going directly to St. Alexius, were given to Henne zum Bildensteder in 1405, after he had served the hospital as legal representative for over a decade.[36] The inclusion of Henne's descendants in the permanent lease agreement is significant, suggestive of the expectation that his family would continue to serve the hospital.[37] Repeated mention of a "house of the tailors" near the hospital suggests a similar multigenerational relationship, with the tailors as tenants, suppliers, or both.[38] The house was located between the hospital and a dyehouse on the Umbach in which St. Agnes also had rights. Though the convent made no such extensive contracts as with Henne and his descendants, St. Agnes did have agreements with the dyers extending over several generations. The first relevant record concerns a contract made during the tenure of Abbess Else with the dyer Bartholomeus, leasing a house adjacent to the dyeworks for his life's term; when Bartholomeus failed to pay his rents, the property reverted to the convent.[39] The convent fought for its rights not only over the dyehouse and adjacent residence, but a garden opposite the dyehouse. In this instance, the women of St. Agnes were apparently anxious enough to maintain their rights over strategic properties that social relationships were deemed to be of secondary importance.

The convent's property, more than that of the Heilig Geist Spital, and certainly more than that of the Cistercian houses of Altmünster, Dalen, or

34 HStAD C1 A Nr. 89 f. 20r–20v.
35 Cf. Dross, "Their Daily Bread," 49–66, passim.
36 Henne is first named as the hospital's legal representative in StAM U / 29 August 1392.
37 StAM U / 3 October 1405.
38 StAM U / 10 July 1454.
39 StAM U / 10 July 1454.

Weißfrauen, remained heavily concentrated in the bustling commercial and residential streets of the growing city. St. Agnes' policies changed not only over time but relative to specific properties, a phenomenon which has been underestimated by historians of hospitals' economic activities as institutions. The recorded property management of St. Agnes shows that strategies of property consolidation and the cultivation of relationships with tenant families coexisted, responding more to the needs of the hospital community than to external economic or social trends. This suggests that the relationships of hospitals with their tenants were more personalized than has hitherto been acknowledged. Adam Davis has recently analyzed multifaceted relationships between hospitals and their donors; I believe considering the plural ways in which tenants interacted with hospitals may also prove fruitful.[40]

The leper hospital of St. Georg, no less than Mainz's multipurpose hospitals, was active in creating and preserving documents relevant to its property rights. Its chartulary includes marginalia indicating when St. Georg, tenants, or officials had possession of the original charters. Charters could function as instruments of authority through having their contents read aloud, or could be used demonstratively in court procedures.[41] Multiple stages of oral debate and affirmation could be involved in their creation, as demonstrated by the 1351 procedure in which Hermann Dam and his wife came before the officials of Astheim and Siegfried, the public scribe, to make a gift to St. Georg. Hermann pledged an annual gift of sixteen measures of grain, from the grain on his good meadow, unless (God forbid!) the Rhine were to flood it. In that case, Hermann promised to fulfill the pledge with other grain, and that he and his heirs would have the responsibility for doing so in perpetuity. This was not viewed as satisfactory by Ortwin, "provisor and representative of Martin, the hospital master, and of the lepers." He demanded that the village officials affirm that the revenue from the grain, worth forty pounds, was adequately supported with pledges. And they answered, as the scribe records, "on oath, unambiguously, and unanimously, one after another, 'Yes, they were well supported.'"[42] And herewith Ortwin seems to have been satisfied, however chaotic the scene that was distilled by the scribe into those emphatic repetitions. This record marks the first

40 Davis, *The Medieval Economy of Salvation: Charity, Commerce, and the Rise of the Hospital* (Ithaca: Cornell University Press, 2019), 187–200.

41 Mary and Robert Rouse, *Authentic Witnesses: Approaches to Medieval Texts and Manuscripts* (Notre Dame, IN: University of Notre Dame Press, 1991), 1–4; Bedos-Resak, "Medieval Identity," 150–159.

42 StAM 32/700 f8–10.

documented appearance of Ortwin as the representative of the lepers in court; he was to fulfill that function at least until 1367. Ortwin's career is illustrative of the close personal ties that could tie staff to the institutions they served, even when not vowed to that service.

Hospital Staff: Their Roles and Relationships

In the contract made in Astheim, Ortwin is identified as "of Kostheim," a toponymic that would fall away in further records of his activities on behalf of the hospital of St. Georg. It is at least a plausible speculation that the identifying moniker in the 1351 document indicates that he had not held his office long. Ortwin's career at the hospital is only incidentally sketched in the surviving records; but piecing together his history of service may be instructive, in view of the paucity of surviving documentation on the men and women who served as hospital staff.[43] Members of Ortwin's family were also associated with St. Georg, within the same generation in which he served the hospital. His brother Jacob, for instance, leased a vineyard from the house.[44]

Ortwin himself is the only named member of staff included on St. Georg's expenses list, included in the hospital's chartulary.[45] The fact that he was a paid rather than a vowed member of hospital staff renders his long service and apparently passionate loyalty to St. Georg particularly interesting. Ortwin's demonstrative advocacy on behalf of the lepers appears in non-formulaic—and occasionally exasperated—language as recorded by the court scribes. To take but one example in addition to that discussed above concerning the fields of Hermann Dam, Ortwin appears as the commissioner of a written document over a grain revenue. The scribe records that Ortwin both presented documents to the court and officials in support of the hospital's claims "and commanded me to describe all of this, and make

43 Meyer and Steffens, *Die spätmittelalterliche Urbare des Heiliggeist-Spitals,* 35–39; Forey, "Women and the Military Orders in the Twelfth and Thirteenth Centuries," 67–71, 89–92; Laqua, *Bruderschaften und Hospitäler,* 48–49; Brodman, "Religion and Discipline in the Hospitals of Thirteenth-Century France," 123–132; Dross, "Their Daily Bread," passim; Knefelkamp, *Das Heilig-Geist-Spital in Nürnberg,* 218–235, 359–362; Georg Schreiber, *Gemeinschaften des Mittelalters: Recht und Verfassung, Kult und Frömmigkeit* (Münster: Regensberg, 1948), 62–71; Timothy S. Miller, *The Birth of the Hospital in the Byzantine Empire* (Baltimore: Johns Hopkins University Press, 1985), 15, 49.

44 StAM 32/701, 2–3.

45 StAM 32/701, f13.

a public instrument concerning it."[46] Ortwin's service was recognized and rewarded by St. Georg in the improvement of his legal status. By 1363, he appears as a freeman, the "former servant" of the hospital.[47] The language of this record also suggests that, just as Ortwin was not the only legal representative of St. Georg (a certain Emmerich fills that role in 1358), he may have filled additional roles in the hospital's service.[48]

There have been calls for more prosopographical exploration of hospital staff, donors, and the resident sick-poor.[49] For all but the wealthiest hospitals, however, such a goal is not easily obtainable. The individuals who served in hospitals are often elusive; rarely do staff lists survive before the fourteenth century. Many donors are known by their first names alone, unconnected with known families; the names of residents are scarcest of all. Reconstructions of hospital networks must use other means. Information from foundation charters or narrative accounts provides some clues; especially in the twelfth century, foundations were often entered by those who provided for their endowment, along with members of their family and household.[50] Franz Josef Felten has cautioned against assuming that such privately founded hospitals must have been essentially elite in culture or social composition.[51] Close ties of noble families to Mainz's hospitals are conspicuous by their absence.[52] This may be partly a consequence of the power held by the archbishops.

Relationships between hospital staff and donors are rarely made explicit, but connections with the inhabitants of particular neighborhoods within the city may be inferred.[53] The extent to which hospital staff remained

46 StAM 32/700 4–5.

47 StAM 32/700 4–5.

48 On Emmerich, see StAM 32/700 1–3, item 1.

49 Alberzoni, "Norditalienische Pilgerhospize," 277–278; Laqua, *Bruderschaften und Hospitäler*, 34–42.

50 Paul Bonenfant, "Les premiers 'hospitia' de Bruxelles au XIIe siècle," in *Annales de la Société belge d'histoire des hôpitaux* 11 (1973), 3–7, 9–13; Alberzoni, "Norditalienische Pilgerhospize," 290–292. Knefelkamp, *Das Heilig-Geist-Spital in Nürnberg*, 58, 64, 134, 219, 374. Laqua, *Bruderschaften und Hospitäler*, finds early thirteenth-century evidence for poor brothers taking vows in the hospitals of Köln and Trier as permanent vowed staff.

51 Franz Josef Felten, "Wie adelig waren Kanonissenstifte (und andere weibliche Konvente) im (frühen und hohen) Mittelalter?" in *Studien zum Kanonissenstifte*, ed. Irene Crusius (Göttingen: Max Planck Institut für Geschichte, 2001), 39–128. Laqua, *Bruderschaften und Hospitäler*, 43–44, discusses how the quality of wine used by hospitals might shed light on their social composition.

52 The Count of Reutlingen appears as a benefactor of the region's earliest leper hospital, but he and his wife form an exception, rather than a rule, among those named individuals associated with Mainz's hospitals. StAM U / 1109 (14/310).

53 On hospitals in particular neighborhoods, see the forthcoming work of Joseph P. Huffman on the hospitals of Köln. Dr. Huffman was kind enough to let me see his work on the hospitals

active outside the hospital, and occupied by interests there, could vary according to region and even according to institution.[54] James Brodman has argued that the strong language of hospital rules prohibiting shared meals or overnight absences in the homes of those outside the hospital should be read in light of inferred familial ties between hospital residents—staff and sick-poor alike—and the surrounding community.[55] Several scholars have analyzed the hospital as a type of double community where the sick-poor and hospital staff lived and worked and worshipped—together.[56] The records from the Rhineland bear out such a picture, of complex and close-knit ties linking hospital staff to their institutions, of staff themselves neither as the potential despoilers envisioned by conciliar legislation, or as persons animated by ahistorical zeal, but as knowledgeable, often canny, and not infrequently passionate individuals.

References to hospital personnel and residents in extant documents usually presume a working knowledge of the community's composition. The disadvantages to modern scholars have been widely lamented.[57] The degree of stratification within the hospital community must remain to some extent a matter of speculation; but the fact that hospital statutes of the thirteenth and fourteenth centuries very often include limitations on

in their parishes while it was in progress.

54 Brodman, "Religion and Discipline," 123–29, offers an overview of conciliar legislation, and its variable application by region. Cf. François-Olivier Touati, *Maladie et Société au Moyen Âge: La lèpre, les lépreux et les léproseries dans la province ecclésiastique de Sens jusqu'au milieu du XIVe siècle* (Bruxelles: De Boeck & Larcier, 1998), 358–62, for tables on the numbers of men and women, healthy and sick, in hospitals from the diocese of Sens. Knefelkamp, *Das Heilig-Geist-Spital in Nürnberg*, 242–74.

55 Brodman, "Religion and Discipline," 129–32. This could apply to staff and sickpoor alike. Brodman argues that such prescriptions, though not themselves constitutive of religious status, were seen as the best method of ensuring that hospitals' essential function was fulfilled.

56 Hyacinthe, *L'Ordre de Saint-Lazare de Jerusalem au Moyen Âge*, 23–41 et passim. Drossbach, "Hospitalstatuten im Spiegel von Norm und Wirklichkeit," 55–7. Concerning the obligations of the staff and sick, Elma Brenner, "The Medical World of Medieval Normandy," presentation at the Institute for Historical Research, London, 2 June 2015, notes that the dietary restrictions in many hospital rules applied equally to the staff and the sick, indicating a shared way of life.

57 Karl Baas, *Mittelalterliche Gesundheitsfürsorge im Gebiet des heutigen Rheinhessens*, Veröffentlichungen aus dem Gebiete der Medizinalverwaltung (Berlin: Richard Schoetz, 1931), 58. Ludwig Falck, "Mainzer Hospitäler im Mittelalter," in *Moguntia Medica: Das medizinische Mainz von Mittelalter bis ins 20. Jahrhundert*, ed. Franz Dumont (Wiesbaden: B. Wylicil, 2002), 410–411; Marie-Anne Saunier, *Le "Pauvre Malade" dans le cadre hospitalier médiéval: France du Nord, vers 1300–1500* (Paris: Editions Arguments, 1993), 119–127; Knefelkamp, *Das Heilig-Geist-Spital in Nürnberg*, 241–264, and Michel Mollat, *The Poor in the Middle Ages: An Essay in Social History*, trans. Arthur Goldhammer (New Haven: Yale University Press, 1986), 150, make tenuously supported assumptions about continuity in the number and duty of staff.

over-familiarity between the staff and the sick suggests that the sharing of living space and liturgical routines counted for more, on a quotidian basis, than differences in roles and responsibilities. The absence of professional medical practitioners from hospital staff has led critics from the early modern period onwards to see in these establishments "nothing worthy of the name of a hospital."[58] Recent interest in medieval hospital history, meanwhile, has coincided with upheaval in and uncertainty regarding contemporary systems of social security and support.[59]

The structures of care in the medieval European hospital did not see the service of doctors as essential to their daily functions in the care of the sick-poor.[60] Licensed physicians became more visible in the later Middle Ages, as their professional prestige grew; Michael McVaugh has argued that this is due far more to the changing status of doctors than to changing policies or functions of hospitals.[61] These patterns hold in the evidence from Mainz; while a number of doctors appear in hospital records, none are identified as being salaried. Despite the absence of licensed practitioners, it is clear that hospitals were dedicated to providing therapeutic care. Largely, this occurred through the regulation of the six non-naturals.[62] Numerous studies have called for the expansion of the definition of medieval medicine to include

58 See Kay Peter Jankrift, "Herren Kranke, arme Siechen. Medizin im spätmittelalterlichen Hospitalwesen," in *Sozialgeschichte mittelalterlicher Hospitäler,* 150–151; Reicke, *Das deutsche Spital,* vol. 2, 73–75, 84–95; Pohl-Resl, *Rechnen mit der Ewigkeit,* 182–185. For an overview of historiographical uncertainty, see Michael Matheus, "Einleitung," in *Funktions- und Strukturwandel spätmittelalterlicher Hospitäler,* i, vii-viii. Rafael Hyacinthe, "De Domo Sancti Lazari Milites Leprosi: Knighthood and Leprosy in the Holy Land," in *The Medieval Hospital and Medical Practice,* ed. Bowers, 209–225.

59 Davis, *The Medieval Economy of Salvation,* 1–4, 241–242, 276–283; Ziegler, *Medieval Healthcare and the Rise of Charitable Institutions,* 8–16.

60 Jankrift, "Herren Kranke, arme Siechen," 149–167.

61 Michael R. McVaugh, *Medicine Before the Plague: Practitioners and their Patients in the Crown of Aragon, 1285–1345* (Cambridge: Cambridge University Press, 2002), 230–245. Raul Villagrasa-Elias, "Sociologia hospitalaria en Castilla la Vieja (1455–1513)" (web presentation, *Salud en cuerpo y alma: el hospital de la Vera Cruz en Medina de Pomar,* Centro de Ciencias Humanas y Sociales, Madrid, November 5, 2020), provides evidence for salaried medical professionals forming part of hospital staff in the late fifteenth century.

62 See Luis García Ballester, "The Origin of the Six Non-Natural Things in Galen," in Galen *and Galenism: Theory and Medical Practice from Antiquity to the European Renaissance,* eds. Jon Arrizabalaga et al (Farnham: Ashgate, 2002), 35–42; Katharine Park, "Healing the Poor: Hospitals and Medical Assistance in Renaissance Florence," in *Medicine and Charity Before the Welfare State,* eds. Jonathan Barry and Colin Jones (London: Routledge, 1991), 37–38; Sharon Strocchia, "Caring for the 'Incurable' in Renaissance Pox Hospitals," in *Hospital Life: Theory and Practice from the Medieval to the Modern,* eds. Laurinda Abreu and Sally Sheard (Oxford: Peter Lang, 2013), 76–77.

the management of hospital atmosphere, dietetics, and the participation of patients and staff in the liturgy and sacraments of the church.[63] Gifts in kind indicate that the provision of warmth and appropriate food and drink to the sick was valued by donors. Medical recipe collections, moreover, indicate that the provision of appropriate care for patients with diverse needs was a task that was taken seriously by many.[64] Hospitals in the archdiocese of Mainz appear to have cultivated relationships with doctors, even though these doctors were not permanently attached to the hospital staff.[65] The 1293 will of one such doctor, Magister Otto, reveals that he had relationships with multiple hospitals in Mainz. He arranges for anniversary Masses to be said for him at St. Agnes, and also gives wheat to women serving at the hospitals of St. Barbara and St. George.[66] He gives the same measure of wheat to the foundation of St. Nicholas, which may also have cared for the sick; the dedication was a common one for leprosaria, and St. Alban, to which St. Nicholas was adjacent, is known to have had a "Siechenmeister."[67] In 1438, another doctor, Johannes de Itzstein, left his possessions "for pious uses" to the dean and chapter of St. Johann, which may have also managed a hospital.[68] To judge by the memorial books of Mainz's religious houses, connections between medical professionals and hospitals were not uncommon in the city, though their presence on hospital staff was rare.[69] The memorial book of Liebfrauen contains an undated commemoration for Master Wilhelm de Leuca, a medical doctor who bequeathed half his goods to a Magister Conrad. This Magister Conrad may be the same man who served as rector

63 Examples of such studies include Jürgen Sydow, "Kanonistische Fragen zur Geschichte des Spitals in Südwestdeutschland," *Historisches Jahrbuch* 83 (1964), 54–68; Knefelkamp, *Das Gesundheits- und Fürsorgewesen der Stadt Freiburg,* 71–74, 115; Alberzoni,"Norditalienische Pilgerhospize," 282–284.

64 Stiftsbibliothek Aschaffenburg MS Perg 26; Bodleian MS Laud MS 237 f203r–228r.

65 Baur, *Hessische Urkunden*, vol 1, Nr. 547, 533–536; Nr. 759, 760; Baas, *Mittelalterliche Gesundheitsfürsorge,* 42–50; StAM Q 63 20, f15r–16v.

66 HStAD A2 168/83 (23 September 1293).

67 HStAD A2 168/83. On St. Alban, see Falck, "Mainzer Hospitäler im Mittelalter," 409, and Ludwig Falck, *Mainz in seiner Blütezeit als Freie Stadt (1244–1328),* Geschichte der Stadt Mainz III (Düsseldorf: Verlag Rau, 1973), 51.

68 HStAD C1 A Nr. 78, 111.

69 StAM Dertsch Zettelkasten: The erstwhile archivist of Mainz compiled the following list of references to an Arzt, medicus, or physicus: Totenbücher St. Agnes Hs. II 11 Johann [...]ürsten; Seelbuch Liebfrauen , StAM 13/284: 1 physicus; Totenbuch Reichklara StAM 13/330: Johann, Arzt zu Reichklara, 22/7; StAM 13/335: 1. Furseler, Peter (note: he appears as a Stiftsherr of Liebfrauen) St. Johann: Magister Heinrich von Kreuznach, 28/1. Identified by Dertsch with Magister H., physicus, 27/8, 2/9; Magister Balzo (physicus) 588 (15/8) Arzt (medicus) see Johann v. Udenheim 32, in StAM 13/370.

of the Heilig Geist Spital, the one hospital staff member in Mainz who may have been a medical professional.

Conrad served as master of the Heilig Geist Spital in the early fourteenth century, and managed a bathhouse after retiring from the post. Both this activity, viewed in Mainz as requiring specialist knowledge, and his consistent appellation as "Magister," suggest that he possessed an unusual degree of medical learning.[70] It is probable that the staff of St. Georg, at least some of whose inmates would have required intensive therapeutic care, included men and women with considerable medical knowledge. Relationships between the leper hospital and medical doctors are treated as a personally dependent custom in the archiepiscopal letter of 1512, concerned with the hospital's (non)provision of a leprosy inspection [*Lepraschau*] for the surrounding area.

According to this letter, issued by Archbishop Uriel von Gemmingen, the lepers of St. Georg had themselves been responsible for such an inspection until Archbishop Berthold von Henneberg (r. 1484–1504) handed over the rights to the university's medical doctors. The process of the inspection itself is referred to as designed for the use and benefit of the sick-poor.[71] This custom is described as having lapsed due to the deaths of the doctors; this is significant because of the implication that the university's medical staff did not merely succeed to such responsibility ex officio, but needed a relationship of trust with the hospital. Archbishop Uriel, seeking to resolve the existing impasse, restores the rights of inspection to the leper hospital, with the proviso that the committee should be composed of two knowledgeable priests of the hospital and a "knowledgeable barber." In difficult cases, "where knowledge is lacking," they should consult—and pay!—a doctor of the university's medical faculty. Notably, the guidelines set up by Archbishop Uriel are not meant to apply to Mainz only, but to the entire region under his administration. This suggests that the archbishop could still claim authority over leper hospitals as religious institutions, even as medical professionals and civic governments sought involvement in their oversight.

The increase of civic involvement in hospital administration has often been over-interpreted as changing the legal status and communal organization of hospitals. Documents such as Archbishop Uriel's letter, attesting the involvement of civic officials and medical professionals in the life of hospitals, have sometimes been tied to the alleged secularization of the late

70 For more on Mainz's bathhouses and their managers, see Barnhouse, "From Helpful Gardens to Hateful Words," 58–59.

71 StAM U 3 October 1512.

medieval hospital.[72] Some scholars have argued that communalization is a more apt label for this process than secularization.[73] Under any name, hospitals' increased connections to civic governments—whether sought or imposed—are often treated as concomitant to a loss of their "original" institutional mission of caring for the sick-poor. Considering hospitals as religious institutions offers an opportunity to reframe the fraught questions of control and secularization. Even into the late Middle Ages, civic and ecclesiastical officials both appear in the records of Mainz's hospitals; and the latter have a stronger claim to authority. Uriel's intervention illustrates some of the tensions between changing medical norms and hospitals' institutional identity at the close of the Middle Ages.

The changing language of hospital rules can be read as responding to evolving understandings of religious status, and how this status bound hospital staff.[74] Through the mid-thirteenth century, hospital rules presume that religious status was the most important shared characteristic of hospital residents, whether clerics or laypersons, healthy or sick, male or female.[75] Blurred boundaries between lay and clerical status, and even between the healthy staff members and those whom they swore to serve, were aided by the fact that the vowed status of the sick paralleled that of religious persons; the inspiration of the Augustine rule was fairly frequent, that of the Benedictine rare but not unheard of. Hospital statutes reflect the reality that the definition of religious status itself was changing from the mid-twelfth to the mid-thirteenth centuries. The vocabulary of hospital rules separated the

72 Brodman, *Charity and Welfare*, 29–46, includes an overview of relevant historiography. Cf. Yearl, "Medieval Monastic Customaries on Minuti and Infirmi," 175–194, on the anachronistic distinction between spiritual and medical care.

73 Liermann, *Handbuch des Stiftungsrechts*, vol. 1, 96–100; Falck, *Mainz in seiner Blütezeit*, 54; Bettina Toson, *Mittelalterliche Hospitäler in Hessen zwischen Schwalm, Eder, und Fulda* (Darmstadt: Hessiche Historische Kommission, 2012), 25–26; Pauly and Uhrmacher, "Die Koblenzer Hospitäler," 341–342, describe a confusing chronology of "communalization" and ""civic control"; civic rectors are only visible in Koblenz from the 1350s, but council members appear as witnesses to hospital transactions in the late 1280s; Nicolas Norbert Huyghebaert, "L'origine ecclésiastique des léproseries en Flandre et dans le Nord de la France," *Revue d'histoire ecclésiastique* 58 (1962), 852–853, uses the terms communalization and secularization interchangeably; Sydow, "Kanonistische Fragen," 54–68, sees the history of the medieval hospital as ending in communalization.

74 Many such rules were penned a century or more after the hospital's date of origin, as in the case of Mainz's Heilig Geist Spital. Laqua, *Bruderschaften und Hospitäler während des hohen Mittelalters*, 238–239. Sommerlechner, "Spitäler in Nord und Mittelitalien," 111.

75 Le Grand, *Statuts d'hotels-dieu*, 22–25, 36–38, et passim; Gisela Drossbach, "Bild und Text im Liber Regulae des roemischen Hospitals von Santo Spirito in Sassia," in *Sozialgeschichte Mittelalterlicher Hospitäler*, ed. Neithard Bulst and Karl-Heinz Spiess (Ostfildern: Jan Thorbecke Verlag, 2007), 125–148; Gilchrist, "Christian Bodies and Souls," 103–104.

sick (including lepers) from the brothers and sisters of the hospital staff with increasing clarity over the course of the thirteenth century.[76] The categories of hospital residents could continue to be labile, however. While Speyer has distinct terminology for the sick and the corrodians (*Siechen, Pfründner,*) the rules for them are conflated in the statutes copied into the hospital's account book in the later fourteenth century.[77] This suggests that a view of the aged as included among the infirm whom hospitals served was far from exceptional, as discussed in the case of Wernher de Indagine, above.

The named staff in charge of hospital administration, who appear in court as recipients of gifts, appear to have been customarily healthy. While the identifying patronymic would not exclude the possibility of leprosy, it is unlikely that no mention would have been made of the illness of these men; moreover, no lepers of St. Georg are known to have appeared in court, being represented there by a hospital servant. Moreover, an agreement from the late fourteenth century survives between named hospital administrators and the lepers as a community. The transaction is a simple one, involving a cash loan; the document's significance lies primarily in the evidence it provides that the interests of the lepers were seen as a significant determinant of hospital policy.[78] Were this claim made in a public document, it might be reasonably claimed that the primacy of the lepers' interests was a rhetorical fiction assumed for legal purposes; the only form in which the agreement survives, however, is in the account book of St. Georg. No mention is made of judges or court officials or even a notary having been involved in the decision; two hospital staff members are described as having come to an agreement between themselves, as witnessed by a representative of the lepers. An addition in a later hand concerning payments made further suggests that the record was created for internal use, attesting to the fact that the leprous residents of St. Georg were involved in decisions about the use of hospital resources, as well as about the admission of new members, as discussed above.

The control of resources and of admission also appears as significant to Mainz's oldest hospital. In the charter of Archbishop Heinrich that provides the first written record of the hospital's existence, a certain Erenfridus is identified as the *praepositus* of the hospital. We do not learn whether or not he is a cleric, but that he is the elected head of an ordered community may be inferred from the language of the charter, which

76 Laqua, *Bruderschaften und Hospitäler,* 109–113, 168–169, 207–209.

77 Stadtarchiv Speyer, Sondersiechenhaus Zinsbuch III 122–123 B.

78 StAM 32/700, 31 June 1392.

delegates the responsibilities of hospital management to him and to his successors. The description of these responsibilities indicates that the therapeutic and liturgical functions of the hospital were taken seriously by the archbishop; their enumeration provided a standard for Erenfridus' successors.[79] The care of the sick is identified as a priority; the equitable division of prebends among new arrivals is listed as a primary way of assuring that care.[80] This suggests both that the hospital patients were socially diverse, and that the hospital community was organized with near parity in status between the sick and those who cared for them. Very little is known about the staff of Mainz's hospital before the very end of the thirteenth century. For the subsequent century and a half, the record is fairly consistent, if incomplete, showing us only those at the head of the hospital's administrative infrastructure.

Fourteenth-century records make clear that both the Heilig Geist Spital and St. Agnes had multiple priests on staff, and that St. Georg had at least one. In the case of St. Agnes, some priests were set to serve particular altars, while other clerical staff were shared with nearby women's monastic houses. The language of St. Georg makes clear that there was at least one priest resident with St. Georg. Another priest resided at Heilig Kreuz with a separate community of lepers; the earliest extant statutes for this community date to the mid-fifteenth century, but there are indications that an informal community was in residence there throughout the later Middle Ages.[81] At St. Agnes, the surprisingly large staff of priests may have been necessary to the hospital's quotidian management. No individual is identified as primarily responsible for the care of the sick, suggesting that such care was seen as the responsibility of the entire community.[82] Ludwig Falck has claimed that St. Jakob, St. Johannes, and Reichklara also managed small hospitals for pilgrims and the sick-poor. While there is certainly suggestive evidence for this in the case of St. Johannes, particularly, none of these hospitals

79 StAM 6/30 (4). See Bedos-Resak, "Medieval Identity," 1507–1509, on the function of such charters as "a space of sacred and secure inscription" (1507) where individual actions and social relationships could be both memorialized and prescribed. On the idea of religious discipline as informing the lives of inmates and carers, see Brodman, "Religion and Discipline," 123–132. Peregrine Horden, "A Discipline of Relevance: The Historiography of the Later Medieval Hospital," *Social History of Medicine* 1 (1988), 365.

80 StAM 6/30 (4).

81 Records of this community are preserved in StAM 13/190.

82 Note the contrast to other religious communities, where masters of the sick are named as presiding over the guesthouses open to the sick-poor of the surrounding area. For St. Alban, in 1331: StAM 13/263, 16; for Altmünster, StAM U 18 February 1367. For detail on St. Agnes and its hospital management, see Chapter 3.

enjoyed legal independence.[83] The Sacraments at the small hospital of St. Barbara were almost certainly provided by the canons of Liebfrauen to whose supervision the hospital was entrusted by its founder.

Mainz's hospital priests, and the privileges granted to them, were of course essential to the hospitals' performance of liturgical functions and provision of the Sacraments, but their activities were also relevant to those beyond the hospital walls. The anticlerical movements of the 1380s were especially violent in both Mainz and Worms, with clerical involvement in the wine trade the direct catalyst. Whether hospital priests were condemned for participating in this trade, as hospitals themselves almost certainly did, is unclear.[84] A clerical chronicler noted with disgust that the burghers of Mainz received the interdict of 1382 with indifference; Jennifer Kolpacoff Deane has convincingly argued that the activities of mendicants may have mitigated the effects of this interdict. Hospital priests, granted special privileges for the celebration of Mass at such times (though without the ringing of bells that would announce it), may have done so no less.[85]

To procure the Sacraments for the sick, and serve the latter humbly and devotedly, are the only prescriptions for hospital staff contained in the 1236 statutes of Mainz's oldest hospital.[86] For the rector, appointed by the archbishop, more specific instructions are given. He is to be answerable to the archbishop for the spiritual affairs of the hospital, and for the care (*cura*) of those under his supervision (*subditorum.*) For the administration of the hospital's temporal affairs, the rector is to be responsible not only to the

83 Falck, *Mainz in seiner Blütezeit*, 51.

84 On the performance of the Sacraments in hospitals in the province of Mainz, see HStAM Urkunde 47 Nr. 9; HStAM Urkunde 47 Nr. 38; BayHStA, Kloster St. Veit Urk 87; HStAD A2 234/49; HStAD A2 186/6; HStAD A2 168/457; HStAD A2 115/48; HStAD 115/36; StAM 013/0005 f9v–11v. For the literature on the subject see Carla Keyvanian, *Hospitals and Urbanism in Rome, 1200–1500* (Leiden: Brill, 2015), 85–90; Bourgeois, *Lépreux et Maladreries du Pas-de-Calais*, 39–47; Jean Imbert, *Histoire des hôpitaux français: contribution à l'étude des rapports de l'église et de l'état dans le domaine de l'Assistance Publique: les hôpitaux en droit canonique du décret de Gratien à la sécularisation de l'administration de l'Hôtel-Dieu de Paris en 1505* (Paris: J. Vrin, 1947), 140–147. On hospitals and wine, see Reinhard Schmid, *Die Abtei St. Alban vor Mainz im hohen und späten Mittelalter: Geschichte, Verfassung und Besitz eines Klosters im Spannungsfeld zwischen Erzbischof, Stadt, Kurie, und Reich* (Mainz: Stadtarchiv Mainz, 1996), 117–118; Peter Linehan, "A Tale of Two Cities: Capitular Burgos and Mendicant Burgos in the Thirteenth Century," in *Church and City, 1000–1500: Essays in Honour of Christopher Brooke*, eds. David Abulafia, Michael J. Franklin, and Miri Rubin (Cambridge: Cambridge University Press, 2002), 81–110; Sonderegger, "Financing Strategy," 216–219; Pohl-Resl, *Rechnen mit der Ewigkeit*, 22–33.

85 Kolpacoff Deane, *Papal Schism*, 97–107.

86 StAM 6/30 (4); printed in Gudenus, vol. 1, 628.

archbishop, but to the other members of the hospital staff.[87] Staff organization appears to have remained egalitarian up until the mid-thirteenth century at least; the *rector* of the hospital is the only post with an official title, and the men named in this position held external offices as well, which may have meant that they did not reside at the hospital.[88] In any case, it is a measure of porous claustration, of ongoing interactions with other groups and spaces within the city. A similar system of administration is attested for the civic hospital of Speyer. A charter of 1261 containing privileges and statutes for the hospital ordained that three burghers (not necessarily council-members) were to be appointed to head the staff. Notably, the same document gives the hospital staff full administrative property. In order to alienate property (a risky move, given the hospital's religious status,) the consent of the council and, not less, the hospital community were prerequisites.[89] Significantly, the council formally affirms in this charter that Speyer's hospital is entitled to the exemptions from taxes and tithes that were the prerogative of religious institutions.[90] Despite the council's claim to authority, it seems reasonable to conclude that, as in the case of Mainz's Heilig Geist Spital, the hospital community itself exercised initiative in obtaining confirmation of its religious status following an expansion of the legal criteria for that status.

In the second half of the thirteenth century, mentions of "all the brothers" of Mainz's oldest hospital vanish; instead, the *Spitalmeister*, who might also be one of the two *Pfleger* appointed by the city council, appear as representatives of the institution and of the sick.[91] The case of Conrad zum Römer, *provisor* around the turn of the fourteenth century, illustrates the possibility for enduring ties to the hospital. Even after he no longer served as Spitalmeister, Conrad zum Römer appears in hospital records as a witness and a donor, and the owner of a steam bath which appears to have been used by the hospital for therapeutic purposes. Although a member of Mainz's urban elite, Meister Conrad appears to have committed his own resources to the welfare of the hospital, rather than exploiting the resources of the hospital in the civic interest.

87 StAM 6/30 (4).

88 StAM U / 1252. Printed in Gudenus I, 627 Nr. 261. StaWu, MBVI 17, CXXII, f. 122r-v. The first named member of staff in the thirteenth century is Fridericus, a canon of the prosperous foundation of St. Stephan, serving as rector in 1252. The Liber Vitae of St. Stephan (StAM 013/310) contains no records of Fridericus' other activities.

89 Alfred Hilgard, ed., *Urkunden zur Geschichte der Stadt Speyer* (Strassburg: Trübner, 1885), no. 98 (1261).

90 Hilgard, ed., *Urkunden zur Geschichte der Stadt Speyer*, no. 98 (1261).

91 StAM 33/1.

It remains to examine the question of who the men and women taking service in Mainz's hospitals were, in order to shed light on the diverse positions of these hospitals in social and ecclesiastical networks.[92] Brigitte Pohl-Resl has observed a transition from clerical to lay leadership beginning in the last third of the thirteenth century.[93] For the Heilig Geist Spital, this appears to have been true—if a slightly later phenomenon—for the hospital *rectores*, but this should not be equated with a laicization of the staff. Daily management was still in the hands of the brothers and the priests. For the claim of Ludwig Falck that "dedicated staff" of Mainz's oldest hospital died out, to be replaced with paid lay servants, I see no justification in the extant medieval records.[94] The religious status of hospital staff was legally fixed; but the social implications of this status could be variable. As work on the religious life has shown, such lability of interpretation was by no means limited to hospitals, and should not be taken as an index of spiritual decline or indifference.[95] Such charters of self-dedication as those known for the leper hospital in Narbonne are unknown in Mainz.[96] It is suggestive, however, that the medieval holdings of both the Heilig Geist Spital and St. Agnes included records concerning properties with no clear link to the hospital in question. Charters and *vidimus* letters issued by the judges of Mainz recording the rights or acquisitions of private persons, and then preserved by these institutions, suggests the possibility that the revenues and properties concerned passed to the hospitals with the vow-taking of staff members. This hypothesis is supported by the fact that the entry of a young woman named Sophia into the community of St. Agnes is indicated only by the fact that documents relating to her own property survive in

92 For examples of such studies on religious institutions, see Heike Reimann, "Cistercian Nuns in the High Middle Ages: The Cistercians of Bergen in the Principality of Rügen (North Germany)," in *Cîteaux: Revue d'histoire cistercienne* 55 (2004), 231–244; Johnson, *Equal in Monastic Profession*, 13–61; Christine Kleinjung, "Nonnen und Personal, Familie und Stifter," in *Norm und Realität: Kontinuität und Wandel der Zisterzienser im Mittelalter*, eds. Franz Josef Gelten and Werner Rösener (Münster: LIT Verlag, 2009), 229–240. Recently, on hospitals, Rehberg, "Die Römer und ihre Hospitäler," Beobachtungen zu den Trägergruppen der Spitalsgründungen in Rom (13.-15. Jahrhundert," in *Hospitäler im Mittelalter*, ed. Drossbach, 225–260.

93 Pohl-Resl, *Rechnen mit der Ewigkeit*, 111–114.

94 Falck, "Mainzer Spitäler," 410–411.

95 Sherri Franks Johnson, *Monastic Women and Religious Orders in Late Medieval Bologna* (Cambridge: Cambridge University Press, 2014), 1–2, 124–125. See also Lester, *Creating Cistercian Nuns*, 7–14, 42–44, et passim; Van Engen, *Sisters and Brothers of the Common Life*, 107–125.

96 Cros-Mayrevieille, *Les Frères Donnés*, 7–9, asserts that the mixed-gender staff of Narbonne's leper hospital were free to leave again as they wished, even in the thirteenth and fourteenth centuries. The two charters of self-dedication attested by Cros-Mayrevieille date to 1275 and 1306.

the house's chartulary.[97] To extrapolate from the documents presumed to be connected to hospital staff, the men and women of Mainz's larger hospital communities were moderately prosperous, if not members of the city's patrician elites.

Of Mainz's hospitals, the Heilig Geist Spital and St. Georg had more known ties to families with civic influence than St. Agnes and St. Barbara. Such ties, however, do not appear to have resulted in disputes or conflicts of interest, as was the case in Nürnberg.[98] The Rosendal family, from whom several overseers of St. Georg were drawn, were burghers of Mainz, and thus of some standing.[99] But their most conspicuous ties in the records of the city are not to municipal administration, but to the city's hospitals, as donors as well as staff members. Wilkin Rosendal served as one of the two *Vormünder* of St. Georg towards the end of the fourteenth century, and a Nese Rosendal was one of the hospital sisters of St. Agnes around the same time.[100] The Medetrost family, less widely connected to the city's institutions of care, served St. Georg for over thirty years; and the first reference to a Medetrost as "the younger" suggests that the connection may have been of even greater duration than explicitly recorded.[101]

The composition of St. Agnes' community remained securely rooted in the social networks of Mainz; an Elsa von Oppenheim, who served as abbess for several decades in the fifteenth century, is the only nun known to have come from outside the city in the late medieval period. The patrician Landecke family maintained close contacts with the convent for several generations.[102] Johannes von Landecke was erroneously commemorated as the founder of the convent in records from the sixteenth century, suggesting that his donation was not only significant in itself, but may have marked the beginning of a new phase in St. Agnes' relationships with its

97 HStAD C1 A Nr. 89, f11v.

98 Knefelkamp, *Das Heilig-Geist-Spital in Nürnberg*, 42–47 on a dispute with heirs.

99 StAM U / 28 August 1352 is a contract between the Clarissans and Peder Rosendal and his wife, directing that water may not be drawn from the nuns' well without express permission; otherwise, the well before the gate should be used. In StAM U / 18 May 1387, a daughter of Gerlach Rosendal appears as the beneficiary of a will, suggesting that she may have entered the religious life.

100 StAM 32/700 32; HStAD C1 A Nr. 78, f38r–39r; a Folke Rosendal witnesses a charter for the new hospital in StAM U /1 September 1403. Intriguingly, there is an Ulrich von Rosendal mentioned as a witness in a 1265 charter conferring valuable properties on the Heilig Geist Spital: StAM 6/30, Urkunden Abschrift 1265.

101 StAM 32/700, 32, contains an entry made by Jakob Medetrost himself for the year 1391. Fields belonging to the Medetrost family appear as an orientation point in StAM 32/701, f1.

102 HStAD C1 A Nr. 89 f14r–15r, f38v–39v; HStAD A2 168/738.

donors.[103] A Katherine zum Landecke appears as abbess in 1395–1396, and Elsa von Landecke, a relative, appears in several positions of authority before being elected abbess herself sometime around 1420; she held the position until her death in 1426.[104] This makes the Landeckes one of the few identifiable families among the named nuns of St. Agnes. From the mid-fourteenth century on, daughters of burgher families begin appearing with more regularity.

People and Property: Types of Donors and Donations

Piety by itself does not found or maintain hospitals; as Carla Keyvanian has observed, "urban hospitals did not appear as if coagulating from a mist of compassionate concerns."[105] The medieval charters belonging to Mainz's hospitals make clear that the language of donation itself could serve as a legal fiction.[106] From the early thirteenth century, hospitals were legally required to receive and use resources exclusively for the needs of the sick. Varied and complicated transactions, covering property, cash, and kind, all used language that acknowledged this, allowing hospital staff to continue managing their resources and relationships in ways that fit the needs and goals of hospital communities. The use of legal fictions exists alongside a range of individualized preambles and prescriptions in testaments and donations that demonstrate donors' appreciation of hospitals as religious institutions, and thereby as providers of spiritual services in many forms. It has been widely suggested that hospitals of all kinds may have been favored recipients of donations, as they were a fixed part of the landscape

103 Fritz Viktor Arens, *Die Kunstdenkmäler der Stadt Mainz* (Berlin: Deutsche Kunstverlag, 1962), 3–10; Simons, *Cities of Ladies*, 24–34, discusses patterns of "retroactive institutionalization" through the crafting of institutional narratives for communities of religious women; something of the sort may have been undertaken by the women of St. Agnes in the fifteenth century.

104 HStAD C1 A Nr. 89 f50v–51r.

105 Keyvanian, *Hospitals and Urbanism in Rome*, 15.

106 See, for example, Sonderegger, "The Financing Strategy of a Major Urban Hospital," 213, as well as, foundationally, Rosenwein, *To Be the Neighbor of St. Peter*, esp. 35–48. Miri Rubin, "Imagining Medieval Hospitals: Considerations on the Cultural Meaning of Institutional Change," in *Medicine and Charity Before the Welfare State*, eds. Jonathan Barry and Colin Jones (London: Routledge, 1991), 15–18. Oliver Auge, "'Ne pauperes et debiles in… domo degentes divinis careant.' Sakralreligiöse Askpete der mittelalterlichen Hospitalgeschichte," in *Sozialgeschichte mittelalterlicher Hospitäler*, eds. Neithard Bulst and Karl-Heinz Spiess (Ostfildern: Jan Thorbecke Verlag, 2007), 92.

of charity.[107] Hospitals' religious status was key to their occupation of such an established place; their legal privileges gave them not only legitimacy, but institutional continuity greater than that of less formal communities. Both the performance of liturgical services such as anniversary Masses for donors, and the provision of care for the sick-poor, were treated as valued tasks, integral to hospital identity.[108]

Hospitals' economic ties to donors were often accompanied by—and indicative of—practical and affective relationships.[109] In 1428, for instance, Jeckel and Clara Landecke bequeathed substantial annual rents in exchange for burial and commemoration in the cloister of St. Agnes; additionally, they made a stipendiary gift to their daughter, a nun of the house.[110] Familial ties may have routinely influenced donors in less prominent cases as well. I have catalogued types of donors, e.g. clerics, widows, spousal couples, and multigenerational groups, for each of Mainz's four independent hospitals. Such an approach facilitates analysis of which types of donors privileged which hospitals, and what they prioritized in making their gifts; for comparative purposes, I have catalogued gifts to Essen's civic hospital using the same criteria. Not enough medieval data survives in the charters of Worms, or even in the account books of Speyer's hospital, to make it possible to extend the analysis to their hospitals.[111] This analysis places hospitals'

107 Daniel Le Blévec, *La Part du Pauvre: l'assistance dans les pays du Bas-Rhône du XIIe siècle au milieu du XVE siècle,* vol. 1 (Rome: École française de Rome, 2000), 187–216, finds percentages and types of donation and donors varying according to region, but with a generally high contribution to hospitals. See also Philippa Maddern, "A Market for Charitable Performances? Bequests to the Poor and their Recipients in Fifteenth-Century Norwich Wills," 93–96; Rawcliffe, *The Hospitals of Medieval Norwich* (Woodbridge: Boydell, 1995), 16–17; Davis, "Hospitals, Charity, and the Culture of Compassion in the Twelfth and Thirteenth Centuries," in *Approaches to Poverty in Medieval Europe: Complexities, Contradictions, Transformations, c. 1100–1500*, ed. Sharon Farmer (Turnhout: Brepols, 2016), 41; John Henderson, *Piety and Charity in Late Medieval Florence* (Oxford: Clarendon Press, 1994), 242; Brodman, "Religion and Discipline," 132.

108 Maddern, "A Market for Charitable Performances," 79–82; James Brodman, *Charity and Religion in Medieval Europe* (Washington, DC: Catholic University of America Press, 2009), 30–41; Anne M. Scott, "Remembering the Poor: Signs of Charity in Late Medieval Images and Texts," 257–274; Davis, "Hospitals, Charity, and the Culture of Compassion," 30–35.

109 Forey, "Women and the Military Orders," 67–71, 89–91, points out the striking discrepancy between statutory exclusion of women and de facto relations they had as donors, assistants, and half-sisters with the Templars and a number of other orders. Cf. Pauly, "Pilgerverkehr," 112–113 on burghers or noble donors wishing to improve their spiritual welfare or temporal prestige by cultivating ties with hospitals.

110 HStAD A2 168/738.

111 StAW Abt. 159 Nr. 431/1 contains excerpts from the inventory of Worms' hospital from 1486 through 1787, compiled in the late eighteenth century. StASp III 122–3 B contains the medieval accounts of Speyer's leper hospital, compiled in 1584, rendering analysis of the institution's

institutional functions in their broader social context. For civic hospitals, smaller institutions, and leper hospitals alike, relationships with donors, landholders, and tenants were shaped by hospitals' religious status. These relationships, in turn, affected how hospitals managed their resources and performed their liturgical and social functions.

The assertion of archiepiscopal influence over the community of St. Agnes in the 1280s, however unwelcome it may have been to the women themselves, may have provided reassurance to those desiring that their donations would have an accepted place in the economy of salvation, supporting a house of unambiguously orthodox religious affiliation.[112] The history of the first major bequest received, in the early fourteenth century—a widow's endowment for the maintenance of priests—suggests that the resources of the convent were thinly spread. This bequest in itself was of such significance that one of Mainz's antiquarians was tempted—by this and perhaps by incredulity at the social and economic independence of a woman at the turn of the fourteenth century—into misidentifying Miltrudis as the first abbess of the community.[113] Miltrudis, widow of the burgher Erkenbold, cultivated connections with the women of St. Agnes, making them monitors of her endowments elsewhere in the city in 1298, before making a gift to the convent itself some years later.[114] Over the course of several months in the winter of 1304–1305, Miltrudis and the convent negotiated the terms of a gift which was to serve for a memorial to herself and her husband, who was buried in the convent.[115] Each of them were to receive prayers on their anniversary, with large and small candles, and with lamps.[116] The latter of these contains an unusually detailed preamble emphasizing the purity of her motives and that she is giving only out of pious zeal and for the good of the souls of herself, and of her friends and relations. This sounds like a response to official suspicion, but nothing in the terms of the gift would seem, in itself, to provoke such suspicion. Perhaps the legitimacy of St. Agnes as a religious institution—and thus its right to receive such gifts—was still in question. The convent also preserved a charter issued by the judges of

medieval account-keeping impossible. Many entries are undated, and few dated entries are given for the late medieval period.

112 Rubin, *Charity and Community in Medieval Cambridge*, 140–142.

113 A note in the StAM copy of *Rerum Moguntine* Vol. II, 875–876, reads: "Magnus benefactor et adjutor fuit Erckenboldus civ. mog. et ejus uxor Miltrudis A. 1304 prima abbatissa."

114 HStAD A2 168/98. 29 June 1298.

115 HStAD A2 115/31.

116 HStAD A2 115/31, 115/32. HStAD A2 168/131 contains the confirmation. Cf. HStAD 168/133 (1306).

Mainz, confirming the gifts. The double confirmation and multigenerational witness groups suggest that the women of St. Agnes were anxious to have ample testimony to the extent of their rights.

Miltrudis' most complicated gift to the convent was made in 1304. She wanted to provide for the maintenance of three priests serving the community of St. Agnes, two of whom were to come from her or her husband's kingroup. In conformity with canon law, the qualifier was added that the priests must be qualified and of good reputation.[117] The convent would, over the course of a little over a twelve-month, repeatedly send legal representatives to petition for the reduction of the number of priests to two, pleading that the income generated by the bequest was insufficient for the support of three men.[118] The visibility of the detail with which the terms of Miltrudis' bequest were negotiated is exceptional; but it appears to have been representative of the interest of men and women in the life of the communities to which they donated properties and income, and of the care with which Mainz's hospitals managed their possessions. The ongoing management of properties is indicated by notes in the margins of all surviving hospital account books and chartularies, making note of when properties were sold, or when their value changed. A typical example from the chartulary of St. Agnes is issued by Heinrich Sander, priest of St. Quintin, and the altar servers, concerning damaged houses. Because the houses were temporarily closed up, "by special request and for friendship's sake" the rent was reduced by six shillings.[119]

By far the largest category of donors to Mainz's hospitals is spouses who made gifts jointly, often together with their heirs; nor does this fully represent the hospitals' multigenerational ties. That hospital staff might be drawn from successive generations of the same family has been discussed above. Moreover, I found seventeen instances—accounting for just over ten percent of St. Agnes' documented interactions with donors—of multigenerational ties with families that were not established through written contracts. The

117 HStAD A2 115/31.

118 HStAD 168/131, printed in Baur, *Hessische Urkunden*, 645–649. Sethina Watson, "A Mother's Past and her Children's Futures: Female Inheritance, Family, and Dynastic Hospitals in the Thirteenth Century," in *Motherhood, Religion and Society in Medieval Europe, 400–1400: Essays Presented to Henrietta Leyser*, eds. Conrad Leyser and Lesley Smith (Farnham: Ashgate, 2011), 227–228, has spoken of such arrangements as unusual. For the legal tensions relevant to this dilemma, see Glenn Warren Olsen, *The Legal Definition of the Ecclesiastical Benefice During the Period of the Appearance of Papal Provisioning* (Ph.D. Diss., University of Wisconsin, 1965), 244–262.

119 HStAD C1 Nr. 89, f100r-v (24 June 1441.)

different record-keeping formats of St. Georg and the Heilig Geist Spital make such connections more difficult to identify, but both of these hospitals also clearly maintained knowledge of those with whom they cultivated ties over the course of several generations. Only eleven of the thirty-nine married couples making gifts to Mainz's hospitals name their heirs as parties to the transaction. In some instances, the children bound by the agreement are also present at its making. The forestalling of possible dispute of a gift's terms in successive generations is often made explicit.[120] Half a dozen records survive of family members making joint gifts, but in only one of these cases is the agreement binding on the heirs.[121]

There are only seven widows on record as having donated to the hospitals of Mainz. They are the donor group with the clearest institutional preference; all, save one, made their gifts exclusively to St. Agnes. One of the outliers, Gisla, gave equal bequests to the sick-poor of Mainz's main hospital, the community of St. Agnes, and "the lepers in the field."[122] The other, Gosta, gave one pound to St. Agnes, which she listed among houses of reform orders, and shared the sum of twenty pounds among a list of religious institutions which included the Heilig Geist Spital and St. Georg.[123] A distinctive characteristic of widows' gifts is that they were usually made with a designation for services: as a memorial for themselves and their loved ones, or for alms to the poor. Gifts from single women were divided nearly evenly between St. Agnes and the Heilig Geist Spital (five to the former; four to the latter). Notably, all of their gifts were explicitly transactions of donation—including three bequests—although not all of their gifts are designated.

There are few clergy on record as hospital donors; those that are appear to have been closely connected to the institutions in question. Several donations suggest firsthand knowledge of hospitals' needs.[124] A cantor of St. Johannes, in 1315, bequeathed his best bed to the poor in the hospital, and his other bed to the lepers; similarly, a chaplain gave sums both to provide clothes and shoes for the city's poor, and for the (unspecified) comforts of

120 HStAD C1 Nr. 89 53r-v, 106r. Cf. Baur, Hessische Urkunden, vol. 2, 744, Nr. 743.

121 StAM U /7 February 1382; HStAD C1 Nr. 89 f51r-v. The account books of the Heilig Geist Spital, StAM 33/1 and StAM 33/2, contain three mentions of siblings coming to court together.

122 HStAD A2 168/67, dated 1283. A 1285 confirmation is copied in HHStAW Abt 22 Nr. 438, f82v–83v.

123 HHStAW Abt 22 Nr. 438, f160v–161v.

124 For other examples of knowledgeable almsgiving, see Alexandra Druzynski v. Boetticher and Marie Ulrike Jaros, "Die representativen Ansprüche der mittelalterlichen Stadt Lüneburg an ihre Leproserie," in *Extra muros: Vorstädtische Räume in Spätmittelalter und früher Neuzeit. Éspaces suburbains au bas Moyen Âge et à l'époque moderne*, eds. Guy Thewes and Martin Uhrmacher (Köln: Böhlau Verlag, 2019), 292–293.

the sick-poor in the hospital. Notably, the latter gift specified that the tunics should be given to "five poor men, of whom three should be lepers."[125] The lepers may be presumed to be those of St. Georg, since they were able to make use of a bed. Gerlacus, a chaplain of St. Boniface, also in the church of St. Johannes, gave gifts to the church itself for memorials and processions, followed by a bequest demonstrating considerable knowledge of the needs of the sick-poor and the provision made for them by the hospital.[126] Similar evidence of familiarity is found in the testament of Emmerich Dyme, made when he believed himself to be mortally ill, and designating revenues "for daily distribution."[127] Evidence from around Europe supports the theory that close social ties between hospitals and their local donors were the norm, not the exception.[128]

Of the four clerics who are known to have donated to Mainz's oldest hospital, at least two appear to have performed sacramental duties there. Godefridus, a scholar (*scolasticus*), made a bequest to the hospital in 1315; he may be identical with another Godefridus identified by his name alone. The Hermann who is known as chaplain in 1366 is likely to have been a permanent member of staff.[129] Two of the four priests donating to St. Agnes made bequests for their own *memoria*, suggesting that it was in that community that they had primary ties to the liturgical round.[130] Of the hospitals of Mainz, St. Agnes is most frequently the recipient of gifts designated for the performance of liturgical functions. The donors making such gifts include, in addition to the aforementioned priests, two married couples (with both the husband and wife named) and a single woman.[131] The Heilig Geist Spital also receives several such gifts.[132] St. Georg receives only one, apparently belying the historiographical truism that the prayers of the leprous were

125 HStAD C1 A Nr. 78, 111v–112r; StAM U 8 August 1427.

126 HStAD C1 A Nr. 78, 112v. See Franz Meffert, *Caritas und Krankenwesen bis zum Ausgang des Mittelalters* (Freiburg im Breisgau: Caritas Verlag, 1927), 295.

127 StAM 13/231, 3–7.

128 Ana Rita Rocha, "Being a Leper in Medieval Portugal"; Rossel, *Urkundenbuch Eberbach*, 622 Nr. 709; Davis, *The Medieval Economy of Salvation*, 115–145; Ziegler, *Medieval Healthcare and the Rise of Charitable Institutions*, 91–95; Anna M. Peterson, "Connotation and Denotation: The Construction of the Leper in Narbonne and Siena Before the Plague," in *Leprosy and Identity in the Middle Ages: From England to the Mediterranean,* ed. Elma Brenner and François-Olivier Touati (Manchester: Manchester University Press, 2021), 327–332.

129 StAM 33/2, StAM 33/4.

130 HStAD A2 115/41 (1345); HStAD A2 115/42; HStAD A2 168/401 (1354); HStAD A2 168/457 (10 November 1367).

131 HStAD A2 168/738 (1428); HStAD C1 A Nr. 89.

132 Regesten III: 2294, 2635. For similar examples, see Rubin, *Charity and Community in Medieval Cambridge*, 259–264; Watson, *Fundatio, Ordinatio, and Statuta*, 212.

particularly prized.[133] The one memorial gift that St. Georg does receive is not for Masses and prayers, but for food and drink. Two artisans set an annual gift in order that the lepers might receive food and drink on St. Martin's Day, and on the anniversary of a named leper, Heine von Eberscheim.[134] This gift also shows that the donors had emotional ties to Heine that ended neither with his diagnosis nor his death.

That St. Georg's distinctive patterns of property-holding were not determined by the fact that it was a leprosarium is demonstrated by comparison with the leper hospital of Worms, also dedicated to St. Georg. Several of the extant records mentioning the hospital refer to it as a point of orientation, indicating its prominence in the neighborhood.[135] St. Georg in Worms received donations in exchange for prayers and often enjoyed the patronage of those who also donated to the city's other hospitals.[136] Extant charters relating to the hospital indicate that it was seen as a religious institution, and that donors were familiar with the therapeutic and liturgical routines of the hospital. A matron from a burgher family of Worms, for instance, organized her gifts by the degree of prestige possessed by the recipient institutions. The cathedral and old foundations appeared first, followed by the mendicants and canons, and "each of the beguine houses." Each of these received a one-time donation. For her anniversary, however, she chose hospital residents as the beneficiaries of her alms: both the lepers and the "sick in the hospital" were given an annual gift of a measure of grain worth five pounds. This suggests that she held a personal preference for the city's hospitals, while recognizing their lack of cachet in the hierarchy of the religious foundations of Worms.[137] A man of modest means bequeathed ten shillings "to the good people [lepers] outside the city here in Worms, to be

133 StAM 700/2, f5r. Cf. for example Gilchrist, "Medieval Bodies in the Material World," 49; Édouard Jeanselme, "Comment l'Europe, au Moyen Âge, se protégea contre la Lèpre," *Bulletin de la Société Française d'Histoire de la Médecine* 25 (1931), 7–8; Jessalynn Lea Bird, "Medicine for Body and Soul: Jacques de Vitry's Sermons to Hospitallers and their Charges," in *Religion and Medicine in the Middle Ages*, eds. Peter Biller and Joseph Ziegler (Rochester, NY: York Medieval Press, 2001), 103–104.

134 StAM 700/01, f25.

135 Heinrich Boos, ed., *Urkundenbuch der Stadt Worms*, vol. 2 (Berlin: Duncker und Humblodt, 1890), 401, 442, 590.

136 Boos, ed., Urkundenbuch der Stadt Worms 199, 32, 41, 240. Ralf Lusiardi, *Stiftung und städtische Gesellschaft: Religiöse und soziale Aspekte des Stiftungsverhaltens im spätmittelalterlichen Stralsund*, Stiftungsgeschichten 2 (Oldenburg: de Gruyter, 2000), 97–113, sees an uptick in hospitals' provision of prayers and Masses in the fifteenth century; similarly, Charlotte A. Stanford, *Commemorating the Dead in Late Medieval Strasbourg: The Cathedral's Book of Donors and its Use (1320–1521)* (Farnham: Ashgate, 2011), 285–291.

137 Boos, ed., Urkundenbuch der Stadt Worms, 112.

on their common table and also on their feast day, and for this they should faithfully pray to God for him and remember his soul in their prayers."[138] The priest of the chapel for the leprous also received a gift on his own account.[139] Outright sales of land to the leper hospital multiply in the later fourteenth and fifteenth centuries, and gifts from this period form the kernel of the rents and properties recorded in the hospital's account book, compiled several centuries later.[140] This, together with the issuing of the leprosarium's first rule in the mid-fifteenth century, suggests that this period saw a change in its institutional fortunes. In view of overall trends in hospital numbers and population, it is unlikely that the expansion of the property base and record-keeping mechanisms of Worms' leper hospital was occasioned by an increase in the number of its residents.[141] Rather, the available evidence points to a new assertion of civic rights over the hospital, paralleled in Mainz.

Those who donated to St. Georg in Mainz were often the hospital's neighbors. While it was usual for hospitals to be connected with their neighbors by contracts as well as by proximity, the concentration of St. Georg's relationships was even more notable than the concentration of its property.[142] Most of St. Georg's donors are referred to as honorable; they were often prosperous, but rarely members of the elite, although a local knight did once use his seal on behalf of the community.[143] The donors and tenants with whom St. Georg and its residents had relationships are geographically concentrated within an approximate twelve kilometer radius of St. Georg. This pattern is consistent with the property consolidation pursued by hospitals and other religious houses in the later Middle Ages. In Mainz, similar policies were followed by the Heilig Geist Spital, St. Barbara, and St. Agnes.[144] In Würzburg, in 1323, the hospital of SS. Agidius and Theodoric

138 Boos, ed., Urkundenbuch der Stadt Worms, 426.

139 Boos, ed., Urkundenbuch der Stadt Worms, 194.

140 Boos, ed., Urkundenbuch der Stadt Worms, 640, 667, 672; the latter gift—of 12.5 acres—comes from a cathedral priest. StAW Bestand 159.3: 0431/1.

141 On the fraught question of the incidence of leprosy in the late medieval period, see Timothy S. Miller and John Nesbitt, *Walking Corpses: Leprosy in Byzantium and the Medieval West* (Ithaca: Cornell University Press, 2014), 44; Picot, "Bona diagnosis, bona curatio," 17–18; Tabuteau, "Vingt mille léproseries au Moyen Âge?," 119–128; François-Olivier Touati, *Archives de la lèpre: Atlas des léproseries entre Loire et Marne au moyen âge* (Paris: Comité des Travaux historiques et scientifiques, 1996), 49–64.

142 See Christianne Jéhanno, "L'emplacement de l'Hotel Dieu de Paris," in *Hôpitaux et maladreries au moyen âge: espace et environnement: actes du colloque international d'AmiensBeauvais, 22, 23 et 24 novembre 2002*, ed. Pascal Montaubin (Rouen: CAHMER, 2004), 35–49.

143 StAM 32/700 11 (1360).

144 StAM U / 11 January 1404 (in U / 12 January 1404); StAM U / 25 September 1410; Richard Dertsch, ed. *Die Urkunden des Stadtarchivs Mainz: Regesten,* vol. 1, nr. 2078; HStAD C1 A Nr. 89

traded territories and revenues with the monastery of Langheim, suggesting that both parties were interested in the consolidation of their respective holdings.[145] These policies may have been intended to cultivate desirable relationships as much as profitable properties.

St. Georg's legal agreements were ordinarily conducted, not in the court of Mainz, nor at the hospital itself, but in the villages where the properties themselves were located.[146] This practice suggests that St. Georg depended on collective memory, as well as on written records, to ensure the stability of their claims. St. Georg's unusually detailed records bear witness to the fact that the hospital was concerned not only with acres and vineyards and measures of grain, but with the process of securing these possessions and revenues; with who came to the place of judgment; and with what was said there. In the resulting charters, even the description of territory invokes relationships—past and future, as well as present—and depends on shared knowledge. St. Georg's records are characterized throughout by an unusual intimacy, as in the item recording that "Contze who lives at the end of [the village of] Trebur has two acres, from which he gives two measures of grain and a half measure of wheat; this is used to light the lamps."[147]

Conclusion: Cultivating Networks, Negotiating Law

The hospitals of Mainz were each embedded in the city's socioeconomic networks, in ways shaped both by their legal status and distinctive institutional priorities. The city's oldest hospital was that with the most extensive properties, and that with the most ties to Mainz's prosperous burghers. It was not, however, a political pawn of civic or familial interests. Rather, the hospital's thirteenth- and fourteenth-century records reveal a staff active in serving the spiritual needs of the sick-poor, and managing the community's valuable properties. Mainz's Heilig Geist Spital appears to have taken its religious status and temporal responsibilities with equal seriousness, contrary to the historiographical truism that attention to the latter must have been given at the expense of the former. Its success in doing so is attested by the many donors of comparatively modest means who entered into contracts and made gifts to the hospital, its staff, and its

folio 26v–27r (1362).

145 Bayrische Akademie der Wissenschaften, *Monumenta Boica* VI, 79.

146 StAM 32/700, 1–3, 4–5, 6–8, 8–10, 12–13, 14–15, 15–17.

147 StAM 700/02 f11.

sick-poor. This required the use of legal rhetoric that would conform to the needs of canon law, with unofficial policy aiding the specific needs of the hospital.[148] The hospital staff, far from being strictly cloistered, enjoyed ongoing relationships with family members and others. "Girkin's mother," for instance, appears as a tenant of the hospital in 1365.[149] Mainz's other hospitals, too, remained connected to the city's socioeconomic networks.

St. Agnes and St. Georg cultivated geographically concentrated properties, enabling them to manage their possessions easily. In the case of St. Georg, it is also clear that they cultivated close multigenerational relationships with many of their donors. Although St. Agnes struggled to acquire lay support in the late thirteenth century, they prospered in the later fourteenth century, as the religious status of their community became more widely accepted. The networks of St. Barbara are less visible, as it was managed by the canonry of Liebfrauen, and was dedicated to a largely transient population of paupers and pilgrims. The alms regularly distributed by Liebfrauen, however, bear witness to the fact that St. Barbara was known as a locus of care for the sick-poor, ranging from lepers to poor scholars, as well as those who were cared for in the hospital itself.

The records from Mainz and elsewhere in the Rhineland confirm that, over the course of the thirteenth and fourteenth centuries, hospital staff became more clearly defined as distinct from the sick they served, as persons bound by religious vows, and as persons with communal responsibilities. These trends can be more clearly connected to the increasingly well-defined parameters of religious status than to any growth—or decline—in pious fervor, or to a growing sense of civic consciousness. While the hospitals of the central Rhineland were embedded in local socioeconomic networks, they also had a clear sense of identity as independent religious institutions.

148 See for example the gift of a married couple, ostensibly of recurring revenues, in StAM 33/3, f29. Within the year, the hospital claims outright ownership of the land because of defaulted rents.

149 StAM 33/3, f29.

Conclusion

As a scribe wrote—repeatedly, and perhaps less than idly—in the margin of the Heilig Geist Spital's account book: *non bene pro toto libertas venditur auro,* liberty is not well sold at any price.[1] The conscientious recordkeeping of Mainz's hospitals indicates that they managed their resources in the service of the sick, and most jealously guarded the economic liberties afforded them by their legal status. As institutions governed by religious rules, though not part of religious orders, independent hospitals enjoyed both the privileges and responsibilities of religious status. As religious institutions, they received donations from their neighbors, indulgences from ecclesiastical officials, and, sometimes, opposition from civic officials. The precise implications of religious status for hospitals were not always clear. Like other religious institutions, they sometimes defended their prerogatives against civic officials; sometimes negotiated their rights in relationship to diocesan authority; and sometimes entered into conflict with lay and parish interests. Such moments of conflict, however, were not the result of legal ambiguity attached to hospitals in particular. Rather, they parallel similar episodes in the institutional histories of monasteries. As hospitals grew in and alongside prosperous cities in the later Middle Ages, debates on their function, location, and regulation were not uncommon. These debates were not the result of a legal vacuum, but of the range of possible meanings attached to religious status in the later Middle Ages.

Analyzing independent hospitals in light of the evolution of canon law makes it possible to identify patterns in their institutional development. Conciliar legislation and local charters alike bear witness to attempts to define both the legal parameters and the practical implications of religious status. To argue that hospitals were places of care rather than religious institutions is to construct a false dichotomy. Rather, providing care for Christ's sick-poor was constructed in legal as well as social terms as the core mission of the men and women who took vows in hospitals, the houses of God.

1 StAM 33/1, 95.

Barnhouse, Lucy C. *Hospitals in Communities of the Late Medieval Rhineland. Houses of God, Places for the Sick.* Taylor & Francis Group, 2023
DOI: 10.5117/9789463720243_CONC

The diversity of vocabulary applied to hospitals has sometimes, paradoxically, led to their invisibility in the historiography of religious institutions. But medieval hospitals were not just *hospitalia* or *leprosaria*, *xenodochia*, *eleemosynaria*, or even *domus dei*, the houses of God. Local documents make clear that hospitals could be referred to as monasteries, and were understood as falling under this broad category for houses dedicated to the communal religious life. Those who took vows in hospitals were bound no less than monks and nuns to poverty, chastity, and obedience. They were bound, too, to the service of the sick in the institutions where they resided, and which they administered. As the evidence from Mainz and the central Rhineland shows, the fact that independent hospitals were not linked to religious orders did not exclude them from religious status. Bishops and archbishops clearly perceived hospitals as necessitating regulation as religious houses. As religious houses, hospitals enjoyed—sometimes controversially—exemptions from taxation. Those who donated to hospitals in the later Middle Ages listed them alongside other religious houses, identifying these institutions as part of a topography of charity and devotion.

Too often, medieval leper hospitals have been studied under the presumption that they were markedly different from multipurpose hospitals, whether in their composition, their location, or in how they were regarded. I have argued that, on the contrary, *leprosaria* can be best understood when studied alongside other hospitals. Like other hospitals, they housed vowed communities of staff providing service to the sick. Like other hospitals, too, they were subject to intervention and regulation by religious authorities. The fact that, unlike multipurpose hospitals, leprosaria served residents who suffered from a single disease, affected these institutions in two ways. First, the identity of the leprous as a clearly identified population in need of assistance meant that leprosaria were less likely than their multipurpose counterparts to have their use of resources questioned. On a social level, the function of these hospitals as religious institutions appears to have been more self-evident. This is connected to the second point: when ecclesiastical regulations were imposed on leper hospitals, this was comparatively late. Civic authorities, meanwhile, might also seek to regulate the activities of the leprous for reasons of public health, without infringing on the religious status conferred on them by their residence in hospitals.

Religious status was, in the later Middle Ages, a dynamic legal category. And the thirteenth-century debates concerning its parameters and implications are particularly visible in the histories of hospitals, legally independent and governed by religious rules, but not connected to religious orders. Particularly in the decades between the Fourth Lateran Council and the

Council of Vienne, hospitals were included in diocesan reform efforts. Hospital communities might counter local opposition to their privileges as religious institutions by appealing to papal authority. Focusing on the central Rhineland, this study has aimed to demonstrate that medieval hospitals were regulated and managed as religious institutions, and integrated as such into the economic and religious networks of Europe. Staffed by vowed men and women, served by priests, and serving the poor, these institutions were understood as both houses of God and places for the sick.

Bibliography

Archival Sources

Aschaffenburg, Stiftsbibliothek MS Perg 26: Fifteenth-century medical miscellany
Darmstadt, Hessisches Staatsarchiv
HStAD A2 115: charters pertaining to St. Agnes
HStAD A2 157/13: closing of a dispute with the Heilig Geist Spital
HStAD A2 168: charters from the city of Mainz
HStAD A2 186/6: charter concerning the hospital in Oppenheim
HStAD A2 197/25: charter concerning the hospital in Oppenheim
HStAD A14 949: charter of donation to the leper hospital of Derneburg
HStAD C1 A Nr. 78: notebooks of Bodmann, Mainz's archivist in the Napoleonic Era
HStAD C1 A Nr. 89: chartulary of St. Agnes
HStAD C2 15/4: list of St. Agnes' possessions in Bischofsheim
HStAD C2 504/1: Heilig Geist Spital income record, ca. 1400
Mainz, Martinus Bibliothek HS 3: Records of the cathedral chapter, 1362–1530
Mainz, Stadtarchiv
StAM 6/30: thirteenth-century statutes of the Heilig Geist Spital in transcription
StAM 13: records of monastic houses
StAM 32: internal records of St. Georg, Mainz's leper hospital
StAM 33: internal records of the Heilig Geist Spital
StAM Dertsch Zettelkasten: notes taken by Richard Dertsch, former archivist
StAM Q 63 20: civic accounts 1459–1460
StAM Urkunden: charters in municipal possession
Marburg, Hessisches Staatsarchiv
HStAM Urkunde 47 Nr. 9: concerning the hospital in Marburg
HStAM Urkunde 47 Nr. 38: concerning the leper hospital in Kassel
HStAM Urkunde 86 Nr 887: concerning the leper hospital in Spangenberg
HStAM Urkunde 86 Nr. 1233: charter of donation to the leper hospital in Kassel
New York, Fordham University, Walsh Library Special Collections: Gemunde Document 16
Oxford, Bodleian Library
MS Laud Misc. 102: Thirteenth-century psalter (bound with hospital account book page)
MS Laud Misc. 237: contents include fourteenth-century medical miscellany
Speyer, Stadtarchiv
Sondersiechenhaus Zinsbuch III 122–3 B: account book of the leper hospital
Strasbourg, Archives de la Ville 1AH 215–217, 1 AH 7432: rules and privileges of the hospital
Wiesbaden, Hessisches Hauptstaatsarchiv
HHStaW Abt. 22: records of the Cistercian cloister of Eberbach
HHStAW Abt. 29 U 3: 1151 charter of Gottesthal
Worms, Stadtarchiv
StAW Abt 1 AI Nr I–0364: rule of the leper hospital
StAW 1B Nr. 2011: account book of the hospital
StAW Abt. 159 Nr. 431/1: excerpts from the hospital inventory from 1486–1787
Würzburg, Bayrisches Staatsarchiv
StAWü Mainzer Bücher Verschiedenen Inhalts 17, 19: civic privileges from Mainz
StAWü MRA Spitäler K 755/14: early modern records from Mainz's hospitals
StAWü Mainzer Urkunden Geistlicher Schrank 22/5: rule of the St. Katherine hospital

Edited Primary Sources

Acht, Peter, ed. *Mainzer Urkundenbuch. Vol 2: 1176–1200.* Darmstadt: Selbstverlag der Hessischen Historischen Kommission Darmstadt, 1971.

Alberigo, Joseph, Joseph A. Dossetti, Pericles Joannou, Claude Leonardi, and Paul Prodi, eds. *Conciliorum Oecumenicorum Decreta.* 3rd ed. Bologna: Istituto per le scienze religiose, 1973.

Aquinas, Thomas. *Summa Theologiae. Corpus Thomisticum*, ed. Roberto Busa. https://www.corpusthomisticum.org/sth3183.html

Banchi, Luciano, ed. *Statuti Volgari de lo Spedale di Santa Maria Vergina di Siena, scritti l'Anno MCCCV.* Siena: I Gati Editori, 1864.

Bannister, A.T., ed. *The Register of Adam de Orleton, Bishop of Hereford (A.D. 1317–1327).* Hereford: Wilson and Phillips, 1907.

Baur, Ludwig, ed. *Hessische Urkunden: Die Provinz Rheinhessen von 963–1325.* Darmstadt: Der historische Verein für das Grossherzogthum Hessen, 1862.

Bayrische Akademie der Wissenschaften. *Monumenta Boica.* Munich: Bayrische Akademie der Wissenchaften, 1763.

Berger, Élie, ed. *Les registres d'Innocent IV (1243–1254): recueil des bulles de ce pape.* 4 vols. Paris: Thorin et Fils, 1881–1919.

Bluhme, Friedrich. *Edictus ceteraeque Langobardorum leges. Cum constitutionibus et pactis principum Beneventanorum.* MGH Fontes Iuris 2. Hanover: Hahn, 1863.

Bodmann, Franz Joseph. *Rheingauische Alterthümer oder Landes und Regimentsverfassung des westlichen oder Niederrheingaues im Mittlern Zeitalter.* Mainz: Florian Kupferberg, 1819.

Böhmer, J.F., and Cornelius Will, eds. *Regesta archiepiscoporum Maguntinensium. Register zur Geschichte der Mainzer Erzbischöfe von Bonifatius bis Heinrich II.* 2 vols. Innsbruck: Wagner, 1886.

Boos, Heinrich, ed. *Urkundenbuch der Stadt Worms.* 2 vols. Berlin: Dunker & Humblot, 1890.

Canivez, Joseph Marie, ed. *Statuta capitulorum generalium ordinis Cisterciensis ab anno 1116 ad annum 1786.* 8 vols. Louvain: Bureaux de la Revue, 1933–1941.

Choppin, René. *Monasticon seu de jure coenobitarum libri duo.* Paris: Michael Sonnius, 1601.

Clement V. *Regestum Clementis papae V: ex vaticanis archetypis sanctissimi domini nostri Leonis XIII pontificis maximi iussu et munificentia.* 6 vols. Rome: Vatican Press, 1887.

Dertsch, Richard, ed. *Die Urkunden des Stadtarchivs Mainz: Regesten.* Beiträge zur Geschichte der Stadt Mainz 20. 3 vols. Mainz: Stadtarchiv, 1962–1963.

Gay, Jules, ed. *Registres et lettres des papes du XIIIe siècle. Les registres de Nicolas III* (1277–1280.) Paris: Thorin et Fils, 1898.

Geoffroy de Vigeois. *Chronica Gaufredi prioris vosiensis.* In *Novae Bibliothecae Manuscriptorum Librorum Tomus Secundus: Rerum Aquitanicarum Presertim Bituricensium Uberrima Collectio. Historias, Chronica, Vitas Sanctorum, ac similia Antiquitatis Monumenta, nunc primum ex MSS Codicibus eruta, copiose repraesentans*, edited by Philippe Labbé, 279–342. Paris: Sebastian & Gabriel Cramoisy, 1657.

Grandjean, Charles. *Le Registre de Benoît XI (1303–1304): recueil des bulles de ce pape.* Paris: Thorin et Fils, 1905.

Gudenus, Valentin Ferdinand, ed. *Codex diplomaticus: exhibens anectoda ab anno DCCCLXXXI ad MCCC Moguntiaca, ius Germanicum, et S.R.I. historiam illustrantia I.* Göttingen: Sumptu Regiae Officinae Librar. Academ., 1743.

Harper-Bill, Christopher, ed. *Charters of the Medieval Hospitals of Bury St. Edmunds.* Woodbridge: Boydell, 1994.

Harper-Bill, Christopher, ed. *English Episcopal Acta 32: Norwich 1244–1266.* Oxford: Oxford University Press, 2007.

Hegel, Karl von, ed. *Die Chroniken der mittelrheinischen Städte: Mainz.* Leipzig: Hirzel, 1881.

Hilgard, Alfred, ed. *Urkunden zur Geschichte der Stadt Speyer.* Strassburg: Trübner, 1885.
Hofmeister, Adolf, ed. *Ottonis Episcopi Frisingensis Chronica: Sive, Historia De Duabus Civitatibus.* MGH SS rer. Germ. 45. Hanover: Hahn, 1912.
Hostiensis. *Summa Aurea.* Venice: n.p., 1574.
Jaffé, Philippe, ed. *Monumenta Moguntina.* Bibliotheca Rerum Germanicarum 3. Berlin: Waidmann, 1866.
Joannis, Georg Christian, ed. *Rerum Moguntiacarum.* 2 vols. Frankfurt am Main: J. M. Sande, 1722.
Kortenkamp, Gottfried, ed. *Urkunden des St. Nikolaus Hospitals in BernkastelKues an der Mosel.* Trier: Kliomedia, 2004.
Le Grand, Léon. *Statuts d'hotels-Dieu et de léproseries: recueil de textes du XIIe au XIVe siècle.* Paris: Alphonse Picard, 1901.
Mansi, Giovan Domenico. *Sacrorum conciliorum nova et amplissima collectio.* 27 vols. Florence: Antonio Zatta, 1759.
Mayer, Ute, and Rudolf Steffens. *Die spätmittelalterlichen Urbare des Heiliggeist Spitals in Mainz.* Stuttgart: Franz Steiner Verlag, 1992.
Odo Rigaldus. *Registers of Eudes of Rouen.* Edited by J. F. Sullivan. Translated by Sydney M. Brown. New York: Columbia University Press, 1964.
Nider, Johannes. *De Morali Lepra.* Louvain: J. de Paderborn de Westphalia, 1485.
Perugi, Massimo. *La Vie de Saint Alexis.* Geneva: Droz, 2000.
Potthast, August, ed. *Regesta Pontificum Romanorum.* 2 vols. Berlin: Rudolf de Decker, 1874.
Pressutti, Pietro. *Regesta Honorii papae III, 1216–1227.* 2 vols. Rome: Vatican Press, 1888–1895.
Romana Repertoria Online, http://www.romanarepertoria.net/993.html
Rossel, Karl, ed. *Urkundenbuch der Abtei Eberbach im Rheingau.* 2 vols. Wiesbaden: Roth, 1862.
Schannat, Johann Friedrich, ed. *Concilia Germaniae: Ab Anno M Ad MCCXC.* Köln: Krakamp & Simon, 1760.
Schunk, Johann Peter, ed. *Beyträge zur Mainzer Geschichte, mit Urkunden.* Vol. 1. Frankfurt: Fleischer, 1788.
Smith, David M., ed. *English Episcopal Acta 30: Carlisle 1133–1292.* Oxford: Oxford University Press, 2005.
Steffens, Rudolf. "Das 'Mainzer Friedgebot' vom Jahre 1300: Neuedition." *Mainzer Zeitschrift* 100 (2005): 1–10.
Stimming, Manfred. *Mainzer Urkundenbuch.* 2 volsHistorischen Vereins für Hessen, 1932.
Tellenbach, Gerd, ed. *Repertorium Germanicum II: Urban VI., Bonifaz IX., Innocenz VII. und Gregor XII. (1378–1415).* Berlin: de Gruyter, 1933.
UCLA Digital Library Program. *Corpus Juris Canonici* (1582), https://digital.library.ucla.edu/canonlaw/.
Urkunden zur Geschichte der Stadt Essen. Essen: Historischer Verein, n.d.
Ut Per Litteras Apostolicas: https://clio.columbia.edu/catalog/4346120
Vogt, Ernst, ed. *Regesten der Erzbischöfe von Mainz.* Leipzig: Veit & Co., 1913.
Wiegand, Wilhelm, ed. *Urkundenbuch der Stadt Strassburg.* Vol. 4. Strassburg: Trübner, 1888.
Würdtwein, Stephan Alexander. *Dioecesis Moguntina.* Vol. I. Mannheim: Typis Academicis, 1768.

Secondary Sources

Abreu, Laurinda and Sally Sheard. "Introduction." In *Hospital Life: Theory and Practice from the Medieval to the Modern*, edited by Laurinda Abreu and Sally Sheard, 1–19. Oxford: Peter Lang, 2013.
Adam, Ingrid. "Eine Äbtissinnenliste aus dem Altmünsterkloster zu Mainz." *Mainzer Zeitschrift* 90/91(1995/1996): 89–109.

Agrimi, Jole, and Chiara Crisciani. "Charity and Aid in Medieval Christian Civilization." In *Western Medical Thought from Antiquity to the Middle Ages*, edited by Mirko D. Grmek, 170–196. Cambridge, MA: Harvard University Press, 1998.

Ahlers, Gerd. *Weibliches Zisterziensertum im Mittelalter und seine Klöster in Niedersachsen*. Berlin: Lukas Verlag, 2003.

Aigrain, René. *L'hagiographie: Ses Sources, Ses Méthodes, Son Histoire*. Brussels: Société des Bollandistes, 2000.

Alberzoni, Maria Pia. "Norditalienische Pilgerhospize im 12. und 13. Jahrhundert." In *Wege zum Heil: Pilger und Heilige Orte an Mosel und Rhein*, edited by Thomas Frank, Michael Matheus, and Sabine Reichert, 277–296. Stuttgart: Franz Steiner Verlag, 2009.

Allen, Peter L. "To Live Outside the Camp: Medieval Leprosy." In *The Wages of Sin: Sex and Disease, Past and Present*." 25–40. Chicago: University of Chicago Press, 2000.

Amulree, Lord. "Monastic Infirmaries." In *The Evolution of Hospitals in Britain*, edited by F. N. L. Poynter, 11–26. London: Pitman Medical Publishing Company Ltd., 1964.

Amundsen, D.W. "Medieval Canon Law on Medical and Surgical Practice by the Clergy." *Bulletin of the History of Medicine* 52 (1978): 22–44.

Andersen, Johannes Gerhard. "The Medieval Diagnosis of Leprosy." In *Human Paleopathology: Current Syntheses and Future Options*, edited by D.J. Ortner and A.C. Aufderheide, 205–208. Washington, DC: Smithsonian, 1991.

Andersen, Johannes Gerhard. "The Osteo-Archaeological Diagnosis of Leprosy." In *Proceedings of the Fourth European Meeting of the Paleopathology Association*, edited by G. T. Haneveld and W. R. K. Perizonius, 221–226. Utrecht: B. V. Elinkwijk, 1982.

Andrews, Frances. "Self-Representation in Times of Crisis: The Case of the Early Humiliati." In *Self-Representation of Medieval Religious Communities: The British Isles in Context*, edited by Anne Müller and Karen Stöber, 221–233. Berlin: LIT Verlag, 2009.

Angers, Denise. "La bourgeoisie de Falaise et ses lepreux à la fin du Moyen Âge." *Florilegium* 6 (1985): 216–245.

Apel, Kathrin. *Caritas und Memoria: Das Hospitalwesen der Stadt Kassel im späten Mittelalter*. Kassel: Universität Kassel Verlag, 2006.

Arens, Fritz Viktor. *Die Kunstdenkmäler der Stadt Mainz*. Berlin: Deutsche Kunstverlag, 1962.

Arens, Fritz Viktor. "St. Martin, der Mainzer Dom und das Erzstift." *Neues Jahrbuch für das Bistum Mainz* (1982): 9–56.

Arlinghaus, Franz-Josef. "The Myth of Urban Unity: Religion and Social Performance in Late Medieval Braunschweig." In *Cities, Texts, and Social Networks, 400–1500: Experiences and Perceptions of Medieval Urban Space*, edited by Caroline Goodson, Anne E. Lester, and Carol Symes, 215–232. Farnham: Ashgate, 2010.

Arlinghaus, Franz-Josef. "Point of Reference: Trust and the Function of Written Agreements in a Late Medieval Town." In *Strategies of Writing: Studies on Text and Trust in the Middle Ages*, edited by Petra Schultert, Marco Mostert, and Irene van Renswoude, 286–299. Turnhout: Brepols, 2008.

Arnold, Harry L. "Leprosy and the Social Class in the Middle Ages." *International Journal of Leprosy and Other Mycobacterial Diseases* 54 (1986): 647–648.

Arnoux, Mathieu. "Aux origines d'une léproserie: la pancarte de la Madeleine d'Orbec (1107–1135)." *Cahiers Leopold Delisle* 44 (1995): 209–222.

Auge, Oliver. "'Ne pauperes et debiles in...domo degentes divinis careant.' Sakralreligiöse Askpete der mittelalterlichen Hospitalgeschichte." In *Sozialgeschichte mittelalterlicher Hospitäler*, edited by Neithard Bulst and KarlHeinz Spiess, 77–125. Ostfildern: Jan Thorbecke Verlag, 2007.

Avril, Jean. "Le troisième concile de Latran et les communautés de lépreux." *Revue Mabillon* 60 (1981): 21–76.

Baas, Karl. *Mittelalterliche Gesundheitsfürsorge im Gebiet des heutigen Rheinhessens.* Sonderdrück. Veröffentlichungen aus dem Gebiete der Medizinalverwaltung. Berlin: Richard Schoetz, 1931.

Bär, Max. "Das vormalige Siechenhaus bei Koblenz." *Mittelrheinische Geschichtsblätter* 4 (1924): 2–3.

Bailey, Michael D. *Battling Demons: Witchcraft, Heresy, and Reform in the Late Middle Ages.* University Park, PA: Pennsylvania State University Press, 2003.

Bailey, Michael D. "Religious Poverty, Mendicancy, and Reform in the Late Middle Ages." *Church History* 72 (2003): 457–483.

Bain, Emmanuel. "Politiques des œuvres de miséricorde dans le discours scolastique (XIIeXIIIe siècles)." In *Politiche di Misericordia tra Teoria e Prassi: Confraternite, ospedali e Monti di Pietà (XIIIXVI secolo)*, edited by Pietro Delcorno, 21–48. Bologna: Il Mulino, 2018.

Barber, Malcolm C. "Lepers, Jews and Moslems: The Plot to Overthrow Christendom in 1321." *History* 66 (1981): 1–17.

Barnhouse, Lucy C. "'A Certain Poor Woman': Vulnerability and Visibility among Hospital Donors and Tenants." *Medieval People: Social Bonds, Kinship, and Networks* 36 (2022): 133–154.

Barnhouse, Lucy C. "Disordered Women? The Hospital Sisters of Mainz and Their Late Medieval Identities." *Medieval Feminist Forum* 55:2 (2020): 60–97.

Barnhouse, Lucy C. "Examining for Leprosy in the Fifteenth Century." In *Medieval Disability Sourcebook: Western Europe,* edited by Cameron Hunt McNabb, 76–93. Earth, Milky Way: punctum books, 2020.

Barnhouse, Lucy C. "From Helpful Gardens to Hateful Words: Moral and Physical Healthscaping in the Late Medieval Rhineland." In *Disease and the Environment in the Medieval and Early Modern Worlds*, edited by Lori Jones, 52–64. London: Routledge, 2022.

Barnhouse, Lucy C. "Good People, Poor Sick: The Social Identities of Lepers in the Late Medieval Rhineland." In *Leprosy and Identity in the Middle Ages: From England to the Mediterranean*, edited by Elma Brenner and François-Olivier Touati, 183–207. Manchester: Manchester University Press, 2021.

Barnhouse, Rebecca. "Leeches and Leprosy: Medieval Medicine in Modern Novels for Young Readers." *Literature and Medicine* 21 (2002): 25–44.

Baron, Françoise. "Le mausolée de saint Elzéar de Sabran à Apt." *Bulletin Monumental* 136 (1978): 267–283.

Barthelemy, M. "Procèsverbal de visite d'un lepreux en 1464 et relation juridique d'une autopsie en 1499." *Actes du comité médical des BouchesduRhone* 20 (1881–1882): 118–120.

Baudot, Marcel, Albert Bourgeois, and Marcel Candille. "Psychologie collective et institutions charitables. Lépreux et maladreries du Pas-de-Calais (Xe-XVIIIe siècles)." *Mémoires de la Commission départementale d'histoire et d'archéologie du Pas*-de-Calais 14 (1972): 1–358.

Beck, Walburga. *Untersuchungen über die frühere Verbreitung des Aussatzes im heutigen Hessen. Eine erste Bestandsaufnahme.* Bochum: Universität Bochum, 1993.

Bedos-Rezak, Brigitte Miriam. "Medieval Identity: A Sign and a Concept." *The American Historical Review* 105 (2000): 1489–1533.

Belker van den Heuvel, Jürgen. "Aussätzige: 'Tückischer Feind' und 'Armer Lazarus.'" In *Randgruppen der Spätmittelalterlichen Gesellschaft,* edited by Bernd-Ulrich Hergemöller, 270–299. Rev. ed. Warendorf: Fahlbusch Verlag, 2001.

Berger, Wilhelm. *Das St. Georgshospital zu Hamburg. Die Wirtschaftsführung eines mittelalterlichen Großhaushaltes.* Hamburg: Hans Christians Verlag, 1972.

Bergman, Fred. "Hoping Against Hope? A Marital Dispute about the Medical Treatment of Leprosy in the Fifteenth-Century Hanseatic Town of Kampen." In *The Task of Healing: Medicine, Religion, and Gender in England and the Netherlands, 1450–1800*, edited by Hilary Marland and Margaret Pelling, 23–48. Rotterdam: Erasmus, 1996.

Bériac, Françoise. *Histoire des lépreux au Moyen Âge. Une société d'exclus*. Paris: Imago, 1988.

Bériac, Françoise. "Les fraternités de lépreux et lépreuses." In *Doppelklöster und andere Formen der Symbiose männlicher und weiblicher Religiosen im Mittelalter*, edited by Kaspar Elm and Michel Parisse, 203–211. Berliner Historische Studien 18: Ordensstudien. Berlin: Duncker und Humblot, 1980.

Bériac, Françoise. "*Mourir au monde*. Les ordines de séparation des lepreux en France aux XVe et XVIe siècles." *Journal of Medieval History* 11 (1985): 245–269.

Bériou, Nicole. "La predication au beguinage de Paris pendant l'année liturgique 1272–1273." *Recherches augustiniennes* 13 (1978): 105–229.

Bériou, Nicole and Francois-Olivier Touati. *Voluntate Dei Leprosus: les lépreux entre conversion et exclusion aux XIIème et XIIIème siècles*. Spoleto: Centro Italiano di studi Sull'altro Medioevo, 1991.

Berkhofer, Robert F. *Day of Reckoning: Power and Accountability in Medieval France*. Philadelphia: University of Pennsylvania Press, 2004.

Berman, Constance Hoffman. "Abbeys for Cistercian Nuns in the Ecclesiastical Province of Sens: Foundation, Endowment, and Economic Activities of the Earlier Foundations." *Revue Mabillon* 69 (1997): 83–113.

Berman, Constance Hoffman. *The Cistercian Evolution: The Invention of a Religious Order in Twelfth-Century Europe*. Philadelphia: University of Pennsylvania Press, 2000.

Bettin, Hartmut. "Von 'den kranken de dar liggen up den bedden'—Krankheit und Kranke in den mittelalterlichen norddeutschen Hansestädten Wahrnehmung, Wertung, Deutung und Umgang, insbesondere im Spiegel der Stralsunder Bürgertestamente." *Historia Hospitalium* 30 (2016–2017): 145–171.

Biller, Peter. "Medicine and Heresy." In *Religion and Medicine in the Middle Ages*, edited by Peter Biller and Joseph Ziegler, 155–174. Rochester, NY: York Medieval Press, 2001.

Bird, Jessalynn Lea. "Medicine for Body and Soul: Jacques de Vitry's Sermons to Hospitallers and their Charges." In *Religion and Medicine in the Middle Ages*, edited by Peter Biller and Joseph Ziegler, 91–108. Rochester, NY: York Medieval Press, 2001.

Bockenheimer, Carl Georg. *Der Gutleuthof bei Mainz*. Mainz: Falk, 1882.

Bodart, Emmanuel. "L'étude des traces matérielles de l'activité hospitalière en Belgique: la rencontre de l'archéologie et l'histoire." In *Einrichtungen der sozialen Sicherung im mittelalterlichen Lotharingien. Actes des 13es Journées Lotharingeinnes (12–15 Oct. 2004)*, edited by Michel Pauly, 19–53. Linden: Section Historie de l'Institut GrandDucal, 2008.

Bodarwé, Katrinette. "Pflege und Medizin in mittelalterlichen Frauenkonventen." *Medizinhistorisches Journal* 37 (2002): 231–263.

Boeckl, Christine M. *Images of Leprosy: Disease, Religion, and Politics in European Art*. Kirksville, MO: Truman State University Press, 2011.

Boetticher, Alexandra Druzynski von, and Marie Ulrike Jaros. "Die representativen Ansprüche der mittelalterlichen Stadt Lüneburg an ihre Leproserie." In *Extra muros: Vorstädtische Räume in Spätmittelalter und früher Neuzeit. Espaces suburbains au bas Moyen Âge et à l'époque moderne*, edited by Guy Thewes and Martin Uhrmacher, 273–299. Köln: Böhlau Verlag, 2019.

Boetticher, Alexandra Druzynski von, and Marie Ulrike Jaros. "'Vorbuwet up sunte Nicolai hove.' Interdisziplinäre Forschungen zur Bau und Sozialgeschichte der Lüneburger Leproserie im Mittelalter." *Historia Hospitalium* 30 (2016–2017): 239–253.

Böhringer, Letha. "Beginen und Schwestern in der Sorge für Kranke, Sterbende und Verstorbene: Eine Problemskizze." In *Organisierte Barmherzigkeit: Armenfürsorge und Hospitalwesen in Mittelalter und früher Neuzeit*, edited by Artur Dirmeier, 127–155. Regensburg: Verlag Friedrich Pustet, 2010.

Bonenfant, Paul. "Les premiers 'hospitia' de Bruxelles au XIIe siècle." *Annales de la Société belge d'histoire des hôpitaux* 11 (1973): 3–25.
Bonenfant-Feytmans, Anne-Marie. "Les organisations hospitalières vues par Jacques de Vitry (1225)." *Annales de la Société belge d'histoire des hôpitaux* 18 (1980): 17–45.
Bonfield, Christopher. "Therapeutic Regimes for Bodily Health in Medieval English Hospitals." In *Hospital Life: Theory and Practice from the Medieval to the Modern*, edited by Laurinda Abreu and Sally Sheard, 21–48. Bern: Peter Lang, 2013.
Bonnin, Luc. "St. Thomas d'Aizier: un exemple de projet de valorisation d'un site archéologique de léproserie médiévale." In *Étude des lépreux et des léproseries au Moyen Âge dans le nord de la France: histoire, archéologie et patrimoine*, edited by Bruno Tabuteau, 35–46. Amiens: Université de Picardie Jules Verne, 2007.
Borradori, Piera. "Etre lépreux autour de 1300." In *Le Pays de Vaud vers 1300*, edited by Piera Borradori and Nadia Pollini, 105–113. Lausanne: Faculté des Lettres, Université de Lausanne, 1992.
Bourgeois, Albert. *Lépreux et Maladreries du Pas-de-Calais*. Arras: Commission Départementale des Monuments Historiques du Pas-de-Calais, 1972.
Braband, Gustav. "Domdekan Johannes Unterschopf (1325–1345): Studien zur Geschichte des Mainzer Domkapitels und seiner Beziehunng zu Papsttum und Reich unter Ludwig dem Bayern." *Archiv für Mittelrheinische Kirchengeschichte* 7 (1955): 22–76.
Braband, Gustav. "Domdekan Johannes Unterschopf (1325–1345): Studien zur Geschichte des Mainzer Domkapitels und seiner Beziehunng zu Papsttum und Reich unter Ludwig dem Bayern: Zweiter Teil." *Archiv für Mittelrheinische Kirchengeschichte* 8 (1956): 94–132.
Brans, Hans Otto. "Leprosorien im früheren Regierungsbezirk Aachen." *Historia Hospitalium* 14 (1981/1982): 17–33.
Brasher, Sally Mayall. *Hospitals and Charity: Religious Culture and Civic Life in Medieval Northern Italy*. Manchester: Manchester University Press, 2017.
Brenner, Elma. "Between Palliative Care and Curing the Soul: Medical and Religious Responses to Leprosy in France and England, c. 1100–c.1500." In *Medicine, Religion and Gender in Medieval Culture*, edited by Naoë Kukita Yoshikawa, 221–236. Cambridge: D.S. Brewer, 2015.
Brenner, Elma. *Leprosy and Charity in Medieval Rouen*. Woodbridge: Boydell, 2015.
Brenner, Elma. "The Medical World of Medieval Normandy." Presentation at the Institute for Historical Research, London, 2 June 2015.
Brenner, Elma. "Outside the City Walls: Leprosy, Exclusion, and Social Identity in Twelfth and Thirteenth-Century Rouen." In *Difference and Identity in Francia and Medieval France*, edited by Meredith Cohen and Judith Firnhaber-Baker, 139–155. Farnham: Ashgate, 2010.
Brenner, Elma. "Recent Perspectives on Leprosy in Medieval Western Europe." *History Compass* 8 (2010): 388–406.
Brocard, Nicole. *Soins, secours, et exclusion: établissements hospitaliers et assistance dans le diocèse de Besançon, XIVe et XVe siècles*. Paris: Presses Universitaires Franc-Comtoises, 1998.
Brodman, James W. *Charity and Religion in Medieval Europe*. Washington, DC: Catholic University of America Press, 2009.
Brodman, James W. *Charity and Welfare: Hospitals and the Poor in Medieval Catalonia*. Philadelphia: University of Pennsylvania Press, 1998.
Brodman, James W. "New Approaches to Written Sources: Religion and Discipline in the Hospitals of Thirteenth-Century France." In *The Medieval Hospital and Medical Practice*, edited by Barbara S. Bowers, 123–132. Farnham: Ashgate, 2007.
Brodman, James W. "Shelter and Segregation: Lepers in Medieval Catalonia." In *On the Social Origins of Medieval Institutions: Essays in Honor of Joseph F. O'Callaghan*, edited by Donald J. Kagay and Theresa M. Vann, 35–45. Leiden: Brill, 1998.

Brody, Saul Nathaniel. *The Disease of the Soul: Leprosy in Medieval Literature*. Ithaca: Cornell University Press, 1974.

Brown, Elizabeth A. R. "Death and the Human Body in the Later Middle Ages: The Legislation of Boniface VIII on the Division of the Corpse." *Viator* 12 (1981): 221–270.

Bruintje, T. D. "The Auditory Ossicles in Human Skeletal Remains from a Leper Cemetery in Chichester, England." *Journal of Archaeological Science* 17 (1990): 627–633.

Brundage, James A. *Law, Sex, and Christian Society in Medieval Europe*. Chicago: University of Chicago Press, 1987.

Brundage, James A. *Medieval Canon Law*. New York: Longman, 1995.

Buckley, Laureen, and Alan Hayden. "Excavations at St. Stephen's Leper Hospital, Dublin: A Summary Account and an Analysis of Burials." In *Medieval Dublin, III: Proceedings of the Friends of Medieval Dublin Symposium 2001*, edited by Sean Duffy, 151–194. Dublin: Four Courts Press, 2002.

Bulst, Neithard, and Karl-Heinz Spiess, eds. *Sozialgeschichte mittelalterlicher Hospitäler*. Ostfildern: Jan Thorbecke Verlag, 2007.

Bundeskonferenz der kirchlichen Archive in Deutschland, ed. *Führer durch die Bistumsarchive der katholischen Kirche in Deutschland*. Siegburg: Franz Schmitt Verlag, 1991.

Burr, David. *The Spiritual Franciscans: From Protest to Persecution in the Century After St. Francis*. University Park, PA: Pennsylvania State University Press, 2001.

Burton, Janet. "Fundator Noster: Roger de Mowbray as Founder and Patron of Monasteries." In *Religious and Laity in Western Europe 1000–1400: Interaction, Negotiation, and Power*, edited by Emilia Jamroziak and Janet Burton, 23–40. Turnhout: Brepols, 2006.

Bynum, Carolyn Walker. *The Resurrection of the Body in Western Christianity, 200–1336*. New York: Columbia University Press, 1995.

Cabré, Montserrat. "Women or Healers? Household Practices and the Categories of Healthcare in Late Medieval Iberia." *Bulletin of the History of Medicine* 82 (2008): 18–51.

Campion, Eleanor. "Bernard and Alice the Leper: An Odor of Life for Some." *Cistercian Studies Quarterly* 39 (2004): 127–139.

Caron, P.G. "L'evoluzione dalla *quarta pauperum* alla pia fundatio a scopo ospedaliero in alcuni testi della letteratura decretistica." *Il diritto ecclesiastico* 73 (1962): 137–159.

Catling, Christopher. "The Archaeology of Leprosy and the Black Death." *Current Archaeology* 236 (2009): 22–29.

Chibnall, Marjorie. "Dating the Charters of the Smaller Religious Houses in Suffolk in the Twelfth and Thirteenth Centuries." In *Dating Undated Medieval Charters*, edited by Michael Gervers, 51–60. Woodbridge: Boydell, 2000.

Chircop, John. "Management and Therapeutic Regimes in Lunatic Asylums." In *Hospital Life: Theory and Practice from the Medieval to the Modern*, edited by Laurinda Abreu and Sally Sheard. 179–208. Bern: Peter Lang, 2013.

Clanchy, Michael T. *From Memory to Written Record: England 1066–1307*. 2nd ed. Oxford: Blackwell, 2006.

Clarke, Catherine A. M., ed. *Mapping the Medieval City: Space, Place, and Identity in Chester c. 1200–1600*. Cardiff: University of Wales Press, 2011.

Clay, Rotha Mary. *The Medieval Hospitals of England*. London: Methuen, 1909.

Cochelin, Isabelle. "Bourgeoisie et léproseries de la principauté de Liège (fin XIIe début XIIIe siècles." *Sources, travaux historiques* 13 (1988): 15–18.

Constable, Giles. "Nudus Nudum Christum Sequi and Parallel Formulas in the Twelfth Century: A Supplementary Dossier." In *Continuity and Discontinuity in Church History: Essays Presented to George Hunston Williams*, edited by F. Forrester Church and Timothy George, 83–91. Leiden: Brill, 1979.

Coomans, Thomas. "Belfries, Cloth Halls, Hospitals, and Mendicant Churches: A New Urban Architecture in the Low Countries around 1300." In *The Year 1300 and the Creation of a New European Architecture*, edited by Alexandra Gajewski, 185–202. Turnhout: Brepols, 2007.

Courtenay, William J. "Curers of Body and Soul: Medical Doctors as Theologians." In *Religion and Medicine in the Middle Ages*, edited by Peter Biller and Joseph Ziegler, 61–77. Rochester, NY: York Medieval Press, 2001.

Crabus, Mirko. "Beginen, Rosen, und Leprosen: Lebten Leprakranke im münsterischen Magdalenenhospital?" *Die Klapper* 20 (2012): 8–10.

Crabus, Mirko. "'Für Arme, Kranke und Pilger.' Die spätmittelalterliche Fürsorgepolitik der Stadt Münster." *Historia Hospitalium* 29 (2014–2015): 493–504

Craemer, Ulrich. *Das Hospital als Bautyp des Mittelalters*. Köln: W. Kohlhammer Verlag, 1963.

Crislip, Andrew T. *From Monastery to Hospital: Christian Monasticism and the Transformation of Healthcare in Late Antiquity*. Ann Arbor: University of Michigan Press, 2005.

Cros-Mayrevieille, Gabriel. *Les frères donnés à la léproserie du bourg de Narbonne*. Toulouse: Privat, 1930.

Cule, John. "Diagnostic et traitement de la lèpre au Moyen Âge au Pays de Galles." In *Colloque international d'histoire de la médecine médiévale, Orléans, 4 et 5 mai 1985*, 83–98. Orleans: Société Orléanaise d'Histoire de la Médecine Centre Jeanne d'Arc, 1985.

Cullum, Patricia H. "Leperhouses and Borough Status in the Thirteenth Century." In *Thirteenth Century England, III: Proceedings of the Newcastle upon Tyne Conference 1989*, edited by P. R. Coss and S. D. Lloyd, 37–46. Woodbridge: Boydell, 1991.

Cyrus, Cynthia J. *The Scribes for Women's Convents in Late Medieval Germany*. Toronto: University of Toronto Press, 2009.

Dadder, Hans. "Die frühe Entwicklung des stadtmainzischen Apothekenwesens bis zur Apothekerordnung Erzbischof Albrechts II. von Brandenburg." In *Das Apothekenwesen von Stadt und Erzstift Mainz: mit der Mainzer Medizinalordnung und grossen Apothekentaxe von 1618*, 13–41. Frankfurt am Main: Govi Verlag, 1961.

Dannenberg, Lars-Arne. *Das Recht der Religiosen in der Kanonistik des 12. und 13. Jahrhunderts*. Berlin: Verlag W. Hopf, 2008.

Davis, Adam J. *The Holy Bureaucrat: Eudes Rigaud and Religious Reform in Thirteenth-Century Normandy*. Ithaca: Cornell University Press, 2006.

Davis, Adam J. "Hospitals, Charity, and the Culture of Compassion in the Twelfth and Thirteenth Centuries." In *Approaches to Poverty in Medieval Europe: Complexities, Contradictions, Transformations, c. 1100–1500*, edited by Sharon Farmer, 23–45. Turnhout: Brepols, 2016.

Davis, Adam J. *The Medieval Economy of Salvation: Charity, Commerce, and the Rise of the Hospital*. Ithaca: Cornell University Press, 2019.

Deane, Jennifer Kolpacoff. "From Case Studies to Comparative Models: Würzburg Beguines and the Vienne Decrees." In *Labels and Libels: Naming Beguines in Northern Medieval Europe*, edited by Letha Böhringer, 53–82. Turnhout: Brepols, 2014.

Deane, Jennifer Kolpacoff. "Geistliche Schwestern: The Pastoral Care of Lay Religious Women in Medieval Würzburg." In *Partners in Spirit: Women, Men, and Religious Life in Germany, 1100–1500*, edited by Fiona J. Griffiths and Julie Hutchin, 237–262. Turnhout: Brepols, 2014.

Deane, Jennifer Kolpacoff. *Papal Schism, Archiepiscopal Politics, and Waldensian Persecution (1378–1396): The Ecclesiopolitical Landscape of Late Fourteenth-Century Mainz*. Ph.D. diss., Northwestern University, 2000.

Dehio, Georg. *Handbuch der deutschen Kunstdenkmäler: Thüringen*. Berlin: Deutscher Kunstverlag, 2003.

De Keyzer, Walter. "Le 'dépistage' de la lèpre en Hainaut. De l'expertise pratiquée par les lépreux à l'examen médical (XIVX-VI siècles)." In *Einrichtungen der sozialen Sicherung im mittelalterlichen Lotharingien. Actes des 13es Journées Lotharingiennes (12–15 Oct. 2004)*, edited by Michel Pauly, 93–136. Linden: Section Historie de l'Institut Grand-Ducal, 2008.

De Keyzer, Walter. "L'évolution interne des léproseries." In *Lépreux et sociabilité du Moyen Âge aux temps modernes,* edited by Bruno Tabuteau, 13–20. Rouen: Publications de l'Université de Rouen, 2000.

De Keyzer, Walter. "Lépreux et léproseries dans le comté de Hainaut au moyen âge." In *Recueil d'études d'histoire Hainuyère offertes à Maurice A. Arnould,* edited by Jean-Marie Cauchies and J. M. Duvosquel, 521–544. Mons: n.p., 1983.

Delaigue, Regis. "L'accueil des malades dans les hôpitaux des Antonins." *Antoniter Forum* 15 (2007): 16–31.

Demaitre, Luke. "The Description and Diagnosis of Leprosy by Fourteenth-Century Physicians." *Bulletin of the History of Medicine* 59 (1985): 327–344.

Demaitre, Luke. *Leprosy in Premodern Medicine: A Malady of the Whole Body*. Baltimore: Johns Hopkins University Press, 2007.

Demaitre, Luke. "The Relevance of Futility: Jordanus de Turre (fl. 1313–1335) on the Treatment of Leprosy." *Bulletin of the History of Medicine* 70 (1996): 25–61.

Demandt, Dieter. *Stadtherrschaft und Stadtfreiheit im Spannungsfeld von Geistlichkeit und Bürgerschaft in Mainz (11–15. Jahrhundert.)* Wiesbaden: Franz Steiner Verlag, 1977.

De Sandre Gasparini, Giuseppina. "L'assistenza ai lebbrosi nel movimento religioso dei primidecenni del Duecento veronese: uomini e fatti." In *Viridarium floridum. Studi di storia veneta offerti dagli allievi a Paolo Sambin*, edited by Maria Chiara Billanovich, Giorgio Cracco, and Antonio Rigon, 25–59. Padua: Editrice Antenore, 1984.

Dethlefs, Günter. "650 Jahre Kinderhaus." In *Lepra--Gestern und Heute: 15 wissenschaftliche Essays zur Geschichte und Gegenwart einer Menschheitsseuche: Gedenkschrift zum 650-jähringen Bestehen des Rektorats Münster-Kinderhaus*, edited by Richard Toellner, 14–28. Münster: Regensberg, 1992.

Diamond, James A. "Maimonides on Leprosy: Illness as Contemplative Metaphor." *Jewish Quarterly Review* 96 (2006): 65–94.

Dobras, Wolfgang. "Münzerhausgenossen und andere Geschlechter. Bemerkungen zur Mainzer Oberschicht in den Bürgerkämpfen des 15. Jahrhunderts." *Mainzer Zeitschrift* 94/95 (1999/2000): 95–109.

Dols, Michael W. "The Leper in Medieval Islamic Society." *Speculum* 58 (1983): 891–916.

Dols, Michael W. "The Origins of the Islamic Hospital, Myth and Reality." *Bulletin of the History of Medicine* 91 (1987): 367–390.

Dora, Cornel. "Der soziale heilige St. Gallens." In *Vater für die Armen: Otmar und die Anfänge des Klosters St. Gallen*. Basel: Schwabe Verlag, 2019.

Doti, Gerardo. "La rete degli *hospitalia* nel Piceno." In *L'accoglienza religiosa tra tardo antico ed età moderna: Luoghi, architetture, percorsi*, edited by Silvia Beltramo and Paolo Cozzo, 47–59. Rome: Viella, 2013.

Douglas, Mary. "Witchcraft and Leprosy: Two Strategies of Exclusion." *Man: Journal of the Royal Anthropological Institute* 26 (1991): 723–736.

Dross, Fritz. "Aussetzen und Einsperren: Zur Integration und Disintegration von Leprosen in Spätmittelalter und früher Neuzeit." In *Verortungen des Krankenhauses*, edited by Arno Görgen and Thorsten Halling, 175–190. Stuttgart: Franz Steiner Verlag, 2014.

Dross, Fritz. "Spitälische und außerspitälische Versorgung von Leprosen im spätmittelalterlichen und frühneuzeitlichen Nürnberg." *Historia Hospitalium* 30 (2016–2017): 277–286

Dross, Fritz. "Vom zuverlässigen Urteilen: Ärztliche Autorität, reichsstädtische Ordnung und der Verlust 'armer Glieder Christi' in der Nürnberger Sondersiechenschau." *Medizin, Gesellschaft, und Geschichte* 29 (2010): 9–46.

Dross, Fritz, and Annemarie Kinzelbach. "'Nit mehr alls sein burger, sonder alls ein frembder.' Fremdheit und Aussatz in frühneuzeitlichen Reichsstädten." *Medizinhistorisches Journal* 46 (2011): 1–23.

Dross, Fritz. "Their Daily Bread: Managing Hospital Finances in Early Modern Germany." In *Hospital Life: Theory and Practice from the Medieval to the Modern, edited* by Laurinda Abreu and Sally Sheard, 49–66. Bern: Peter Lang, 2013.

Drossbach, Gisela. "Bild und Text im Liber Regulae des roemischen Hospitals von Santo Spirito in Sassia." In *Sozialgeschichte Mittelalterlicher Hospitäler*, edited by Neithard Bulst and Karl-Heinz Spiess, 125–148. Ostfildern: Jan Thorbecke Verlag, 2007.

Drossbach, Gisela. *Christliche caritas als Rechtsinstitut: Hospital und Orden von Santo Spirit in Sassia (1198–1378)* Paderborn: Ferdinand Schöningh, 2005.

Drossbach, Gisela. "Das Hospital—eine kirchenrechtliche Institution? (ca. 1150–1350)" *Zeitschrift der Savigny-Stiftung für Rechtsgeschichte. Kanonistische Abteilung* 118 (2001): 510–522.

Drossbach, Gisela, ed. *Hospitäler in Mittelalter und Früher Neuzeit: Frankreich, Deutschland und Italien. Eine Vergleichende Geschichte*. Munich: Oldenbourg, 2007.

Drossbach, Gisela. "Hospitäler in Patrimonium Petri." In *Europäisches Spitalwesen. Institutionelle Fürsorge in Mittelalter und Früher Neuzeit*, edited by Martin Scheutz, Andrea Sommerlechner, Herwig Weigl, and Alfred Stefan Weiß, 91–104. Munich: R. Oldenbourg Verlag, 2008.

Drossbach, Gisela. "Hospitalstatuten im Spiegel von Norm und Wirklichkeit." In *Hospitäler in Mittelalter und Früher Neuzeit: Frankreich, Deutschland und Italien. Eine Vergleichende Geschichte*, edited by Gisela Drossbach, 55–106. Munich: Oldenbourg, 2007.

Dubourg, Ninon. "Clerical Leprosy and the Ecclesiastical Office: Dis/Ability and Canon Law." In *New Approaches to Disease, Disability, and Medicine in Medieval Europe*, edited by Erin Connelly and Steffi Künzel, 62–77. Oxford: Archaeopress, 2018.

Dumont, Franz, Ferdinand Scherf, and Friedrich Schütz, eds. *Mainz: die Geschichte der Stadt*. Mainz: Philipp von Zabern, 1998.

Ebel, Friedrich. "Ein Fragment eines kirchlichen Rechtsbuches aus dem 14. Jh. in deutscher Sprache." *Zeitschrift der Savigny-Stiftung für Rechtsgeschichte* 62 (1976): 373–382.

Eberl, Immo. "Die Frauenzisterzen des Zisterzienserordens. Entstehung und Entwicklung des weiblichen Ordenszweiges im Umfeld des Ordens." In *Fromme Frauen-unbequeme Frauen? Weibliches Religiosentum im Mittelalter*, edited by Edeltraud Klueting, 45–66. Hildesheim: Georg Olms Verlag, 2006.

Eckert, Christian. "Der Mainzer Rat vom 13. Nov 1244 bis 28 Oct 1462." *Archiv für Hessische Geschichte und Altertumskunde* 2 (1899): 321–357.

Eibach, Joachim. "Burghers or Town Council: Who Was Responsible for Urban Stability in Early Modern German Towns?" *Urban History* 34 (2007): 14–26.

Eichbauer, Melodie H. and Danica Summerlin. "Introduction." In *The Use of Canon Law in Ecclesiastical Administration, 1000–1234*, edited by Melodie H. Eichbauer and Danica Summerlin, 1–22. Leiden: Brill, 2019.

Ell, Stephen. "Blood and Sexuality in Medieval Leprosy." *Janus* 71 (1984): 153–164.

Ell, Stephen. "Diet and Leprosy in the Medieval West: The Noble Leper." *Janus* 72 (1985): 113–129.

Elm, Kaspar. "Vita regularis sine regula. Bedeutung, Rechtsstellung und Selbstverständnis des mittelalterlichen und frühneuzeitlichen Religiosentums." In *Häresie und vorzeitige Reformation im Spätmittelalter*, edited by František Šmahel, 239–273. Munich: Oldebourg, 1998.

Engel, Ute, and Alexandra Gajewski, eds. *Mainz and the Middle Rhine Valley: Mainz and the Middle Rhine Valley*. Leeds: British Archaeological Association, 2007.

Erhard, Heinrich August. "Konstitutionen einer Mainzer Synode aus der Zeit des Erzbischofs Wernher von Eppenstein." *Zeitschrift des Vereins für Geschichte und AlterthumsKunde Westfalens* 10 (1847): 284–299.

Eschner-Apsner, Monika. "Geistliche Institutionen und Hospitäler." In *Caritas im Bistum Trier: Eine Geschichte des Helfens und Heilens*, edited by Roland Ries and Werner Marzi, 77–85. Trier: Kliomedia Verlag, 2006.

Eschner-Apsner, Monika. "Karitativsoziale Leistungen bruderschaftlicher Organisationen im hohen und späten Mittelalter." In *Einrichtungen der sozialen Sicherung im mittelalterlichen Lotharingien, Actes des 13es Journées Lotharingeinnes (12–15 Oct. 2004)*, edited by Michel Pauly, 137–180. Linden: Section Historie de l'Institut Grand-Ducal, 2008.

Euler, Karl Friedrich. "Die Geschichte des Gießener AussätzigenHospitals." *Mitteilungen des oberhessischen Geschichtsvereins Gießen* 73 (1988): 53–62.

Faber, Karl-Georg. "Was ist eine Geschichtslandschaft?" In *Festschrift Ludwig Petry, Teil 1*, 1–28. Wiesbaden: F. Steiner, 1968.

Falck, Ludwig. "Die Erzbischöfliche Metropole, 1011–1244." In *Mainz: Die Geschichte der Stadt*, edited by Franz Dumont, Friedrich Schütz, and Ferdinand Scherf, 111–137. Mainz: Philipp von Zabern, 1998.

Falck, Ludwig. "Die Freie Stadt in ihre Blütezeit." In *Mainz: Die Geschichte der Stadt*, edited by Franz Dumont, Friedrich Schütz, and Ferdinand Scherf, 143–170. Mainz: Philipp von Zabern, 1998.

Falck, Ludwig. "Klosterfreiheit und Klosterschutz. Die Klosterpolitik der Mainzer Erzbischöfe von Adalbert I. bis Heinrich I (1100–1153)." *Archiv für Mittelrheinische Kirchengeschichte* 8 (1958): 21–75.

Falck, Ludwig. *Mainz im frühen und hohen Mittelalter* Geschichte der Stadt Mainz II. Düsseldorf: Richter Verlag, 1972.

Falck, Ludwig. *Mainz in seiner Blütezeit als Freie Stadt (1244–1328)* Geschichte der Stadt Mainz III. Düsseldorf: Verlag Rau, 1973.

Falck, Ludwig. "Mainzer Hospitäler im Mittelalter." In *Moguntia Medica: Das medizinische Mainz vom Mittelalter bis ins 20. Jahrhundert*, edited by Franz Dumont, 409–417. Wiesbaden: B. Wylicil Verlag, 2002.

Falck, Ludwig. "Sammlung und Erschliessung der Quellen zur Mainzer Geschichte, vornehmlich des Mittelalters. Ein Zwischenbericht." *Mainzer Zeitschrift* 96/97 (2001/2002): 49–53.

Falkenstein, Ludwig. "Alexander III. und der Schutz unheilbar Kranker. Zu einem Streit in Épernay." *Francia* 38 (2011): 33–60.

Farley, Michael, and Keith Manchester. "The Cemetery of the Leper Hospital of St. Margaret, High Wycombe, Buckinghamshire." *Medieval Archaeology* 1 (1989): 82–89.

Farmer, Sharon. "The Beggar's Body." In *Monks and Nuns, Saints and Outcasts: Religion in Medieval Society*, edited by Sharon Farmer and Barbara Rosenwein, 153–171. Ithaca: Cornell University Press, 2000.

Farmer, Sharon. "The Leper in the Master Bedroom: Thinking Through a Thirteenth-Century Exemplum." In *Framing the Family: Narrative and Representation in the Medieval and Early Modern Periods*, edited by Rosalynn Voaden and Diane Wolfthal, 79–100. Temple, AZ: Arizona Center for Medieval and Renaissance Studies, 2005.

Febert, Heidi. *Between the Law and the World: Defining Women's Religious Identity in the Later Middle Ages*. PhD. Diss., Fordham University, 2012.

Febert, Heidi. "The Poor Sisters of Söflingen: Religious Corporations as Property Litigants, 1310–1317." *Traditio* 68 (2013): 327–340.

Felskau, Christian-Frederik. "Von Brabant bis Böhmen und darüber hinaus. Zu Einheit und Vielfalt der 'religiösen Frauenbewegung' des 12. und des 13. Jahrhunderts." In *Fromme Frauen-unbequeme Frauen? Weibliches Religiosentum im Mittelalter*, edited by Edeltraud Klueting, 67–104. Hildesheim: Georg Olms Verlag, 2006.

Felten, Franz Josef. "Abwehr, Zuneigung, Pflichtgefühl. Reaktionen der frühen Zisterzienser auf den Wunsch religiöser Frauen, zisterziensisch zu leben." In *Female vita religiosa between Late Antiquity and the High Middle Ages: Structures, Developments, and Spatial Contexts*, edited by Gert Melville and Anne Müller, 391–416. *Vita Regularis* 47. Berlin: LIT Verlag, 2011.

Felten, Franz Josef. "Die Zisterzienserorden und die Frauen." In *Vita religiosa sanctimonialium: Norm und Praxis des weiblichen religiösen Lebens vom 6. bis zum 13. Jahrhundert*, edited by Christine Kleinjung, 199–274. Korb: Didymos Verlag, 2011.

Felten, Franz Josef. "Wie adelig waren Kanonissenstifte (und andere weibliche Konvente) im (frühen und hohen) Mittelalter?" In *Studien zum Kanonissenstifte*, edited by Irene Crusius, 39–128. Göttingen: Max Plank Institut für Geschichte, 2001.

Felten, Franz Josef, Harald W. Müller, and Heidrun Ochs, eds. *Landschaft(en): Begriffe, Formen, Implikationen. Geschichtliche Landeskunde* 68. Stuttgart: Franz Steiner Verlag, 2012.

Felten, Franz Josef and Werner Rösener, eds. *Norm und Realität: Kontinuität und Wandel der Zisterzienser im Mittelalter. Vita Regularis* 42. Berlin: LIT Verlag, 2009.

Felten, Sebastian. "Mittendrin statt außen vor? Ein neuer Ort für Melaten bei Köln und der Paradigmenwechsel in der Leprageschichtsschreibung." *Geschichte in Köln: Zeitschrift für Stadt und Regionalgeschichte* 57 (2010): 11–37.

Flug, Brigitte. *Äußere Bindung und innere Ordnung. Das Altmünsterkloster in Mainz in seiner Geschichte und Verfassung von den Anfängen bis zum Ende des 14. Jahrhunderts.* Stuttgart: Franz Steiner Verlag, 2006.

Flug, Brigitte. "Mainz, Altmünster." *Die Männer- und Frauenklöster der Benediktiner in Rheinland-Pfalz und Saarland*, edited by Friedhelm Jürgensmeier, 398–425. *Germania Benedictina* vol. 9. St. Ottilien: EOS Verlag, 1999.

Flug, Brigitte.. "Mainz, Dalen." *Die Männer und Frauenklöster der Benediktiner in Rheinland-Pfalz und Saarland*, edited by Friedhelm Jürgensmeier, 426–444. *Germania Benedictina*, vol. 9. St. Ottilien: EOS Verlag, 1999.

Flug, Brigitte. "Vom Kloster in der Stadt zum städtischen Kloster. Innere und äußere Bindungen des Altmünsterklosters in Mainz von den Anfängen bis ins 14. Jahrhundert." In *Bausteine zur Mainzer Stadtgeschichte*, edited by Michael Matheus and Walter Rödel, 1–12. Stuttgart: Franz Steiner Verlag, 2002.

Forey, Alan. "Women and the Military Orders in the Twelfth and Thirteenth Centuries." In *Miltary Orders and Crusades*, 67–91. Aldershot: Variorum, 1994.

Fouquet, Gerhard. "Zwölf-Brüder-Häuser und die Vorstellung vom verdienten Ruhestand im Spätmittelalter." In *Sozialgeschichte mittelalterlicher Hospitäler*, edited by Neithard Bulst and Karl-Heinz Spiess, 37–77. Ostfildern: Jan Thorbecke Verlag, 2007.

Frank, Isnard W. "Die Bettelorden im mittelalterlichen Mainz." *Mainzer Zeitschrift* 84/85 (1989/1990): 129–142.

Frank, Thomas. "Bruderschaften und Armenfürsorge im spätmittelalterlichen Italien." In *Mittelalterliche Bruderschaften in europäischen Städten*, edited by Monika Eschner-Apsner, 293–319. Frankfurt am Main: Peter Lang, 2009.

Frank, Thomas. *Heilsame Wortgefechte: Reformen europäischer Hospitäler vom 14. bis 16. Jahrhundert.* Berlin: Vandenhoek & Ruprecht, 2014.

Frank, Thomas. "Spätmittelalterliche Hospitalreformen und Kanonistik." *Reti Medievali Rivista* 11 (2010): 1–40.

Fransen, Gérard. "La Lexicographie du Droit Canonique Medieval." In *Lexicographie du latin médiéval et ses rapports avec les recherches actuelles sur la civilisation du Moyen âge*, 191–196. Paris: Éditions du CNRS, 1981.

Franzolin, Monia. "Gli ospizi lungo il tratto bellunese della Strada Regia di Alemagna." In *L'accoglienza religiosa tra tardo antico ed età moderna: Luoghi, architetture, percorsi*, edited by Silvia Beltramo and Paolo Cozzo, 129–134. Rome: Viella, 2013.

Fray, Jean-Luc. "Hospitäler, Leprosenhäuser und mittelalterliches Straßennetz in Lothringen (ca. 1200–ca. 1500)." In *Auf den Römerstraßen ins Mittelalter: Beiträge zur Verkehrsgeschichte zwischen Maas und Rhein von der Spätantike bis ins 19. Jahrhundert*, edited by Friedhelm Burgard and Alfred Haverkamp, 407–426. Mainz: Philipp Von Zabern, 1997.

Fray, Jean-Luc. "Institutions hospitalières médiévales et problématique historienne de la centralité." In *Zwischen Maas und Rhein: Beziehungen, Begegnungen und Konflikte in einem europäischen Kernraum von der Spätantike bis zum 19. Jahrhundert: Versuch einer Bilanz*, edited by Franz Irsigler, 349–361. Trier: Kilomedia Verlag, 2006.

Frohn, Wilhelm. *Der Aussatz im Rheinland: sein Vorkommen und seine Bekämpfung*. Jena: G. Fischer, 1933.

Frölich, Karl. "Um die mittelalterlichen Straßennamen. Ein Beitrag zur Problematik und Methodik der Straßennamenforschung." *Nachrichten der Gießener Hochschulgesellschaft* 18 (1949): 118–151.

Fuhrmann, Bernd. "Norm und Praxis der Armenfürsorge in Spätmittelalter und früher Neuzeit – Eine Einleitung." In *Norm und Praxis in der Armenfürsorge in Spätmittelalter und früher Neuzeit*, edited by Sebastian Schmidt and Jens Aspelmeier, 1–20. Stuttgart: Steiner Verlag, 2006.

Gabler, Leona C. *Benefit of Clergy in England in the Later Middle Ages*. New York: Octagon, 1969.

García Ballester, Luis. "The Origin of the Six Non-Natural Things in Galen." In *Galen and Galenism: Theory and Medical Practice from Antiquity to the European Renaissance*, edited by Jon Arrizabalaga, Montserrat Cabré, and Lluis Cifuentes, 35–42. Farnham: Ashgate, 2002.

Geltner, Guy. "Social Deviancy: A Medieval Approach." In *Why the Middle Ages Matter: Medieval Light on Modern Injustice*, edited by Celia Chazelle, Simon Doubleday, Felice Lifshitz, and Amy G. Remensnyder, 29–40. New York: Routledge, 2012.

Génestal, Robert. *Le Privilegium fori en France: du Décret de Gratian à la fin du XIVe siècle*. Paris: Éditions Ernest Leroux, 1921.

Gilchrist, Roberta. "Christian Bodies and Souls: The Archaeology of Life and Death in Later Medieval Hospitals." In *Death in Towns: Urban Responses to the Dying and the Dead, 100–1600*, edited by Steven Bassett, 101–118. Leicester, UK: Leicester University Press, 1992.

Gilchrist, Roberta. "Medieval Bodies in the Material World: Gender, Stigma, and the Body." In *Framing Medieval Bodies*, edited by Sarah Kay and Miri Rubin, 43–61. Manchester: Manchester University Press, 1994.

Gilchrist, Roberta. *Requiem: The Medieval Monastic Cemetery in Britain*. London: Museum of London Archaeology Service Monograph, 2005.

Gill, Katherine. "Scandala: Controversies Concerning Clausura and Women's Religious Communities in Late Medieval Italy." In *Christendom and its Discontents: Exclusion, Persecution, and Rebellion, 1000–1500*, edited by Peter D. Diehl and Scott L. Waugh, 177–203. Cambridge: Cambridge University Press, 1996.

Gilomen-Schenkel, Elsanne. "Mittelalterliche Spitäler und Leprosorien im Gebiet der Schweiz." In *Stadt und Landmauern: Abgrenzungen-Ausgrenzungen in der Stadt und um die Stadt*, edited by Brigitte Siegel, 117–124. Zürich: VDF Hochschulverlag, 1999.

Götz, Werner. "Tamquam mortuus. Auf den Spuren des mittelalterlichen Aussatzes." *Notabene medici* 1 (1990): 30–35.

Grandin, Jean. "Recherches sur les maladreries dans l'Orne au Moyen Âge." *Cahiers Léopold Delisle* 23 (1974): 3–20.

Green, Monica H. "Books as a Source of Medical Education for Women." *Dynamis* 20 (2000): 331–369.

Griffiths, Fiona J., and Julie Hotchin, eds. *Partners in Spirit: Women, Men, and Religious Life in Germany, 1100–1500*. Turnhout: Brepols, 2014.

Grmek, Mirko D., ed. *Western Medical Thought from Antiquity to the Middle Ages*. Cambridge, MA: Harvard University Press, 1998.

Gros, Beate Sophie. *Das Hohe Hospital in Soest (ca. 1178–1600): Eine prosopographische und sozialgeschichtliche Untersuchung*. Münster: Aschendorff, 1999.

Grundmann, Herbert. *Religious Movements in the Middle Ages: The Historical Links Between Heresy, the Mendicant Orders, and the Women's Religious Movement in the Twelfth and Thirteenth Centuries, with the Historical Foundations of German Mysticism*. Translated by Steven Rowan. Notre Dame, IN: University of Notre Dame Press, 1995.

Guidera, Christine. "The Role of the Beguines in Caring for the Ill, the Dying, and the Dead." In *Death and Dying in the Middle Ages*, edited by Edelgard E. DuBruck and Barbara I. Gusick, 51–72. New York: Peter Lang, 1999.

Günther, Barbara. "100 Jahre Totenregister St. Barbara Hospital in Mainz (1700–1798)." *Archiv für mittelrheinische Kirchengeschichte* 40 (1988): 333–385.

Guy, John R. "Of the Writing of Hospital Histories There Is No End." *Bulletin of the History of Medicine* 59 (1985): 415–420.

Härtel, Reinhard. "Additamenta zur Enumeratio bonorum in päpstlichen Privilegien." In *Päpste, Privilegien, Provinzen: Beiträge zur Kirchen-, Rechts- und Landesgeschichte. Festschrift für Werner Maleczek zum 65. Geburtstag*, edited by Johannes Gießauf, Rainer Murauer, and Martin P. Schennach, 103–122. Oldenbourg: Böhlau Verlag, 2010.

Hartmann, Helmut. "Die Domherren der zweiten Hälfte des 15. Jahrhunderts in Mainz, Worms und Speyer." *Mainzer Zeitschrift* 70 (1975): 148–160.

Hartmann, Wilfried, and Kenneth Pennington, eds. *The History of Medieval Canon Law in the Classical Period, 1140–1234: From Gratian to the Decretals of Pope Gregory IX*. Washington, DC: Catholic University of America Press, 2008.

Harvey, John. "Westminster Abbey: The Infirmarer's Garden." *Garden History* 20 (1992): 97–115.

Hedtke, Britta, and Christoph Winterer. "Mainz." In *Schreiborte des deutschen Mittelalters: Skriptorien – Werke – Mäzene*, edited by Martin Schubert, 347–372. Berlin: de Gruyter, 2013.

Hehl, Ernst-Dieter. "Goldenes Mainz und Heiliger Stuhl." In *Mainz: die Geschichte der Stadt*, edited by Franz Dumont, Friedrich Schütz, and Ferdinand Scherf, 838–857. Mainz: Philipp von Zabern, 1998.

Helmrath, Johannes. "Partikularsynoden und Synodalstatuten des späteren Mittelalters im europäischen Vergleich: Vorüberlegungen zu einem möglichen Projekt." In *Das europäische Mittelalter im Spannungsbogen des Vergleichs. Zwanzig internationale Beiträge zu Praxis, Problemen und Perspektiven der historischen Komparatistik*, edited by Michael Borgolte, 135–169. Berlin: Akademie Verlag, 2001.

Helmrath, Johannes. "Theorie und Praxis der Kirchenreform im Spätmittelalter." *Rottenburger Jahrbuch für Kirchengeschichte* 11 (1992): 41–70.

Henderson, John. "Medizin für den Körper und Medizin für die Seele-Hospitäler im Florenz der Renaissance." In *Funktions- und Strukturwandel spätmittelalterlicher Hospitäler im europäischen Vergleich*, edited by Michael Matheus, 29–57. Geschichtliche Landeskunde 56. Stuttgart: Franz Steiner Verlag, 2005.

Henderson, John. *Piety and Charity in Late Medieval Florence*. Oxford: Clarendon Press, 1994.

Henderson, John. *The Renaissance Hospital: Healing the Body and Healing the Soul*. New Haven: Yale University Press, 2006.

Henderson, John, Peregrine Horden, and Alessandro Pastore. *The Impact of Hospitals 300–2000*. Oxford: Lang, 2007.

Henn, Karl Heinz. "Mittelalterliche Spitäler in Ingelheim: Krankheiten und Nöte lassen Standesschranken fallen." *Heimat am Mittelrhein* 47 (2002): 2–3.

Heuser, Rita. *Namen der Mainzer Straßen und Örtlichkeiten. Sammlung, Deutung, sprach und motivgeschichtliche Auswertung*. Stuttgart: Franz Steiner Verlag, 2008.

Heyden, Helmut. "Hospitäler St. Georg und St. Gertrud in Pommern." *Blätter für Kirchengeschichte Pommerns* 20/21 (1939): 14–36.

Heyden, Karl W. "Die Hospitäler in Oppenheim." *Oppenheimer Hefte* 1 (1990): 1–14.

Higl, Andrew. "Henryson's Textual and Narrative Prosthesis onto Chaucer's Corpus: Cresseid's Leprosy and her Schort Conclusioun." In *Disability in the Middle Ages: Rehabilitations, Reconsiderations, Reverberations*, edited by Joshua Eyler, 167–81. Aldershot: Ashgate, 2010.

Hillebrandt, Maria. "Social Groups as Recognition Patterns: A Means of Dating Medieval Charters." In *Dating Undated Medieval Charters*, edited by Michael Gervers, 163–176. Woodbridge: Boydell, 2002.

Hinkel, Erich. *Das Gau-Algesheimer Hospital. Beiträge zur Geschichte des Gau-Algesheimer Raumes*. Carl-Brilmayer-Gesellschaft: Gau-Algesheim, 1987.

Hirschmann, Frank G. "Frauenklöster und Beginenhöfe im Maas-Mosel-Raum des 12. und 13. Jh." In *Landschaft(en): Begriffe, Formen, Implikationen*, edited by Franz Josef Felten, Harald Müller, and Heidrun Ochs, 245–278. Stuttgart: Franz Steiner Verlag, 2012.

Homolka, Anita. "Die Lebensgewohnheiten der Leprakranken im Spätmittelalter." In *Aussatz-Lepra-Hansen-Krankheit: ein Menschheitsproblem im Wandel*, 151–162. Edited by Jörn Henning Wolf. Würzburg: Deutsches Aussätzigen-Hilfswerk, 1986.

Horden, Peregrine. "A Discipline of Relevance: The Historiography of the Later Medieval Hospital." *Social History of Medicine* 1 (1988): 359–374.

Horden, Peregrine. "A Non-Natural Environment: Medicine without Doctors and the Medieval European Hospital." In *The Medieval Hospital and Medical Practice*, edited by Barbara S. Bowers, 133–147. Farnham: Ashgate, 2007.

Horden, Peregrine. "Religion as Medicine: Music in Medieval Hospitals." In *Religion and Medicine in the Middle Ages*, edited by Peter Biller and Joseph Ziegler, 135–153. Rochester, NY: York Medieval Press, 2001.

Hotchin, Julie. "Reformatrices and Their Books: Religious Women and Reading Networks in Fifteenth-Century Germany." In *Communities of Learning: Networks and the Shaping of Intellectual Identity in Europe, 1100–1500*, edited by Constant J. Mews and John N. Crossley, 251–291. Turnhout: Brepols, 2011.

Huffman, Joseph P. "*Potens et pauper*: Charity and Authority in Jurisdictional Disputes over the Poor in Medieval Cologne." In *Plenitude of Power: The Doctrines and Exercise of Authority in the Middle Ages: Essays in Honor of Robert Louis Benson*, edited by Robert C. Figueira, 122–139. Aldershot: Ashgate, 2006.

Huyghebaert, Nicolas-Norbert. "L'origine ecclésiastique des léproseries en Flandre et dans le Nord de la France." *Revue d'histoire ecclésiastique* 58 (1962): 848–856.

Hyacinthe, Rafael. "*De Domo Sancti Lazari Milites Leprosi*: Knighthood and Leprosy in the Holy Land." In *The Medieval Hospital and Medical Practice*, edited by Barbara S. Bowers, 209–225. Farnham: Ashgate, 2007.

Hyacinthe, Rafael. *L'Ordre de Saint-Lazare de Jerusalem au Moyen Âge: Milites Christi*. Millau: Conservatoire Larzac Templier et Hospitalier, 2003.

Imbert, Jean. *Histoire des hôpitaux français: contribution à l'étude des rapports de l'église et de l'état dans le domaine de l'Assistance Publique: les hôpitaux en droit canonique (du décret de Gratien à la sécularisation de l'administration de l'Hôtel-Dieu de Paris en 1505.)* Paris: J. Vrin, 1947.

Imbert, Jean. "Le régime juridique des établissements hospitaliers du Nord de la France au Moyen Âge." *Revue du Nord* 29 (1947): 195–204.

Irsigler, Franz. "Matriculae, xenodochia, hospitalia und Leprosenhäuser im Frühmittelalter." In *Einrichtungen der sozialen Sicherung im mittelalterlichen Lotharingien. Actes des 13es Journées Lotharingiennes (12–15 Oct. 2004)*, edited by Michel Pauly, 323–338. Linden: Section Historie de l'Institut Grand-Ducal, 2008.

Isenmann, Eberhard. *Die deutsche Stadt im Mittelalter, 1150–1500. Stadtgestalt, Recht, Stadtregiment, Kirche, Gesellschaft, Wirtschaft*. Stuttgart: Böhlau Verlag, 2012.

Jamroziak, Emilia. "Spaces of Lay-Religious Interaction in Cistercian Houses of Northern Europe." *Parergon: Journal of the Australian and New Zealand Association for Medieval and Early Modern Studies* 27 (2010): 37–58.

Jankrift, Kay Peter. "Herren Kranke, arme Siechen. Medizin im spätmittelalterlichen Hospitalwesen." In *Sozialgeschichte mittelalterlicher Hospitäler,* edited by Neithard Bulst and Karl-Heinz Spiess, 149–167. Ostfildern: Jan Thorbecke Verlag, 2007.

Jankrift, Kay Peter. "Hospitäler und Leprosorien im Nordwesten des mittelalterlichen Regnum Teutonicum unter besonderer Berücksichtigung rheinischwestfälischer Städte." In *Europäisches Spitalwesen. Institutionelle Fürsorge in Mittelalter und Früher Neuzeit,* edited by Martin Scheutz, Andrea Sommerlechner, Herwig Weigl, and Alfred Stefan Weiß, 295–305. Munich: R. Oldenbourg Verlag, 2008.

Jankrift, Kay Peter. *Im Angesicht der 'Pestilenz': Seuchen in westfälischen und rheinischen Städten (1349–1600)*. Stuttgart: Franz Steiner Verlag, 2020.

Jankrift, Kay Peter. *Mit Gott und schwarzer Magie: Medizin im Mittelalter.* Stuttgart: Konrad Theiss Verlag, 2005.

Jankrift, Kay Peter. "Moses und die Schlangen oder ein Blick auf die Beziehung von Macht und Heilkunde im Zeitalter der 'Klostermedizin.'" In *Der Dienst am Kranken. Krankenversorgung zwischen Caritas, Medizin und Ökonomie vom Mittelalter bis zur Neuzeit. Geschichte und Entwicklung der Krankenversorgung im sozioökonomischen Wandel,* edited by Gerhard Aumüller, Cornelia Grundmann, and Christina Vanja, 53–64. Marburg: Elwert, 2007.

Jankrift, Kay Peter. "Vieillir parmi les morts vivants. La léproserie, hospice pour habitants non lépreux?" In *Lépreux et sociabilité du Moyen Âge aux temps modernes,* edited by Bruno Tabuteau, 31–37. Rouen: Publications de l'Université de Rouen, 2000.

Jaron Lewis, Gertrud. *By Women, for Women, about Women: The Sister-Books of Fourteenth-Century Germany.* Toronto: Pontifical Institute for Medieval Studies, 2006.

Jáuregui, Clara. "Inside the *Leprosarium*: Illness in the Daily Life of Fourteenth-Century Barcelona." In *New Approaches to Disease, Disability, and Medicine in Medieval Europe,* edited by Erin Connelly and Steffi Künzel, 78–93. Oxford: Archaeopress, 2018.

Jeanne, Damien. "Le groupe de lépreux de Saint Lazare de Falaise." In *Lépreux et sociabilité du Moyen Âge aux temps modernes,* edited by Bruno Tabuteau, 39–62. Rouen: Publications de l'Université de Rouen, 2000.

Jeanne, Damien. "Leprosy, Lepers, and Leper-Houses: Between Human Law and God's Law, Sixth-Fifteenth Centuries." In *Social Dimensions of Medieval Disease and Disability,* edited by Sally Crawford and Christina Lee, 69–79. Oxford: Archaeopress, 2014.

Jeanselme, E. "Comment l'Europe, au Moyen Âge, se protégea contre la Lèpre." *Bulletin de la Société Française d'Histoire de la Médecine* 25 (1931): 1–155.

Jéhanno, Christine. "L'Alimentation hospitalière à la fin du Moyen Âge: l'exemple de l'HotelDieu de Paris." In *Hospitäler in Mittelalter und Früher Neuzeit: Frankreich, Deutschland und Italien. Eine Vergleichende Geschichte,* edited by Gisela Drossbach, 107–130. Munich: Oldenbourg, 2007

Jéhanno, Christine. "L'emplacement de l'Hotel-Dieu de Paris." In *Hôpitaux et maladreries au moyen âge: espace et environnement: actes du colloque international d'AmiensBeauvais, 22, 23 et 24 novembre 2002,* edited by Pascal Montaubin, 35–49. Rouen: CAHMER, 2004.

Johnson, Penelope. *Equal in Monastic Profession: Religious Women in Medieval France.* Chicago: University of Chicago Press, 2009.

Johnson, Sherri Franks. *Monastic Women and Religious Orders in Late Medieval Bologna.* Cambridge: Cambridge University Press, 2014.

Jolly, Karen Louise. *Popular Religion in Late Saxon England: Elf Charms in Context.* Chapel Hill: University of North Carolina Press, 1996.

Jones, Peter Murray. "Image, Word, and Medicine in the Middle Ages." In *Visualizing Medieval Medicine and Natural History, 1200–1550,* edited by Jean A. Givens, 1–24. Farnham: Ashgate, 2006.

Jordan, Mark D. "The Very Idea of Disease." In *Death, Sickness, and Health in Medieval Society and Culture,* edited by Susan J. Ridyard, 55–76. Sewanee, TN: University of the South Press, 2000.

Jordan, Erin L. "Pro remedio anime sue: Cistercian Nuns and Space in the Low Countries." In *Women in the Medieval Monastic World,* edited by Janet Burton and Karen Stöber, 279–298. Turnhout: Brepols, 2015.

Jucker, Michael. "Trust and Mistrust in Letters: Late Medieval Diplomacy and Its Communication Practices." In *Strategies of Writing: Studies on Text and Trust in the Middle Ages,* edited by Petra Schultert, Marco Mostert, and Irene van Renswoude, 213–236. Turnhout: Brepols, 2008.

Juckes, Tim. *The Parish and Pilgrimage Church of St. Elizabeth in Košice: Town, Court, and Architecture in Late Medieval Hungary.* Turnhout: Brepols, 2011.

Jürgensmeier, Friedhelm. "Das Erzbistum Mainz." In *Die Bistümer des Heiligen Römischen Reiches von ihren Anfängen bis zur Säkularisation,* edited by Erwin Gatz, 400–426. Freiburg im Breisgau: Herder, 2003.

Jürgensmeier, Friedhelm. *Germania Benedictina: Die Männerund Frauenklöster der Benediktiner in RheinlandPfalz und Saarland.* St. Ottilien: EOS Verlag, 1999.

Jürgensmeier, Friedhelm, ed. *Die Mönchsund Nonnenklöster der Zisterzienser in Hessen und Thüringen.* St. Ottilien: EOS Verlag, 2011.

Jürgensmeier, Friedhelm, ed. *Handbuch der Mainzer Kirchengeschichte: Christliche Antike und Mittelalter.* 2 vols. Würzburg: Echter Verlag, 2000.

Just, Thomas, and Herwig Weigl. "Spitäler im südöstlichen Deutschland und in den österreichischen Ländern im Mittelalter." In *Europäisches Spitalwesen. Institutionelle Fürsorge in Mittelalter und Früher Neuzeit,* edited by Martin Scheutz, Andrea Sommerlechner, Herwig Weigl, and Alfred Stefan Weiß, 149–184. Munich: R. Oldenbourg Verlag, 2008.

Jütte, Robert. "The Social Construction of Illness in the Early Modern Clinic." In *The Social Construction of Illness,* edited by Jens Lachmund and Gunnar Stollberg, 23–38. Stuttgart: Franz Steiner Verlag, 1992.

Jütte, Robert. "Stigma-Symbole: Kleidung als identitätstiftendes Merkmal bei spätmittelalterlichen und frühneuzeitlichen Randgruppen (Juden, Dirnen, Aussätzige, Bettler)." *Saeculum* 44 (1993): 65–89.

Kaelber, Lutz. *Schools of Asceticism: Ideology and Organization in Medieval Religious Communities.* University Park, PA: Pennsylvania State University Press, 1998.

Kealey, Edward J. *Medieval Medicus: Physicians and Health Care in England, 1100–1154.* Baltimore: Johns Hopkins University Press, 1981.

Kehrberger, Eduard Otto. *Provinzial und Synodalstatuten des Spätmittelalters. Eine quellenkritische Untersuchung der Mainzer Provinzialgesetze des 14. und 15. Jahrhunderts und der Synodalstatuten der Diözesen Bamberg, Eichstätt und Konstanz.* Ph.D. Diss., Universität Tübingen, 1938.

Kejr, Jiri. "Die Urkunde als Beweismittel im Gerichtsverfahren in mittelalterlichen Böhmen." In *The Development of Literate Mentalities in East Central Europe*, edited by Anna Adams and Marco Mostert, 51–59. Utrecht Studies in Medieval Literacy 4. Turnhout: Brepols, 2004.

Kerr, Julie. *Monastic Hospitality: The Benedictines in England, c.1070–c.1250.* Woodbridge: Boydell, 2007.

Kerr, Julie. "The Symbolic Significance of Hospitality." In *Self-Representation of Medieval Religious Communities: The British Isles in Context*, edited by Anne Müller and Karen Stöber, 125–142. Berlin: LIT Verlag, 2009.

Kéry, Lotte. "Verbrechen und Strafen im kanonischen Recht des Mittelalters." In *Kriminalität in Mittelalter und früher Neuzeit: Soziale, Rechtliche, Philosophische und Literarische Aspekte*, edited by Sylvia Kesper-Biermann and Diethelm Klippel, 13–34. Wiesbaden: Harrassowitz Verlag, 2007.

Keyvanian, Carla. *Hospitals and Urbanism in Rome, 1200–1500.* Leiden: Brill, 2015.

Kinzelbach, Annemarie. "'An jetzt grasierender kranckheit sehr schwer darnider.' Schau und Kontext in süddeutschen Reichsstädten der frühen Neuzeit." In *Seuche und Mensch. Herausforderung in den Jahrhunderten*, edited by Carl Christian Wahrmann, Martin Buchsteiner, and Antje Strahl, 269–282. Rostock: Universität Rostock, 2010.

Kläger, Michael. "Das Stadtbild im Wandel." *Beiträge zur Mainzer Geschichte* 28 (1988): 13–25.

Kleemann, Jasmin. "Die Neuordnung des Heiliggeist-Hospitals im Jahre 1502." In *Himmel-Hölle-Fegefeuer: Jenseitsvorstellungen und Sozialgeschichte im spätmittelalterlichen Dortmund*, edited by Thomas Schilp, 135–141. Dortmund: Stadtarchiv Dortmund, 1996.

Kleinjung, Christine. *Frauenklöster als Kommunikationszentren und soziale Räume. Das Beispiel Worms vom 13. bis zum Beginn des 15. Jahrhunderts.* Korb: Didymos Verlag, 2008.

Kleinjung, Christine. "Nonnen und Personal, Familie und Stifter." In *Norm und Realität: Kontinuität und Wandel der Zisterzienser im Mittelalter*, edited by Franz Josef Felten and Werner Rösener, 225–264. Münster: LIT Verlag, 2009.

Knefelkamp, Ulrich. *Das Gesundheits und Fürsorgewesen der Stadt Freiburg im Breisgau im Mittelalter.* Freiburg im Breisgau: Herder, 1981.

Knefelkamp, Ulrich. *Das Heilig-Geist-Spital in Nürnberg vom 14–17. Jahrhundert: Geschichte, Struktur, Alltag.* Nürnberger Forschungen 26. Nürnberg: Verein für Geschichte der Stadt Nürnberg, 1989.

Knefelkamp, Ulrich. "Stadt und Spital." In *Städtisches Gesundheits und Fürsorgewesen vor 1800*, edited by Peter Johanek, 19–40. Cologne: Böhlau Verlag, 2000.

Knefelkamp, Ulrich. "Über den Funktionswandel von Spitälern vom Spätmittelalter zur Frühen Neuzeit, aufgezeigt an Beispielen aus Deutschland, England und Italien." *Historia Hospitalium* 22 (2000–2001): 9–34

Koch, Wilfred Maria. "Archäologischer Bericht 1988/1989: Das Leprosorium AachenMelaten. Vorbericht der Ausgrabungen 1988/1989." *Zeitschrift des Aachener Geschichtsvereins* 96 (1989): 409–419.

Koenig, Harold G. *Medicine, Religion, and Health: Where Science and Spirituality Meet.* West Conshohocken: Templeton Press, 2008.

Kolling, Hubert. "Die Sorge für die Kranken." In: *Der Dienst am Kranken. Krankenversorgung zwischen Caritas, Medizin und Ökonomie vom Mittelalter bis zur Neuzeit. Geschichte und Entwicklung der Krankenversorgung im sozioökonomischen Wandel*, edited by Gerhard Aumüller, Cornelia Grundmann, and Christina Vanja, 65–86. Marburg: Elwert, 2007.

Konietzny, Thomas. "Stiftung des Dortmunder Patriziers Arnd Kalf an des HeiliggeistSpital und die Nikolaikirche (1410)." In *Himmel-Hölle-Fegefeuer: Jenseitsvorstellungen und Sozialgeschichte im spätmittelalterlichen Dortmund*, edited by Thomas Schilp, 105–111. Dortmund: Stadtarchiv Dortmund, 1996.

Krolikoski, Courtney. "Saints and Sinners: The Role of the Saint in the Life of the Leper Before the Thirteenth Century." *Annual of Medieval Studies at CEU* 18 (2012): 66–78.

Kurz, Christiane Ulrike. *"Ubi et est habitatio sororum et mansio fratrum": Doppelklöster und ähnliche Klostergemeinschaften im mittelalterlichen Österreich* (*Diözese Passau in den Ausdehnungen des 13. Jahrhunderts*). Kiel: Solivagus Verlag, 2015.

Kuttner, Stephan. "The Scientific Investigation of Medieval Canon Law: The Need and the Opportunity." *Speculum* 24 (1949): 493–501.

Kuttner, Stephan and Antonio García y García. "A New Eyewitness Account of the Fourth Lateran Council." *Traditio* 20 (1964): 115–178.

Lambert, Malcolm. *Medieval Heresy: Popular Movements from the Gregorian Reform to the Reformation*. Oxford: Blackwell, 2002.

Landau, Peter. "Die Leprakranke im mittelalterlichen kanonischen Recht." In *Staat, Kirche, Wissenschaft in einer pluralistischen Gesellschaft: Festschrift zum 65. Geburtstag von Paul Mikat,* edited by Dieter Schwab, Dieter Giesen, Joseph Liste, and Hans-Wolfgang Strätz, 565–578. Berlin: Duncker und Humblot, 1989.

Lang, Jane. "The Reform Work of the Episcopate on the Lines Laid Down by the Lateran Council of 1215." In *Bishops and Reform, 1215–1272: With Special Reference to the Lateran Council of 1215*, edited by Marion Gibbs and Jane Lang, 94–179. Oxford: Oxford University Press, 1934.

Laqua, Benjamin. *Bruderschaften und Hospitäler während des hohen Mittelalters: Kölner Befunde im westeuropäisch-vergleichende Perspektive*. Stuttgart: Hiersemann, 2011.

Laqua, Benjamin. "Erzbischof, Bruderschaft und Hospital in Köln. Die Luxusbrüder während des hohen Mittelalters." In *Mittelalterliche Bruderschaften in europäischen Städten*, edited by Monika Eschner-Apsner, 111–142. Frankfurt am Main: Peter Lang, 2009.

Le Blévec, Daniel. "Infirmes et infirmités dans la société médiévale, d'après les sources méridionales." In *Handicaps et sociétés dans l'Histoire. L'estropié, l'aveugle et le paralytique de l'Antiquité aux temps modernes*, edited by Franck Collard and Evelyne Samama, 145–156. Paris: L'Harmattan, 2010.

Le Blévec, Daniel. *La Part du Pauvre: l'assistance dans les pays du BasRhône du XIIe siècle au milieu du XVE siècle*. 2 vols. Rome: École française de Rome, 2000.

Le Blévec, Daniel. "Les lépreux peuventils vivre en société? Réflexions sur l'exclusion sociale dans les villes du Midi à la fin du Moyen Âge." In *Vivre en société au Moyen Âge,* edited by Claude Carozzi and Huguette Taviani-Carozzi, 281–291. Aix-en-Provence: Publications de l'Université de Provence, 2008.

Lee, Gerard A. *Leper Hospitals in Medieval Ireland*. Dublin: Four Courts Press, 1996.

Leistikow, Dankwart. "Die Leproserie als Sonderform des städtischen Hospitals." *Architectura: Zeitschrift für Geschichte der Baukunst* 16 (1986): 114–129.

Lester, Anne E. "Cares Beyond the Walls: Cistercian Nuns and the Care of Lepers in Twelfth and Thirteenth-Century Northern France." In *Religious and Laity in Western Europe, 1000–1400: Interaction, Negotiation, and Power,* edited by Emilia Jamroziak and Janet Burton, 197–224. Turnhout: Brepols, 2006.

Lester, Anne E. "Crafting a Charitable Landscape: Urban Topographies in Charters and Testaments from Medieval Champagne." In *Cities, Texts, and Social Networks, 400–1500: Experiences and Perceptions of Medieval Urban Space,* edited by Caroline Goodson, Anne E. Lester, and Carol Symes, 125–148. Farnham: Ashgate, 2010.

Lester, Anne E. *Creating Cistercian Nuns: The Women's Religious Movement and Its Reform in Thirteenth-Century Champagne*. Ithaca: Cornell University Press, 2011.

Liebeherr, Irmtraud. *Der Besitz des Mainzer Domkapitels im Spätmittelalter*. Mainz: Gesellschaft für Mittelrheinische Kirchengeschichte, 1971.

Lieber, Elinor. "Old Testament 'Leprosy,' Contagion and Sin." In *Contagion: Perspectives from Premodern Societies*, edited by Lawrence I. Conrad and Dominik Wujastyk, 99–136. Aldershot: Ashgate Press, 2000.

Liermann, Hans. *Handbuch des Stiftungsrechts. Vol. 1: Geschichte des Stiftungsrechts*. Tübingen: J. C. B. Mohr, 1963.

Lilley, Keith. *City and Cosmos: The Medieval World in Urban Form*. Chicago: University of Chicago Press, 2009.

Lilley, Keith. "Mapping the Medieval City: Plan Analysis and Urban History." *Urban History* 27 (2000): 5–30.

Löther, Andrea. "Grenzen und Möglichkeiten weiblichen Handelns im 13. Jahrhundert: Die Auseinandersetzung um die Nonnenseelsorge der Bettelorden." *Rottenburger Jahrbuch für Kirchengeschichte* 11 (1992): 223–240.

Lohmann, Clemens. "Vom mittelalterlichen Spital zum modernen Klinikum: Die Entwicklungen bis 1945."In: *Eine Stadt im Spiegel der Heilkunst: Streiflichter zu 850 Jahren Fritzlarer Hospitalwesen: Festschrift des Hospitals zum Heiligen Geist, Fritzlar*, edited by Sabine Trosse, 34–71. Kassel: LWV Hessen, 1998.

Louth, Andrew. "The Body in Western Catholic Christianity." In *Religion and the Body*, edited by Sarah Coakley, 111–130. Cambridge: Cambridge University Press, 1997.

Lusiardi, Ralf. *Stiftung und städtische Gesellschaft. Religiöse und soziale Aspekte des Stiftungsverhaltens im spätmittelalterlichen Stralsund*. Berlin: Akademie Verlag, 2000.

Mackay, Dorothy Louise. *Les Hôpitaux et la Charité a Paris au XIIIe Siècle*. Paris: E. Champion, 1923.

Maddern, Philippa. "A Market for Charitable Performances? Bequests to the Poor and their Recipients in Fifteenth-Century Norwich Wills." In *Experiences of Charity, 1250–1650*, edited by Anne M. Scott, 79–103. Farnham: Ashgate, 2015.

Makowski, Elizabeth. *A Pernicious Sort of Woman: Quasi-Religious Women and Canon Lawyers in the Later Middle Ages*. Washington, DC: Catholic University of America Press, 2005.

Makowski, Elizabeth. "When is a Beguine not a Beguine? Names, Norms, and Nuance in Canonical Literature." In *Labels and Libels: Naming Beguines in Northern Medieval Europe*, edited by Letha Böhringer, 83–98. Turnhout: Brepols, 2014.

Maleczek, Werner. "Der Mittelpunkt Europas im frühen 13. Jahrhundert: Chronisten, Fürsten, und Bischöfe an der Kurie our Zeit Papst Innocenz' III." *Römische Historische Mitteilungen* 49 (2007): 89–97.

Manco, Jean. "The Heritage of Mercy." *Medieval History Magazine* 3 (2003): 22–29.

Martin, José Luis Martin. *Documentación medieval de la iglesia catedral de Coria*. Acta Salmanticensia 12. Salamanca: Universidad de Salamanca, 1989.

Matheus, Michael, ed. *Funktions- und Strukturwandel spätmittelalterlicher Hospitäler im europäischen Vergleich*. Geschichtliche Landeskunde 56. Stuttgart: Franz Steiner Verlag, 2005.

Matheus, Michael. "Vom Bistummstreit zur Stiftsfehde: Mainz 1328–1459." In *Mainz: die Geschichte der Stadt*, edited by Franz Dumont, Friedrich Schütz, and Ferdinand Scherf, 171–204. Mainz: Philipp von Zabern, 1998.

McNamara, Jo Ann Kay. *Sisters in Arms: Catholic Nuns Through Two Millennia*. Cambridge, MA: Harvard University Press, 1996.

McVaugh, Michael Rogers. *Medicine Before the Plague: Practitioners and their Patients in the Crown of Aragon, 1285–1345*. Cambridge: Cambridge University Press, 2002.

Meffert, Franz. *Caritas und Krankenwesen bis zum Ausgang des Mittelalters*. Freiburg im Breisgau: Caritas Verlag, 1927.

Meinert, Ernst-Adolf. *Die Hospitäler Holsteins im Mittelalter: Ein Beitrag zur mittelalterlichen Stadtgeschichte*. Neumünster: Wachholtz Verlag, 1997.

Melville, Gert. "Construction and Deconstruction of Religious Symbols in the Middle Ages." In *Self-Representation of Medieval Religious Communities: The British Isles in Context*, edited by Anne Müller and Karen Stöber, 3–20. Berlin: LIT Verlag, 2009.

Melville, Gert. "Nuove Tendenze della storiografia monastica di area tedesca." In *Dove va la storiografia monastica in Europa? temi e metodi di ricerca per lo studio della vita monastica e regolare in età medievale alle soglie del terzo millennio: atti del convegno internazionale BresciaRodengo, 23–25 marzo 2000*, edited by Giancarlo Andenna, 35–52. Milan: Vita e Pensiero, 2001.

Melville, Gert. "Ordensstatuten und allgemeines Kirchenrecht: Eine Skizze zum 12./13. Jahrhundert." In *Proceedings of the 9th International Congress of Medieval Canon Law*, edited by Peter Landau, 693–712. Città del Vaticano: Biblioteca Apostolica Vaticana, 1997.

Mercier, Charles. *Leper Houses and Medieval Hospitals*. London: H. K. Lewis, 1919.

Merzbacher, Friedrich. "Die Leprosen im alten kanonischen Recht." *Zeitschrift der Savigny-Stiftung für Rechtsgeschichte. Kanonistische Abteilung* 84 (1967): 27–45.

Metzler, Irina. "Liminality and Disability: Spatial and Conceptual Aspects of Physical Impairment in Medieval Europe." In *Medicine and Space: Body, Surroundings, and Borders in Antiquity and the Middle Ages*, edited by Patricia A. Baker, Han Nijdam, and Karine van 't Land, 273–296. Leiden: Brill, 2012.

Metzler, Irina. "Speechless: Speech and Hearing Impairments as Problem of Medieval Normative Texts—Theological, Natural-Philosophical, Legal." In *Social Dimensions of Medieval Disease and Disability*, edited by Sally Crawford and Christina Lee, 59–68. Oxford: Archaeopress, 2014.

Meyer, Andreas. "Lepra und Lepragutachten aus dem Lucca des 13. Jahrhunderts." In *Gesund und Krank im Mittelalter: Marburger Beiträge zur Kulturgeschichte der Medizin*, edited by Andreas Meyer and Jürgen Schulz-Grobert, 145–201. Leipzig: Eudora Verlag, 2007.

Meyvaert, Paul. "The Medieval Monastic Garden." In *Medieval Gardens*, edited by Elisabeth Blair Macdougall, 23–53. Dumbarton Oaks Colloquium on the History of Landscape Architecture 9. Cambridge, MA: Harvard University Press, 1986.

Militzer, Klaus. *Das Markgröninger Heilig-Geist-Spital im Mittelalter. Ein Beitrag zur Wirtschaftsgeschichte des 15. Jahrhunderts*. Sigmaringen: Jan Thorbecke Verlag, 1975.

Miller, Timothy S. *The Birth of the Hospital in the Byzantine Empire*. Baltimore: Johns Hopkins University Press, 1985.

Miller, Timothy S. and John W. Nesbitt. *Walking Corpses: Leprosy in Byzantium and the Medieval West*. Ithaca: Cornell University Press, 2014.

Miramon, Charles de. *Les 'donnés' au Moyen Âge: une forme de vie religieuse laïque, v. 1180–v. 1500*. Paris: Cerf, 1999.

Mitchell, Piers. "The Myth of the Spread of Leprosy with the Crusades." In *The Past and Present of Leprosy: Archaeological, Historical, Palaeopathological, and Clinical Approaches*, edited by Charlotte A. Roberts, Mary E. Lewis, and Keith Manchester, 171–178. Oxford: Archaeopress, 2000.

Mollat, Michel. *The Poor in the Middle Ages: An Essay in Social History*. Translated by Arthur Goldhammer. New Haven: Yale University Press, 1986.

Mone, Franz Joseph. „Kirchenverordnungen der Bistümer Mainz und Konstanz aus dem 13. und 16. Jh." *ZGO* 4 (1853): 257–274.

Mone, Franz Joseph. „Kirchenverordnungen der Bistümer Mainz und Strassburg." *ZGO* 3 (1852): 129–150.

Monsees, Yvonne. *Das Zisterzienserinnenkloster Gottesthal im Rheingau*. Wiesbaden: Selbstverlag der Historischen Kommission für Nassau, 1986.

Montford, Angela. *Health, Sickness, Medicine, and the Friars in the Thirteenth and Fourteenth Centuries*. Aldershot: Ashgate, 2004.

More, Alison. *Fictive Orders and Feminine Religious Identities, 1200–1600*. Oxford: Oxford University Press, 2018.

Moritz, Werner. *Die Bürgerlichen Fürsorgeanstalten der Reichsstadt Frankfurt a.M. im späten Mittelalter*. Frankfurt am Main: W. Kramer, 1981.

Mortimer, Richard. "The Prior of Butley and the Lepers of West Somerton." *Bulletin of the Institute of Historical Research* 53 (1980): 99–103.

Mülsner, Dirk. "Bruderschaften und caritative Werke." In *Caritas im Bistum Trier: Eine Geschichte des Helfens und Heilens*, edited by Roland Ries and Werner Marzi, 91–98. Trier: Kliomedia Verlag, 2006.

Mundy, John H. "Charity and Social Work in Toulouse 1100–1250." *Traditio* 22 (1966): 203–287.

Mundy, John H. "Hospitals and Leproseries around 1400." In *Studies in the Ecclesiastical and Social History of Toulouse in the Age of the Cathars*, edited by John H. Mundy, 225–234. Aldershot: Ashgate, 2006.

Murken, Axel Hinrich. "Die Geschichte des Leprosoriums Melaten in Aachen vom Mittelalter bis zum Beginn der Neuzeit–300 Jahre geschlossene Anstaltspflege für die Aussätzigen." In *Lepra-Gestern und Heute: 15 wissenschaftliche Essays zur Geschichte und Gegenwart einer Menschheitsseuche: Gedenkschrift zum 650jahrigen Bestehen des Rektorats Munster-Kinderhaus*, edited by Richard Toellner, 189–207. Münster: Regensberg, 1992.

Murray, Alexander. "Religion Among the Poor in Thirteenth-Century France: The Testimony of Humbert de Romans." *Traditio* 30 (1974): 284–325.

Muschel, Heinz. *Das Spital der reichen Siechen zu St. Katharina in Ulm: eine rechtsgeschichtliche Untersuchung zur Inkorporation der Wohlfahrtsanstalten durch die Reichsstadt am ausgehenden Mittelalter*. Ulm: Stadtarchiv, 1965.

Navon, Liona. "Beggars, Metaphors, and Stigma: A Missing Link in the Social History of Leprosy." *Social History of Medicine* 11 (1998): 89–105.

Neeb, Ernst. "Zur Baugeschichte des Hospitals zum Heiligen Geist und der mittelalterlichen Stadtmauer der Rheinseite zu Mainz." *Mainzer Zeitschrift* 15/16 (1920/1921): 56–61.

Nelson, Amy. "Soror nostra: Religious Identity among Premonstratensians and their Patrons." Presentation at the Medieval Academy of America annual meeting, Boston, MA, February 25–27, 2016.

Neumann, Eva Gertrud. *Rheinisches Beginen- und Beghardenwesen: Ein Mainzer Beitrag zur religiösen Bewegung am Rhein*. Mainzer Abhandlungen zur mittleren und neueren Geschichte 4. Meisenheim am Glan: A. Hain, 1960.

Ober, William B. "Can the Leper Change His Spots? The Iconography of Leprosy." *American Journal of Dermatopathology*, Part I, 5/1 (1983): 43–58, Part II, 5/2 (1983): 173–186.

Oberste, Jörg. "Donaten zwischen Kloster und Welt. Das Donatenwesen der religiösen Ritterorden in Südfrankreich und die Entwicklung der städtischen Frömmigkeitspraxis im 13. Jahrhundert." *Zeitschrift für historische Forschung: Halbjahresschrift für die Erforschung des Spätmittelalters und der frühen Neuzeit* 29 (2002): 1–37.

Oexle, Gerhard. "Armut, Armutsbegriff, und Armenfürsorge." In *Soziale Sicherheit und soziale Disziplinierung: Beiträge zu einer historischen Theorie der Sozialpolitik*, edited by Christoph Sachse and Florian Tennstedt, 73–100. Frankfurt am Main: Suhrkamp, 1986.

Oliva, Marilyn. *The Convent and the Community in Late Medieval England: Female Monasteries in the Diocese of Norwich, 1350–1540*. Woodbridge: Boydell,1998.

Olsen, Glenn Warren. *The Legal Definition of the Ecclesiastical Benefice During the Period of the Appearance of Papal Provisioning (1140–1230)*. Ph.D., University of Wisconsin, 1965.

Orlemanski, Julie. "How to Kiss a Leper." *Postmedieval* 3 (2012): 142–157.

Orme, Nicholas, and Margaret Webster. *The English Hospital 1070–1570*. New Haven: Yale University Press, 1995.

Osborn, Marijane. "Anglo-Saxon Ethnobotany: Women's Reproductive Medicine in Leechbook III." In *Health and Healing from the Medieval Garden*, edited by Peter Dendle and Alain Touwaide, 145–161. Woodbridge: Boydell, 2008.

Palmer, Richard. "The Church, Leprosy, and Plague in Medieval and Early Modern Europe." *Studies in Church History* 19 (1982): 79–99.

Park, Katharine. "Healing the Poor: Hospitals and Medical Assistance in Renaissance Florence." In *Medicine and Charity Before the Welfare State*, edited by Jonathan Barry and Colin Jones, 26–45. London: Routledge, 1991.

Parkes, Malcolm. "Folia librorum quaerere: Medieval Experience of the Problems of Hypertext and the Index." In *Fabula in tabula: Una storia degli indici dal manoscritto al testo elettronico: Atti Del Convegno Di Studio Della Fondazione Ezio Franceschini e Della Fondazione IBM Italia: Certosa Del Galluzzo, 21–22 Ottobre 1994*, edited by Claudio Leonardi, Marcello Morelli, and Francesco Santi, 23–41. Florence: Fondazione Ezio Franceschini, 1995.

Patrico, Ryan. "Frauenklöster in Württemberg zur Zeit der Reformation." Presentation at the annual meeting of the Arbeitskreis Geistliche Frauen im Europäischen Mittelalter, Dhaun, Germany, February 22, 2014.

Paulus, Nikolaus. "Die ältesten Ablässe für Almosen und Kirchenbesuch." *Zeitschrift für katholische Theologie* 33:1 (1909): 1–40.

Pauly, Michel. "Für eine raumbezogene Hospitalgeschichte: Einführende Bemerkungen." In *Einrichtungen der sozialen Sicherung im mittelalterlichen Lotharingien. Actes des 13es Journées Lotharingeinnes (12–15 Oct. 2004)*, edited by Michel Pauly, 1–14. Linden: Section Historie de l'Institut Grand-Ducal, 2008.

Pauly, Michel. "Hospitäler im Mittelalter-wann und wo gehörte das Hospital zur Stadt?" In *Was machte im Mittelalter zur Stadt?: Selbstverständnis, Außensicht und Erscheinungsbilder mittelalterlicher Städte*, edited by Christhard Schrenk, 245–269. Heilbronn: Stadtarchiv Heilbronn, 2007.

Pauly, Michel. *Peregrinorum, pauperum ac aliorum transeuntium receptaculum: Hospitäler zwischen Maas und Rhein im Mittelalter.* Stuttgart: Franz Steiner Verlag, 2007.

Pauly, Michel. "Pilgerverkehr und Hospize." In *Wege zum Heil: Pilger und Heilige Orte an Mosel und Rhein*, edited by Thomas Frank, Michael Matheus, and Sabine Reichert, 229–239. Stuttgart: Franz Steiner Verlag, 2009.

Pauly, Michel. "Das Versorgungsgebiet der Stadt Luxemburg im späten Mittelalter." In *Städtische Wirtschaft im Mittelalter: Festschrift für Franz Irsigler zum 70. Geburtstag*, edited by Rudolf Holbach and Michel Pauly, 211–254. Cologne: Böhlau Verlag, 2011.

Pauly, Michel, and Martin Uhrmacher. "Die Koblenzer Hospitäler in zentralörtlicher Perspektive." In *Zwischen Maas und Rhein: Beziehungen, Begegnungen und Konflikte in einem europäischen Kernraum von der Spätantike bis zum 19. Jahrhundert: Versuch einer Bilanz*, edited by Franz Irsigler, 331–347. Trier: Kilomedia Verlag, 2006.

Paxton, Frederick S. "Anointing the Sick and Dying in Christian Antiquity and the Early Medieval West." In *Health, Disease, and Healing in Medieval Culture*, edited by Sheila Campbell, Bert Hall, and David Klausner, 93–102. New York: St. Martin's Press, 1992.

Pennington, Kenneth. "The Decretalists 1190 to 1234." In *The History of Medieval Canon Law in the Classical Period, 1140–1234: From Gratian to the Decretals of Pope Gregory IX*, edited by

Wilfried Hartmann and Kenneth Pennington, 211–245. Washington, DC: Catholic University of America Press, 2008.

Pennington, Kenneth. "Gregory IX, Emperor Frederick II, and the Constitutions of Melfi." In *Popes, Teachers, and Canon Law in the Middle Ages*, edited by James Ross Sweeney and Stanley Chodorow, 53–61. Ithaca: Cornell University Press, 1989.

Pennington, Kenneth. *Pope and Bishops: The Papal Monarchy in the Twelfth and Thirteenth Centuries*. Philadelphia: University of Pennsylvania Press, 1984.

Peterson, Anna M. "A Comparative Study of the Hospitals and Leprosaria in Narbonne, France and Siena, Italy (1080–1348)." PhD diss., University of St. Andrews, 2017.

Peterson, Anna M. "Connotation and Denotation: The Construction of the Leper in Narbonne and Siena Before the Plague." In *Leprosy and Identity in the Middle Ages: From England to the Mediterranean,* edited by Elma Brenner and François-Olivier Touati, 323–343. Manchester: Manchester University Press, 2021.

Peyroux, Catherine. "The Leper's Kiss." In *Monks and Nuns, Saints and Outcasts: Religion in Medieval Society*, edited by Sharon Farmer and Barbara Rosenwein, 172–188. Ithaca: Cornell University Press, 2000.

Phillips, Dayton. *Beguines in Medieval Strasbourg: A Study of the Social Aspects of Beguine Life*. Palo Alto: Stanford University Press, 1941.

Pichon, Genevieve. "Essai sur la lèpre du Haut Moyen Âge." *Le Moyen Âge: Revue d'histoire et de philologie* 90 (1984): 331–356.

Pichon, Genevieve. "Quelques reflexions sur l'affaire des lepreux de 1321." *Sources: Travaux Historiques* 13 (1988): 25–30.

Picot, John. "Bona Diagnosis, Bona Curatio: Lèpre, Justice, et Société." In *Lieux et pratiques de santé du Moyen Âge à la Première Guerre mondiale*, edited by M. C. Dinet and S. Beauvalet, 17–35. Amiens: Encrage Editions, 2013.

Picot, John. "Dans le secret des archives: Le testament de Jean Potinhat, forgeron lépreux de Saint-Germain-l'Herm (1456)." *Bulletin Historique et Scientifique de l'Auvergne* 113 (2012): 127–137.

Pilsworth, Clare. *Healthcare in Early Medieval Northern Italy*. Turnhout: Brepols, 2014.

Pitz, Ernst. *Papstreskript und Kaiserreskript im Mittelalter*. Tübingen: Niemeyer Verlag, 1971.

Pixton, Paul B. *The German Episcopacy and the Implementation of the Decrees of the Fourth Lateran Council 1216–1245: Watchmen on the Tower*. Leiden: Brill, 1995.

Poeck, Dietrich W. *Rituale der Ratswahl: Zeichen und Zeremoniell der Ratssetzung in Europa*. Cologne: Böhlau Verlag, 2003.

Pohl-Resl, Brigitte. *Rechnen mit der Ewigkeit: Das Wiener Bürgerspital im Mittelalter*. Munich: Oldenbourg Verlag, 1996.

Prior, Lindsay. "The Local Space of Medical Discourse: Disease, Illness, and Hospital Architecture." In *The Social Construction of Illness*, edited by Jens Lachmund and Gunnar Stollberg, 67–85. Stuttgart: Franz Steiner Verlag, 1992.

Probst, Christian. "Das Hospitalwesen im hohen und späten Mittelalter und die geistliche und gesellschaftliche Stellung des Kranken." In *Medizin im mittelalterlichen Abendland*, edited by Gerhard Baader and Gundolf Keil, 260–274. Darmstadt: Wissenschaftliche Buchgesellschaft, 1982.

Puth, Andreas. "'Our and the Empire's Free City on the Rhine': Visualizing the Empire in the Mainz Kaufhaus Reliefs." In *Mainz and the Middle Rhine Valley*, edited by Ute Engel and Alexandra Gajewski, 89–124. Leeds: British Archaeological Association, 2007.

Quigley, Maureen. "Appropriating the Hospital: The Crusading Identity of a Hospitaller of St. Jacques du Haut Pas." Presentation at the International Medieval Congress, Leeds, July 4–7, 2016.

Rabe, Horst. "Frühe Stadien der Ratsverfassung in den Reichslandstädten bzw. Reichsstädten Oberdeutschlands." In *Beiträge zum spätmittelalterlichen Städtewesen*, edited by Bernhard Diestelkamp, 1–17. Cologne: Böhlau Verlag, 1982.

Racinet, Philippe. "Les infirmeries monastiques: perspectives de recherche." In *Hôpitaux et maladreries au moyen âge: espace et environnement: actes du colloque international d'Amiens-Beauvais, 22, 23 et 24 novembre 2002*, edited by Pascal Montaubin, 21–34. Rouen: CAHMER, 2004.

Ramsay, Nigel, and James M. W. Willoughby, eds. *Hospitals, Towns, and the Professions.* London: British Library, 2009.

Ranft, Patricia. "An Overturned Victory: Clare of Assisi and the Thirteenth-Century Church." *Journal of Medieval History* 17 (1991): 123–134.

Rankin, Alisha. *Panaceia's Daughters: Noblewomen as Healers in Early Modern Germany.* Chicago: University of Chicago Press, 2013.

Rasmussen, Linda. "Monastic Benefactors in England and Denmark: Their Social Background and Gender Distribution." In *Religious and Laity in Western Europe 1000–1400: Interaction, Negotiation, and Power*, edited by Emilia Jamroziak and Janet Burton, 77–91. Turnhout: Brepols, 2006.

Rausch, Ute. *Das Medizinal und Apothekenwesen der Landgrafschaft Hessen-Darmstadt und des Grossherzogtums Hessen: unter besonderer Berücksichtigung der Provinz Starkenburg.* Darmstadt: Hessische Historische Kommission, 1978.

Rawcliffe, Carole. *The Hospitals of Medieval Norwich.* Woodbridge: Boydell, 1995.

Rawcliffe, Carole. "Isolating the Medieval Leper: Ideas—and Misconceptions—about Segregation in the Middle Ages." In *Freedom of Movement in the Middle Ages: Proceedings of the 2003 Harlaxton Symposium*, edited by Peregrine Horden, 229–248. Donington: Shaun Tyas, 2007.

Rawcliffe, Carole. *Leprosy in Medieval England.* Woodbridge: Boydell, 2006.

Rehberg, Andreas. "Die Römer und ihre Hospitäler: Beobachtungen zu den Trägergruppen der Spitalsgründungen in Rom (13.–15. Jahrhundert)." In *Hospitäler in Mittelalter und Früher Neuzeit: Frankreich, Deutschland und Italien. Eine Vergleichende Geschichte*, edited by Gisela Drossbach, 225–260. Munich: Oldenbourg, 2007.

Reicke, Siegfried. *Das deutsche Spital und sein Recht im Mittelalter.* 2 vols. Stuttgart: Enke, 1932.

Reifenberg, Hermann. "Die 'Ansprache' bei der Krankensalbung nach Mainzer Diözesanbrauch seit dem Mittelalter." *Mainzer Zeitschrift* 60/61 (1965/1966): 61–69.

Reimann, Heike. "Cistercian Nuns in the High Middle Ages: The Cistercians of Bergen in the Principality of Rügen (North Germany)." *Cîteaux: Revue d'histoire cistercienne* 55 (2004): 231–244.

Resnick, Irven M. "The Jews and Leprosy." In *Marks of Distinction: Christian Perceptions of Jews in the High Middle Ages*, 93–143. Washington, DC: Catholic University of America Press, 2012.

Rexroth, Frank. "Armenhäuser—eine neue Institution der sozialen Fürsorge im späten Mittelalter." In *Funktions und Strukturwandel mittelalterlicher Hospitäler*, edited by Michael Matheus, 1–14. Geschichtliche Landeskunde 56. Stuttgart: Franz Steiner Verlag, 2005.

Rexroth, Frank. "Zweierlei Bedürftigkeit. Armenhäuser und selektive caritas im England des 14. bis 16. Jahrhundert." In *Sozialgeschichte Mittelalterlicher Hospitäler*, edited by Neithard Bulst and Karl-Heinz Spiess, 11–37. Ostfildern: Jan Thorbecke Verlag, 2007.

Reyerson, Kathryn L. "Medieval Walled Space: Urban Development vs. Defense." In *City Walls: The Urban Enceinte in Global Perspective*, edited by James D. Tracy, 88–116. Cambridge: Cambridge University Press, 2000.

Richards, Peter. *The Medieval Leper and His Northern Heirs.* Woodbridge: Boydell, 2000.

Riddle, John. "Research Procedures in Evaluating Medieval Medicine." In *The Medieval Hospital and Medical Practice*, edited by Barbara S. Bowers, 3–18. Aldershot: Ashgate, 2007.

Riegel, Martin. *Lepra, Pest, und andere Seuchen: Krankheit und Krankenpflege in Kitzingen am Main zwischen Mittelalter und früher Neuzeit.* Hamburg: Krämer, 2002.

Riha, Ortrun. "Aussatz als Metapher. Aus der Geschichte einer sozialen Krankheit." In *Medizin in Geschichte, Philologie und Ethnologie: Festschrift für Gundolf Keil*, edited by Dominik Gross and Monika Reininger, 89–104. Würzburg: Königshausen & Neumann, 2003.

Risse, Gunther. *Mending Bodies, Saving Souls: A History of Hospitals.* Oxford: Oxford University Press, 1999.

Ritchey, Sara. *Acts of Care: Recovering Women in Late Medieval Health.* Ithaca: Cornell University Press, 2021.

Roberts, Charlotte A. "The Antiquity of Leprosy in Britain: The Skeletal Evidence." In *The Past and Present of Leprosy: Archaeological, Historical, Palaeopathological, and Clinical Approaches*, edited by Charlotte A. Roberts, Mary E. Lewis, and Keith Manchester, 213–222. Oxford: Archaeopress, 2000.

Roberts, Simon. *Order and Dispute: An Introduction to Legal Anthropology.* London: Penguin, 1979.

Rocha, Ana Rita. "Being a Leper in Medieval Portugal: The Lepers and the Leper House of Coimbra, Twelfth-Sixteenth Centuries." Presentation at the International Medieval Congress, Leeds, July 4–7, 2016.

Roffey, Simon. "Medieval Leper Hospitals in England: An Archaeological Perspective." *Medieval Archaeology* 56 (2012): 203–233.

Roffey, Simon. "Treating Leprosy: St. Mary Magdalen, Winchester." *Current Archaeology* 267 (2012): 12–18.

Rohmann, Gregor. *Tanzwut: Kosmos, Kirche und Mensch in der Bedeutungsgeschichte eines mittelalterlichen Krankheitskonzepts.* Göttingen: Vandenhoeck & Ruprecht, 2013.

Rörig, Reinhold. *Die Mainzer Spitäler und Krankenhäuser: ein Rückblick auf 2000 Jahre Krankenhaus Geschichte.* Mainz: Verlag des Bischöflichen Stuhles, 1989

Rosenwein, Barbara. *To Be the Neighbor of St. Peter: The Social Meaning of Cluny's Property, 909–1049.* Ithaca: Cornell University Press, 1989.

Rosenwein, Barbara. "Views from Afar: North American Perspectives on Medieval Monasticism." In *Dove va la storiografia monastica in Europa? Temi e metodi di ricerca per lo studio della vita monastica e regolare in età medievale alle soglie del terzo millennio: atti del convegno internazionale BresciaRodengo, 23–25 marzo 2000*, edited by Giancarlo Andenna, 67–84. Milan: Vita e pensiero, 2001.

Rouse, Mary A. and Richard H. Rouse. *Authentic Witnesses: Approaches to Medieval Texts and Manuscripts.* Notre Dame, IN: University of Notre Dame Press, 1991.

Rovinksi, Jacques. "L'isolement du lépreux au Moyen Âge (Genèse et réalisation)." *Razo: Cahiers du Centre d'études médiévales de Nice* 4 (1984): 75–94.

Rubin, Miri. *Charity and Community in Medieval Cambridge.* Cambridge: Cambridge University Press, 1988.

Rubin, Miri. "Imagining Medieval Hospitals: Considerations on the Cultural Meaning of Institutional Change." In *Medicine and Charity Before the Welfare State*, edited by Jonathan Barry, 14–25. London: Routledge, 1994.

Rubin, Miri. "Religious Culture in Town and Country: Reflections on a Great Divide." In *Church and City, 1000–1500: Essays in Honour of Christopher Brooke*, edited by David Abulafia, Michael Franklin, and Miri Rubin, 3–22. Cambridge: Cambridge University Press, 1992.

Rückert, Maria Magdalena. "Fromme Frauen, weltliche Stifter und geistliche Förderer." In *Landschaft(en): Begriffe, Formen, Implikationen*, edited by Franz Josef Felten, Harald Müller, and Heidrun Ochs, 223–244. Stuttgart: Franz Steiner Verlag, 2012.

Rückert, Maria Magdalena. "Zur Inkorporation südwestdeutscher Frauenklöster in den Zisterzienserorden. Untersuchungen zu Zisterzen der Maulbronner Filiation im 12. und 13.

Jahrhundert." *Studien und Mitteilungen zur Geschichte des BenediktinerOrdens und seiner Zweige* 111 (2000): 381–410.

Saalwächter, Andreas. "Ingelheimer Armen- und Krankenfürsorge im Mittelalter." In *AltIngelheim: Kulturgeschichtliche Bilder aus der Vergangenheit Ingelheims und des Ingelheimer Grundes in gesammelten Schriften*, 93–97. Ingelheim: Historischer Verein, 1958.

Salvadori, Patrizia. "La Peste e la Lebbra in 'Medioevo Latino': Un Prospetto Bibliogeografico." In *The Regulation of Evil: Social and Cultural Attitudes to Epidemics in the Late Middle Ages*, edited by Agostino Paravicini Bagliani and Francesco Santi, 177–193. Florence: Sismei Edizioni del Galluzzo, 1998.

Saunier, Marie-Anne. *"Le pauvre malade" dans le cadre hospitalier médiéval: France du Nord, vers 1300–1500*. Paris: Éditions Arguments, 1993.

Schaab, Karl Anton. *Die Geschichte der Stadt Mainz*. 4 vols. Mainz: Kupferberg, 1844–1851.

Schelberg, Antje. "Unification des recherches sur la lepre et les lepreux sous le nom de 'leprographie'? Une reponse." In *Lépreux et sociabilité du Moyen Âge aux temps modernes*, edited by Bruno Tabuteau, 93–98. Rouen: GRHIS, 2000.

Schenk, Winfried. *Historische Geographie*. Darmstadt: Wissenschaftliche Buchgesellschaft, 2011.

Schilp, Thomas. "Totengedenken des Mittelalters und kulturelles Gedächtnis: Überlegungen zur Perspektive der Memoriaforschung für das Frauenstift Essen." In *Pro Remedio et Salute Anime Peragemus: Totengedenken am Frauenstift Essen im Mittelalter*, edited by Thomas Schilp, 19–36. Essen: Klartext Verlag, 2008.

Schlösser, Susanne. "Armen- und Krankenfürsorge in städtischen Hospitälern im Gebiet des heutigen Rheinhessen. Ein Beitrag zur mittelalterlichen und frühneuzeitlichen Geschichte des Hospitalwesens von Alzey, Mainz, Oppenheim, und Worms." *Archiv für hessische Geschichte* 43 (1991): 61–84.

Schlösser, Susanne. *Den Armen und Elenden zu Troste und Frommen ...600 Jahre Hospital zu Alzey*. Alzeyer Geschichtsblätter, Sonderheft 12. Alzey: Altertumsverein, 1987.

Schlösser, Susanne. "Das Bacharacher Hospital. Ein Beitrag zu seiner mittelalterlichen und frühneuzeitlichen Geschichte." In *Bacharach und die Geschichte der Viertälerorte Bacharach, Steeg, Siebach und Manubach*, edited by Friedrich Ludwig Wagner, 327–332. Bacharach: Verein für die Geschichte der Stadt Bacharach, 1996.

Schmid, Reinhard. *Die Abtei St. Alban vor Mainz im Hohen und Späten Mittelalter: Geschichte, Verfassung und Besitz eines Klosters im Spannungsfeld zwischen Erzbischof, Stadt, Kurie, und Reich*. Mainz: Stadtarchiv Mainz, 1996.

Schmidt, Charles. "Notice sur l'Église rouge et la Léproserie de Strasbourg." *Bulletin de la Société pour la Conservation des Monuments Historiques d'Alsace* 2 (1879): 236–269.

Schmidt, Marie Ulrike. "Das Nikolaihospital. Untersuchungen zum mittelalterlichen Leprosorium der Stadt Lüneburg (1251–1530)." *Historia Hospitalium* 29 (2014–2015): 553–558.

Schneider, Jean. "Lexicographie du Latin Mediévale et Vocabulaire des Institutions." In *La Lexicographie du latin médiéval et ses rapports avec les recherches actuelles sur la civilisation du Moyen âge*, edited by Yves Lefèvre, 197–213. Paris: Centre nationale de la recherche scientifique, 1981.

Schneider, Walter. "Die Hospitäler im Raum AltTirol: Probleme einer Pass- und Übergangsregion." In *Funktions- und Strukturwandel spätmittelalterlicher Hospitäler im europäischen Vergleich*, edited by Michael Matheus, 59–100. Geschichtliche Landeskunde 56. Stuttgart: Franz Steiner Verlag, 2005.

Schreiber, Georg. *Gemeinschaften des Mittelalters: Recht und Verfassung, Kult und Frömmigkeit*. Münster: Regensberg, 1948.

Schürle, Wolfgang W. *Das Hospital zum Heiligen Geist in Konstanz: ein Betrag zur Rechtsgeschichte des Hospitals im Mittelalter*. Sigmaringen: Jan Thorbecke Verlag, 1970.

Schütz, Friedrich. "Zum Beyhülf und Trost der Erkrankten: Jüdische Ärzte in Mainz vom Mittelalter bis zum 19. Jh." In *Moguntia Medica: Das medizinische Mainz vom Mittelalter bis ins 20. Jahrhundert*, edited by Franz Dumont, 213–221. Wiesbaden: B. Wylicil Verlag, 2002.

Schulz, Ilse. *Schwestern, Beginen, Meisterinnen: Hygieias christliche Töchter im Gesundheitswesen einer Stadt: ein Beitrag zur Geschichte der Pflege und Heilkunde*. Ulm: Universität Verlag Ulm, 1992.

Schulze, Olaf. "Institutionen der Krankenpflege: Kloster, Spital, Leprosen, Seel und Pesthaus." In *Pforzheim zur Zeit der Pest*, edited by the Löblicher Singergesellschaft von 1501, 75–168. Pforzheim: Ubstadt-Weiher Verlag, 1993.

Scott, Anne M. "Remembering the Poor: Signs of Charity in Late Medieval Images and Texts." In *Experiences of Charity, 1250–1650*, edited by Anne M. Scott, 257–274. Farnham: Ashgate, 2015.

Seymour, Margaret A. "The Organization, Personnel, and Functions of the Hospital in the Later Middle Ages." *The Bulletin of the Institute for Historical Research* 21 (1948): 249–250.

Shahar, Shulamith. "Des lépreux pas comme les autres. L'ordre de Saint-Lazare dans le royaume latin de Jérusalem." *Revue historique* 267 (1982): 19–41.

Sherman, Irwin W. "Leprosy, The Striking Hand of God." In *The Power of Plagues*, 303–312. Washington, DC: ASM Press, 2006.

Shoham-Steiner, Ephraim. *On the Margins of a Minority: Leprosy, Madness, and Disability among the Jews of Medieval Europe*. Translated by Haim Watzman. Detroit: Wayne State University Press, 2014.

Sieben, Hermann Josef. *Die Partikularsynode: Studien zur Geschichte der Konzilsidee*. Frankfurter theologische Studien. Frankfurt am Main: Knecht, 1990.

Simon-Muscheid, Katharina. *Die Dinge im Schnittpunkt sozialer Beziehungsnetze: Reden und Objekte im Alltag (Oberrhein, 14. bis 16. Jahrhundert.)* Göttingen: Vandenhoeck und Ruprecht, 2004.

Simon-Muscheid, Katharina. "Sozialer Abstieg im Mittelalter." In *The Sign Languages of Poverty: International Roundtable Discussion, Krems an der Donau, October 10 and 11, 2005*, edited by Gerhard Jaritz, 95–117. Vienna: Österreichische Akademie der Wissenschaften, 2007.

Simons, Walter. "Beginnings: Naming Beguines in the Southern Low Countries, 1200–1250." In *Labels and Libels: Naming Beguines in Northern Medieval Europe*, edited by Letha Böhringer, 9–52. Turnhout: Brepols, 2014.

Simons, Walter. *Cities of Ladies: Beguine Communities in the Medieval Low Countries, 1200–1565*. Philadelphia: University of Pennsylvania Press, 2001.

Siraisi, Nancy. *Medieval and Early Renaissance Medicine: An Introduction to Knowledge and Practice*. Chicago: University of Chicago Press, 1990.

Siraisi, Nancy. *Taddeo Alderotti and his Pupils: Two Generations of Italian Medical Learning*. Princeton: Princeton University Press, 1981.

Skevington, Fay. "The Unhal and the Semantics of Anglo-Saxon Disability." In *Social Dimensions of Medieval Disease and Disability*, edited by Sally Crawford and Christina Lee, 7–14. Oxford: Archaeopress, 2014.

Sommerlechner, Andrea. "Spitäler in Nordund Mittelitalien vom 11. bis zum Beginn des 14. Jahrhunderts." In *Europäisches Spitalwesen. Institutionelle Fürsorge in Mittelalter und Früher Neuzeit*, edited by Martin Scheutz, Andrea Sommerlechner, Herwig Weigl, and Alfred Stefan Weiß, 105–134. Munich: R. Oldenbourg Verlag, 2008.

Sonderegger, Stefan. "The Financing Strategy of a Major Urban Hospital in the Late Middle Ages (St. Gallen, 15th Century.)" In *Assistenza e solidarità in Europa Secc. XIIIXVIII = Social Assistance and Solidarity in Europe from the 13th to the 18th centuries: at della "Quarantaquattresima Settimana di Studi," 22–26 aprile 2012*, edited by Francesco Ammannati, 209–226. Florence: Firenze University Press, 2013.

Sonderegger, Stefan. "Zum eignen und zum Nutzen anderer. Gedenkstiftungen in hoch und spätmittelalterlichen St. Galler Urkunden." In *Bücher des Lebens—Lebendige Bücher*, edited by Peter Erhart and Jakob Kuratli, 226–233. St. Gallen: Stiftarchiv St. Gallen, 2010.

Sontag, Susan. *Illness as Metaphor*. New York: Farrar, Strauss, and Giroux, 1978.

Spiegeler, Pierre de. *Les Hôpitaux et l'assistance à Liège (Xe-XVe siècles): aspects institutionnels et sociaux*. Paris: Belles Lettres, 1987.

Staab, Franz. "Reform und Reformgruppen im Erzbistum Mainz. Vom 'Libellus de Willigisi consuetudinibus' zur 'Vita domnae Juttae inclusae'." In *Reformidee und Reformpolitik im SpätsalischFrühstaufischen Reich: Vorträge der Tagung der Gesellschaft für Mittelrheinische Kirchengeschichte vom 11. bis 13. September 1991 in Trier*, edited by Stefan Weinfurter, 172–196. Trier: Gesellschaft Mittelrheinische Kirchengeschichte, 1992.

Stadtarchiv Mainz. *Digitales Häuserbuch Mainz*. http://www.mainz.de/microsite/digitale-shaeuserbuch/kartenteil/index.php. 2016.

Staerk, Dieter. "Gutleuthäuser und Kotten im südwestdeutschen Raum. Ein Beitrag zur Erforschung der städtischen Wohlfahrtspflege in Mittelalter und Frühneuzeit." In *Die Stadt in der europäischen Geschichte: Festschrift Edith Ennen*, edited by Franz Irsigler, 529–553. Bonn: Röhrscheid Verlag, 1972.

Stanford, Charlotte A. *Commemorating the Dead in Late Medieval Strasbourg: The Cathedral's Book of Donors and its Use (1320–1521)*. Farnham: Ashgate, 2011.

Stemmle, Jennifer. "From Cure to Care: Indignation, Assistance, and Leprosy in the High Middle Ages." In *Experiences of Charity, 1250–1650*, edited by Anne M. Scott, 43–62. Farnham: Ashgate, 2015.

Stöber, Karen. *Late Medieval Monasteries and their Patrons: England and Wales, c. 1300–1540*. Woodbridge: Boydell, 2007.

Stoob, Heinz. "Die Stadtbefestigung. Vergleichende Überlegungen zur bürgerlichen Siedlungs und Baugeschichte, besonders der frühen Neuzeit." In *Europäische Städte im Zeitalter des Barock: Gestalt, Kultur, Sozialgefüge*, edited by Kersten Krüger, 25–56. Cologne: Böhlau Verlag, 1988.

Strocchia, Sharon. "Caring for the 'Incurable' in Renaissance Pox Hospitals." In *Hospital Life: Theory and Practice from the Medieval to the Modern*, edited by Laurinda Abreu and Sally Sheard, 67–92. Oxford: Peter Lang, 2013.

Sudhoff, Karl. "Was geschah mit den (nach erneuter Schau) als 'leprafrei' Erklärten und aus den Leprosorien wieder Entlassenen, von behördlicher und ärztlicher Seite?" In *Archiv für Geschichte der Medizin* 6 (1912/13): 149–154.

Summerlin, Danica. *The Canons of the Third Lateran Council of 1179, Their Origins and Reception*. Cambridge: Cambridge University Press, 2019.

Sweeney, James Ross. "Innocent III, Canon Law, and Papal Judges Delegate in Hungary." In *Popes, Teachers, and Canon Law in the Middle Ages*, 26–52. Ithaca: Cornell University Press, 1989.

Sweet, Victoria. *God's Hotel: A Doctor, A Hospital, and a Pilgrimage to the Heart of Medicine*. New York: Riverhead, 2012.

Sweetinburgh, Sheila. *The Role of the Hospital in Medieval England: Gift-Giving and the Spiritual Economy*. Dublin: Four Courts Press, 2004.

Sweetinburgh, Sheila. "Royal Patrons and Local Benefactors: The Experience of the Hospitals of St. Mary at Ospringe and Dover in the Thirteenth Century." In *Religious and Laity in Western Europe 1000–1400: Interaction, Negotiation, and Power*, edited by Emilia Jamroziak and Janet Burton, 111–130. Turnhout: Brepols, 2006.

Sydow, Jürgen. "Kanonistische Fragen zur Geschichte des Spitals in Südwestdeutschland." *Historisches Jahrbuch* 83 (1964): 54–68.

Sydow, Jürgen. "Landesherrliche Städte des deutschen Südwestens in Nachstaufischer Zeit." In *Beiträge zum spätmittelalterlichen Städtewesen*, edited by Bernhard Diestelkamp, 18–33. Köln: Böhlau Verlag, 1982.

Sydow, Jürgen. "Spital und Stadt in Kanonistik und Verfassungsgeschichte des 14. Jahrhunderts." In *Der deutsche Territorialstaat im 14. Jahrhundert*, edited by Hans Patze, 175–195. Frankfurt am Main: Thorbecke, 1970.

Tabuteau, Bruno. "Combien de lépreux au Moyen Âge? Essai d'étude quantitative appliquée à la lèpre: les exemples de Rouen et de Bellencombre au XIIIe siècle." *Sources, travaux historiques* 13 (1988): 19–23.

Tabuteau, Bruno. "De l'expérience érémétique à la normalisation monastique: étude d'un processus de formation des léprosies aux XIIeXIIIe siècles. Le cas d'Evreux." In *Fondations et œuvres charitables au Moyen Âge: Actes du 121e congrès national des sociétés historiques et scientifiques, section histoire médiévale et philologie, Nice, 1996*, edited by Jean Dufour and Henri Platelle, 89–96. Paris: CTHS, 1999.

Tabuteau, Bruno, ed. *Lépreux et sociabilité du Moyen Âge aux temps modernes*. Rouen: Publications de l'Université de Rouen, 2000.

Tabuteau, Bruno. "Vingt mille léproseries au Moyen Âge? Tradition française d'un poncif historiographique." *Memini: Travaux et documents* 15 (2011): 119–128.

Talbot, C. H. *Medicine in Medieval England*. London: Oldbourne, 1955.

Thompson, Benjamin. "From 'Alms' to 'Spiritual Services:' The Function and Status of Monastic Property in Medieval England." In *Monastic Studies, II. The Continuity of Tradition*, edited by Judith Loades, 227–261. Bangor, Gwynedd: Headstart History, 1991.

Thompson, Benjamin. "Habendum et Tenendum: Lay and Ecclesiastical Attitudes to the Property of the Church." In *Religious Belief and Ecclesiastical Careers in Late Medieval England*, edited by Christopher Harper-Bill, 197–238. Studies in the History of Medieval Religion 3. Woodbridge: Boydell, 1991.

Tierney, Brian. *Foundations of the Conciliar Theory: The Contribution of the Medieval Canonists from Gratian to the Great Schism*. Cambridge: Cambridge University Press, 1955.

Tierney, Brian. *Medieval Poor Law: A Sketch of Canonical Theory and its Application in England.* Berkeley: University of California Press, 1959.

Toellner, Richard. *Lepra, gestern und heute: 15 wissenschaftliche Essays zur Geschichte und Gegenwart einer Menschheitsseuche: Gedenkschrift zum 650jahrigen Bestehen des Rektorats Munster-Kinderhaus*. Münster: Regensberg, 1992.

Toson, Bettina. *Mittelalterliche Hospitäler in Hessen zwischen Schwalm, Eder, und Fulda*. Darmstadt: Hessische Historische Kommission, 2012.

Touati, François-Olivier. *Archives de la lèpre: Atlas des léproseries entre Loire et Marne au moyen âge*. Paris: Comité des Travaux historiques et scientifiques, 1996.

Touati, François-Olivier. "La géographie hospitalière Médiévale." In *Hôpitaux et maladreries au moyen âge: espace et environnement: actes du colloque international d'Amiens-Beauvais, 22, 23 et 24 novembre 2002*, edited by Pascal Montaubin, 7–20. Rouen: CAHMER, 2004.

Touati, François-Olivier. "Les groupes de laïcs dans les hôpitaux et les léproseries au Moyen Âge." In *Les Mouvances laïques des ordres religieux: Actes du troisième colloque international du CERCOR, Tournus, 17–20 juin 1992*, 137–162. Saint-Etienne: Publications de l'Université de Saint-Etienne, 1996.

Touati, François-Olivier. "Histoire des maladies, histoire totale? L'exemple de la Lèpre et de la Société au Moyen Âge." *Sources et Travaux d'Histoire Haut-Pyrenéenne* 13 (1988): 3–14.

Touati, François-Olivier. *Maladie et Société au Moyen Age: la lèpre, les lépreux et les léproseries dans la province ecclésiastique de Sens jusqu'au milieu du XIVe siècle*. Brussels: De Boeck & Larcier, 1998.

Touati, François-Olivier. "Les traités sur la lèpre des médecins montpelliérains: Bernard de Gordon, Henri de Mondeville, Arnaud de Villeneuve, Jourdain de Turre et Guy de Chauliac." In *L'Université de médecine de Montpellier et son rayonnement (XIIIe-XVe siècles)*, edited by Daniel le Blévec and Thomas Granier, 205–231. Turnhout: Brepols, 2004.

Trenery, Claire. *Madness, Medicine, and Miracle in Twelfth-Century England.* Abingdon: Routledge, 2019.

Truempy, Hans. "Die Aussätzigen in der mittelalterlichen Gesellschaft." In *Beiträge zur Geschichte der Lepra*, edited by Huldrych Koelbing, 84–93. Zürich: Juris Druck und Verlag, 1972.

Uhrmacher, Martin. "Entstehung und Verbreitung von Leprosorien im Westen des Reiches." In *Einrichtungen der sozialen Sicherung im mittelalterlichen Lotharingien. Actes des 13es Journées Lotharingeinnes (12–15 Oct. 2004)*, edited by Michel Pauly, 461–477. Linden: Section Historie de l'Institut Grand-Ducal, 2008.

Uhrmacher, Martin. *Lepra und Leprosorien im rheinischen Raum vom 12. bis zum 18. Jahrhundert.* Trier: Porta Alba Verlag, 2011.

Uhrmacher, Martin. *Leprosorien in Mittelalter und früher Neuzeit.* Köln: Rheinland Verlag, 2000.

Uhrmacher, Martin. "Norm und Praxis in Leprosorien des 15. Jh. im Spiegel Ihrer Statuten. Trier." In *Norm und Praxis in der Armenfürsorge in Spätmittelalter und früher Neuzeit,* edited by Sebastian Schmidt and Jens Aspelmeier, 147–167. Stuttgart: Steiner Verlag, 2006.

Unger, Stefanie. *Generali concilio inhaerentes statuimus: die Rezeption des Vierten Lateranum (1215) und des Zweiten Lugdunense (1274) in den Statuten der Erzbischöfe von Köln und Mainz bis zum Jahr 1310.* Mainz: Gesellschaft für mittelrheinische Kirchengeschichte, 2004.

Van Houts, Elisabeth. "Nuns and Goldsmiths: The Foundation and Early Benefactors of St. Radegund's Priory at Cambridge." In *Church and City, 1000–1500: Essays in Honour of Christopher Brooke*, edited by David Abulafia, Michael Franklin, and Miri Rubin, 59–80. Cambridge: Cambridge University Press, 1992.

Vanja, Christine. "Offene Fragen und Perspektiven der Hospitalgeschichte." In *Europäisches Spitalwesen. Institutionelle Fürsorge in Mittelalter und Früher Neuzeit*, edited by Martin Scheutz, Andrea Sommerlechner, Herwig Weigl, and Alfred Stefan Weiß, 19–41. Munich: R. Oldenbourg Verlag, 2008.

Varanini, Gian Maria, and Giuseppina de Sandre Gasparini. "Gli ospedali dei 'malsani' nella società veneta del XII-XIII secolo. Tra assistenza e disciplinamento urbano." In *Città e servizi sociali nell'Italia dei secoli XII-XV: Dodicesimo convegno di studi, Pistoia, 9–12 ottobre 1987*, edited by Emilio Cristiani and Enrica Salvatori, 141–200. Pistoia: Centro italiano di studi di storia e d'arte, 1990.

Vauchez, André. *The Laity in the Middle Ages: Religious Beliefs and Devotional Practices*, edited by Daniel E. Bornstein. Translated by Margery J. Schneider. Notre Dame, IN: University of Notre Dame Press, 1993.

Vauchez, André. "Lay People's Sanctity in Western Europe: Evolution of a Pattern (Twelfth and Thirteenth Centuries)." In *Images of Sainthood in Medieval Europe*, edited by Renate Blumenfeld Kosinski and Timea Szell, 21–32. Ithaca: Cornell University Press, 1991.

Venarde, Bruce L. *Women's Monasticism and Medieval Society: Nunneries in France and England, 890–1215*. Ithaca: Cornell University Press, 1997.

Villagrasa-Elias, Raul. "Sociologia hospitalaria en Castilla la Vieja (1455–1513)." Salud en cuerpo y alma: el hospital de la Vera Cruz en Medina de Pomar, Centro de Ciencias Humanas y Sociales, Madrid, November 5, 2020. Web presentation.

Villinger, Carl Johann Heinrich. "Wormser Hospitäler. Ein Beitrag zur Geschichte der Wormser Caritas im Mittelalter." *Jahrbuch für das Bistum Mainz* 2 (1947): 162–186.

Virchow, Rudolf. "Der HospititaliterOrden des Heiligen Geist, zumal in Deutschland." *Monatsberichte der Königlich Preussischen Akademie der Wissenschaften zu Berlin* 43 (1878): 349–377.

Von Steynitz, Jesko. *Mittelalterliche Hospitäler der Orden und Städte als Einrichtungen der sozialen Sicherung.* Berlin: Duncker und Humblot, 1970.

Wagner, Willi. "Das Aufsichtsrecht Eberbachs über die ihm unterstellten Zisterzienserinnenklöster mit besonderen Berücksichtigung von Kumbd." *Landeskundliche Vierteljahrsblätter* 10 (1964): 160–172.

Walker, David. "The Organization of Material in Medieval Chartularies." In *The Study of Medieval Records: Essays in Honour of Kathleen Major*, edited by D. A. Bullough and R. L. Storey, 132–150. Oxford: Clarendon Press, 1971.

Wann, Wolfgang. "Die alten Mainzer Archive." *Archivalische Zeitschrift* 60 (1964): 100–130.

Warren, Nancy Bradley. *Spiritual Economies: Female Monasticism in Later Medieval England.* Philadelphia: University of Pennsylvania Press, 2001.

Watson, Sethina C. *Fundatio, Ordinatio, and Statuta: The Statutes and Constitutional Documents of English Hospitals to 1300.* D.Phil. Oxford, 2003.

Watson, Sethina C. *On Hospitals: Welfare, Law, and Christianity in Western Europe, 400–1320.* Oxford: Oxford University Press, 2020.

Watson, Sethina C. "A Mother's Past and her Children's Futures: Female Inheritance, Family, and Dynastic Hospitals in the Thirteenth Century." In *Motherhood, Religion, and Society in Medieval Europe, 400–1400: Essays Presented to Henrietta Leyser,* edited by Conrad Leyser and Lesley Smith, 213–249. Farnham: Ashgate, 2011.

Watts, Sheldon J. "Dark Hidden Meanings: Leprosy and Lepers in the Medieval West and in the Tropical World under the European Imperium." In *Epidemics and History: Disease, Power, and Imperialism*, 40–83. New Haven: Yale University Press, 1999.

Weigl, Herwig. "Städte und Spital, Arme und Almosen: Beobachtungen aus dem späten Mittelalter: Ein Vorspann." In *Orte der Stadt im Wandel vom Mittelalter zur Gegenwart*, edited by Lukas Morscher, Martin Scheutz, and Walter Schuster, 407–446. Innsbruck: Studien Verlag, 2013.

Weigl, Herwig. "What to Write in Court: Literacy and Lawsuits in Late Medieval Austria." In *Charters and the Use of the Written Word in Medieval Society*, edited by Karl Heidecker, 63–80. Turnhout: Brepols, 2000.

Weinert, Franz-Rudolf. *Mainzer Domliturgie zu Beginn des 16. Jahrhunderts: Der Liber Ordinarius der Mainzer Domkirche.* Tübingen: A. Francke Verlag, 2009.

Weingärtner, Elke. *Das Medizinal und Fürsorgewesen der Stadt Trier im Mittelalter und der frühen Neuzeit.* Trier: Porta Alba Verlag, 1981.

Wernher, Carl. "Das Hospital zum Heiligen Geiste." In *Oppenheim: Geschichte einer alten Reichsstadt*, 306–309. Oppenheim am Rhein: Oppenheimer Druckhaus, 1975.

Wetter, Johannes. "Die Kirche zum heiligen Geist in Mainz, ein Denkmal der Baukunst im romanischen Styl lombardischer Art, aus der Mitte des dreizehnten Jahrhunderts." *Zeitschrift des Vereins zur erforschung der rheinischen Geschichte und Alterthümer in Mainz* 2 (1859–1864): 427–442.

Widmann, Hans-Peter. "Das Spitalwesen." In *Spätmittelalter am Oberrhein. Große Landessausstellung BadenWürttemberg, Staatliche Kunsthalle Karlsruhe, 29. September 2001– 3. Februar 2002*, edited by Sönke Lorenz and Markus Dekiert, 491–496. Stuttgart: Jan Thorbecke Verlag, 2002.

Wiegand, Peter. *Diözesansynoden und bischöfliche Statutengesetzgebung im Bistum Kammin.* Köln: Böhlau Verlag, 1998.

Wilhelmy, Winfried. "Ein unbekanntes Krönungsrelief der Mainzer Erzbischöfe: Bonifatius und die Bildpropaganda der sedes Moguntiae im Zeitalter der Goldenen Bulle." *Mainzer Zeitschrift* 99 (2004): 17–30.

Wimmer, Otto and Hartmann Melzer. *Lexikon der Namen und Heiligen.* Innsbruck: Tyrolia Verlag, 1982.

Winckelmann, Otto. *Das Fürsorgewesen der Stadt Strassburg vor und nach der Reformation bis zum Ausgang des sechzehnten Jahrhunderts: ein Beitrag zur deutschen Kultur und Wirtschaftsgeschichte*. Leipzig: Heinsius, 1922.

Windemuth, Marie-Louise. *Das Hospital als Träger der Armenfürsorge im Mittelalter*. Sudhoffs Archiv Beihefte 36. Stuttgart: Franz Steiner Verlag, 1995.

Wolf, Jörn Henning. "Einführung." In *Aussatz-Lepra-Hansen-Krankheit: ein Menschheitsproblem im Wandel*, edited by Jörn Henning Wolf, 1–16. Würzburg: Deutsches Aussätzigen-Hilfswerk, 1986.

Wollasch, Joachim. "Anmerkungen zur Gemeinschaft des Heiliggeistspitals zu Freiburg i.Br. im Spätmittelalter." In *Civitatum communitas: Studien zum europäischen Städtewesen. Festschrift Heinz Stoob zum 65. Geburtstag*, edited by Helmut Jäger, Friedrich Bernhard Fahlbusch, and Bernd-Ulrich Hergemöller, 606–621. Cologne: Böhlau Verlag, 1984.

Wood, Susan Meriel. *English Monasteries and their Patrons in the Thirteenth Century*. Oxford: Oxford University Press, 1955.

Wray, Shona Kelly. "Instruments of Concord: Making Peace and Settling Disputes Through a Notary in the City and Contado of Late Medieval Bologna." *Journal of Social History* 42 (2009): 733–760.

Yearl, M. K. "Medieval Monastic Customaries on Minuti and Infirmi." In *The Medieval Hospital and Medical Practice*, edited by Barbara S. Bowers, 175–194. Aldershot: Ashgate, 2007.

Zechlin, Erich. *Lüneburgs Hospitäler im Mittelalter*. Forschungen zur Geschichte Niedersachsens I. Hannover: Hahn, 1907.

Ziegler, Tiffany A. *Medieval Healthcare and the Rise of Charitable Institutions: The History of the Municipal Hospital*. London: Palgrave Macmillan, 2018.

Zimmerman, Susan. "Leprosy in the Medieval Imaginary." *Journal of Medieval and Early Modern Studies* 38 (2008): 559–587.

Zitzmann, Mirjam. *Das Jahrzeitbuch des Heiliggeist-Hospitals Kaufbeuren*. Thalhofen: Bauer Verlag, 2009.

Index

For Product Safety Concerns and Information please contact our EU representative GPSR@taylorandfrancis.com
Taylor & Francis Verlag GmbH, Kaufingerstraße 24, 80331 München, Germany

www.ingramcontent.com/pod-product-compliance
Ingram Content Group UK Ltd.
Pitfield, Milton Keynes, MK11 3LW, UK
UKHW021722240926
475702UK00029BA/1783

9781041181019